MEDICAL AND CARE COMPUNETICS 6

Studies in Health Technology and Informatics

This book series was started in 1990 to promote research conducted under the auspices of the EC programmes' Advanced Informatics in Medicine (AIM) and Biomedical and Health Research (BHR) bioengineering branch. A driving aspect of international health informatics is that telecommunication technology, rehabilitative technology, intelligent home technology and many other components are moving together and form one integrated world of information and communication media. The complete series has been accepted in Medline. Volumes from 2005 onwards are available online.

Volume 156

Recently published in this series

Vol. 155. B. Blobel, E.Þ. Hvannberg and V. Gunnarsdóttir (Eds.), Seamless Care – Safe Care – The Challenges of Interoperability and Patient Safety in Health Care – Proceedings of the EFMI Special Topic Conference, June 2–4, 2010, Reykjavik, Iceland

Vol. 154. B.K. Wiederhold, G. Riva and S.I. Kim (Eds.), Annual Review of Cybertherapy and Telemedicine 2010 – Advanced Technologies in Behavioral, Social and Neurosciences

Vol. 153. W.B. Rouse and D.A. Cortese (Eds.), Engineering the System of Healthcare Delivery

Vol. 152. T.C. Lee and P.F. Niederer (Eds.), Basic Engineering for Medics and Biologists – An ESEM Primer

Vol. 151. E.J.S. Hovenga, M.R. Kidd, S. Garde and C. Hullin Lucay Cossio (Eds.), Health Informatics – An Overview

Vol. 150. K.-P. Adlassnig, B. Blobel, J. Mantas and I. Masic (Eds.), Medical Informatics in a United and Healthy Europe – Proceedings of MIE 2009 – The XXIInd International Congress of the European Federation for Medical Informatics

Vol. 149. R.G. Bushko (Ed.), Strategy for the Future of Health

Vol. 148. R. Beuscart, W. Hackl and C. Nøhr (Eds.), Detection and Prevention of Adverse Drug Events – Information Technologies and Human Factors

Vol. 147. T. Solomonides, M. Hofmann-Apitius, M. Freudigmann, S.C. Semler, Y. Legré and M. Kratz (Eds.), Healthgrid Research, Innovation and Business Case – Proceedings of HealthGrid 2009

ISSN 0926-9630 (print)
ISSN 1879-8365 (online)

Medical and Care Compunetics 6

Edited by

Lodewijk Bos

ICMCC, The Netherlands

Bernd Blobel

eHealth Competence Center, University Hospital Regensburg, Germany

Stephen Benton

University of Westminster, UK

and

Denis Carroll

ICMCC, University of Westminster, UK

IOS
Press

Amsterdam • Berlin • Tokyo • Washington, DC

ISBN 978-1-60750-564-8 (print)
ISBN 978-1-60750-565-5 (online)
Library of Congress Control Number: 2010927838

Publisher
IOS Press BV
Nieuwe Hemweg 6B
1013 BG Amsterdam
Netherlands
fax: +31 20 687 0019
e-mail: order@iospress.nl

Distributor in the USA and Canada
IOS Press, Inc.
4502 Rachael Manor Drive
Fairfax, VA 22032
USA
fax: +1 703 323 3668
e-mail: iosbooks@iospress.com

PRINTED IN THE NETHERLANDS

Medical and Care Compunetics 6
L. Bos et al. (Eds.)
IOS Press, 2010

Preface

This volume contains the proceedings of the seventh annual Event of the International Council on Medical and Care Compunetics (ICMCC), which will be held in London, UK, from 8–11 June 2010. ICMCC is an international foundation which acts as the knowledge centre for medical and care compunetics, i.e. for the field of the social, societal and ethical implications of computing and networking in health. In contrast to conferences addressing technology, dedicated scientific domains or specialized professionals, ICMCC follows a multidisciplinary approach by nature. Therefore, it addresses all entities involved in health issues such as health professionals, politicians, supporting specialist, administrators, researchers and developers, but primarily the subject of care – the patient or the citizen before they become a patient. ICMCC is unique on the global scene in this bridging and embracing functionality.

The theme of the 2010 annual event is "Personal Health – Intelligent solutions to serve empowered patients". The seventh ICMCC annual event addresses *the active participation of the citizen in his or her health and care pathway with the interactive use of Information and Communication Technologies*, in other words; Patient 2.0 Empowerment as defined by ICMCC in 2008. The 2010 Event intends to combine ontology-driven health information system design for advanced interoperability with the paradigm change towards pervasive person-centric care, including prevention, home care and wellness, together forming adaptive distributed health information systems solutions. Important issues to be considered are virtual Electronic Health Records and Personal Health Records acting as a semantically interoperable communication and cooperation platform for personalized ubiquitous health services in a reliable environment.

The scientific topics presented in the proceedings comprise System Design and Evaluation, Computer-Assisted Learning, Knowledge Representation and Ontologies, Electronic Health Records and Patient Empowerment. 82 researchers, residing in 17 different countries from Europe, North and South America, and Asia, have reported their results in this volume. A comprehensive overview and in-depth, first hand information on new developments, advanced systems, technologies and applications will be introduced to an international audience.

The ICMCC has been supported by the European Federation for Medical Informatics (EFMI), notably by the EFMI Working Groups "Electronic Health Records", "Security, Safety and Ethics" and "Personal Portable Devices".

The editors would like to thank the scientific board for their assistance and all the authors for their excellent work as well as the reviewers for lending their expertise to the conference. Last but not least the local organizers, for their contribution to the final achievements.

Lodewijk Bos (Event Chair)
Bernd Blobel (Scientific Chair)

List of Reviewers

Dr. Rajeev Bali
Prof. Stephen Benton
Prof. Bernd Blobel
Drs. Lodewijk Bos
Dr. Brian Fisher
Dr. Fleur Fisher
Dr. Rajaram Lakhsminarayan
Prof. Andrew Marsh
Prof. Manuel Prado-Velasco
Dr. Stef Verlinden
Dr. Amol Wagholikar
Prof. Kanagasingam Yogesan
Dr. Qing Zhang

ICMCC Event Scientific Board

ICMCC Event Organizing Board

ICMCC Executive Board

ICMCC Advisory Board

Contents

Computer-Assisted Learning

Knowledge Representation and Ontologies

Electronic Health Records

Patient Empowerment

Keynotes

Medical and Care Compunetics 6
L. Bos et al. (Eds.)
IOS Press, 2010

doi:10.3233/978-1-60750-565-5-3

What is Missing in Health Informatics Standardization for pHealth?

Bernd BLOBEL[a,1], Frank OEMIG[b], Carolina GONZÁLES[a,c], Diego LÓPEZ[a,d]
[a] *eHealth Competence Center, University Hospital Regensburg, Germany*
[b] *Agfa Healthcare GmbH, Bonn, Germany*
[c] *Software Engineering Research Group, University of Cauca, Colombia*
[d] *Telematics Engineering Group, University of Cauca, Colombia*

Abstract. Health systems turn everywhere, but with different speed, from organization-centered to personalized eHealth or pHealth, i.e. ubiquitous care delivery independent of time and location of the resources involved. As interoperability is an important issue in such distributed, fully integrated, intelligent and individualized environment, pHealth solutions have to comply with advanced architectural solutions based on international standards. Representing concepts and their interrelations, such architectural framework perspectives' system architecture, domains, and development process can be described by the domains' ontologies. Therefore, advanced interoperability approaches have to refer to ontology principles, finally resulting in ontology-driven approaches to semantically interoperable and sustainable health information systems. The paper investigates functional requirements, interoperability levels, architectural approaches to pHealth systems, thereby analyzing and classifying related existing or emerging standards.

Keywords. Personalized health, HIS architecture, Interoperability, Ontologies, Knowledge representation, Standards

Introduction

For improving safety and quality of care as well as efficiency and efficacy of care processes within the challenging constraints framework of demographic changes with multi-morbid and frequently chronically ill subjects of care, consumer expectations, progress in medicine and biomedical engineering, shortage of funds and globalization of the health business, health systems undertake paradigm changes towards personalized eHealth or in short pHealth. pHealth as ubiquitous care is individual care delivery independent of time and location of the resources involved. Because interoperability is an important issue in such distributed, fully integrated, intelligent and individualized environment, pHealth solutions have to comply with international standards. The paper investigates functional requirements, interoperability levels, and architectural approaches to pHealth systems, in that context offering a taxonomy for analyzing and classifying related existing or emerging standards.

---

[1] Corresponding Author: Bernd Blobel, PhD, Associate Professor; eHealth Competence Center, Regensburg University Hospital; Franz-Josef-Strauss-Allee 11, D-93053 Regensburg, Germany; Phone: +49-941-944-6769. Fax: +49-941-944-6766. Email: bernd.blobel@klinik.uni-regensburg.de; http://www.ehealth-cc.de

1. Methods

Cooperation in job sharing environments between specialized, distributed actors usually requires first communication, thereafter negotiation, agreed harmonization, contracted interrelations and finally collaboration. All those steps are based on information. After an evaluation of the cooperation outcome, the cycle runs again. In a technical environment, such cooperation is called interoperability. Meanwhile, the term interoperability has been introduced in other domains (a systematic definition of domains follows later on) such as social, organizational, or legal ones as well [1].

Interoperability starts with common interest between the principals involved. Otherwise, there would not be any communication and cooperation. Principals, according to the OMG/CORBA definition, include any actors such as persons, organizations, systems, devices, and applications [2, 3]. The common interest is defined by joined business objectives to be supported by that interoperability. The business needs must be defined and the business process for meeting them must be negotiated. For the correct reflection of the environment as well as meaningful communication, common knowledge and its representation to derive the right information from data and to take the right action for meeting the aforementioned business objectives, common reference models, an agreed set of coordinated reference ontologies and terminologies as well as a common development process for analyzing, designing, specifying, implementing, running and maintaining the appropriate solution is inevitable. All steps have to be based on an architectural framework. All the basics and requirements for interoperability mentioned have to be harmonized and fixed, and their use and fulfillment must be enforced. This is the intention behind standards. Following, the collaborative system described will be explained in some detail

1.1. Personal Health

For realizing ubiquitous care, pHealth solutions have to comprise three technical paradigms: mobile computing, pervasive computing and autonomic computing. Mobile computing enables the permanent, location and time independent accessibility of the principals involved, providing, for example, teleconsultation services. Pervasive computing enables remote and pervasive service provision through any type of principals, thereby bridging the gap between the physical and the informational world and so directly integrating the subject of care in communication and cooperation networks using sensors, actuators, body area networks, or home networks [4]. These services are commonly called telemedicine services. For providing personalized care, services have to be flexible for responding to the special subject of care's individual status, needs and wishes. They cannot be rigidly predefined. Such adaptive health information system design, which is directed towards a self-organizing environment, is realized by autonomic computing. Furthermore, information delivered through the "omics" disciplines and characterizing the individual has to be appropriately reflected. With the combination of those paradigms, ubiquitous care is provided.

For combining those paradigms comprehensively and consistently towards a multi-disciplinary pHealth interoperability framework, the pHealth services delivering system has to follow a harmonized architectural model which defines structure and behavior of the system by describing all system's components, their functions and their interrelationships.

1.2. Interoperability levels

Interoperability covers communication and collaboration of actors to achieve a business goal. The outcome of the overall business process of those actors defines the interoperability level required for the facilitating infrastructure deployed (Table 1). From an information cycle viewpoint, this means that interoperability comprises a successful information cycle from investigating the business process' internal and external variables, interpreting the information carried by those data, and deriving the right action for meeting the business needs. Interpretation and the derivation of actions depend on knowledge about the domain the component deals with. Commonly, domains are defined as groupings of common characteristics such as business objectives, methodologies, principles, etc. As any characteristic has to be described, ontologies are a natural way of grouping components to a domain from a knowledge representation perspective. Such strategy can best be exemplified at personalized health. Beside medicine, sensors, actuators and other biomedical devices monitoring a person, genomics individually tailoring diagnosis and therapy, legal affairs such as legislation, regulations, especially security and privacy issues, defining administrative as well as operational rules and conditions, and finally social and ethical aspects setting additional humanistic principles have to be implemented in an ICT environment. All aforementioned domains are represented by domain experts using their specific terminologies based on the domains' ontologies. Representing one dimension of a component-based system model (see the next section), domains can be aggregated to super-domains or separated into sub-domains. If cooperating actors share the entire knowledge required for running the full cycle, the exchange of the observed data is sufficient. If the knowledge about the actions (services) and their integration in the delivery chain is a priori established, just the information exchange in the sense of semantic interoperability between the domain experts is needed. In other words, all interoperability levels defined in Table 1 above the technical interoperability are sufficient if knowledge (competence), ability (capability), and skills for the higher level of interoperability are given by deploying shared data/information provided at the lower levels.

Table 1. Interoperability levels

Interoperability Level	**Instances**
Organizations/Service interoperability	Common business process
Semantic interoperability	Advanced messaging, common information models and terminology
Syntactic interoperability	Messages, clinical documents, agreed vocabulary
Structural interoperability	Simple EDI, envelopes
Technical interoperability	Technical plug&play, signal- & protocol compatibility

1.3. Architectural approach to pHealth

As the pHealth system consists of components, their composition/decomposition forms one dimension of a reasonable architectural approach. The aforementioned aggregation of different domains to a multi-domain pHealth system provides its domain dimension isolating and combining domains. The development process covering requirement analysis, design, implementation, evaluation, use, and maintenance according to ISO/IEC 10746 "Information Technology – Reference Model Open Distributed Processing" (RM-ODP) or the Rational Unified Process (RUP) finally completes the dimensions of the comprehensive architectural model. The described architectural framework complies with the Generic Component Model (GCM), which has been developed in the early nineties by the German OMG/CORBA Chapter and furthermore improved by the Magdeburg Medical Informatics Department [5]. The GCM combines a system theoretical and biocybernetic approach applicable to any kind of system (IT, technical, living, social, etc.) with unified processes for IT systems' development. It enables structural and behavioral system modeling in a multi-dimensional concept representation space deploying different languages and related grammars [6, 7, 8]. Thereby, the limitations of formally representing systems components have to be considered carefully.

As mentioned already, domain components' concepts, their functions and their interrelationships representing the domain knowledge have to be formally described, thereby considering all three architectural dimensions. Figure 1 demonstrates specializations according to the aggregation hierarchy as well as associations at aggregations level within and between domains, all together matter of constraints. Components can communicate their concepts if they are interconnected. Not connected components must share their concepts a priory. It must be mentioned that only neighbored components can be interconnected.

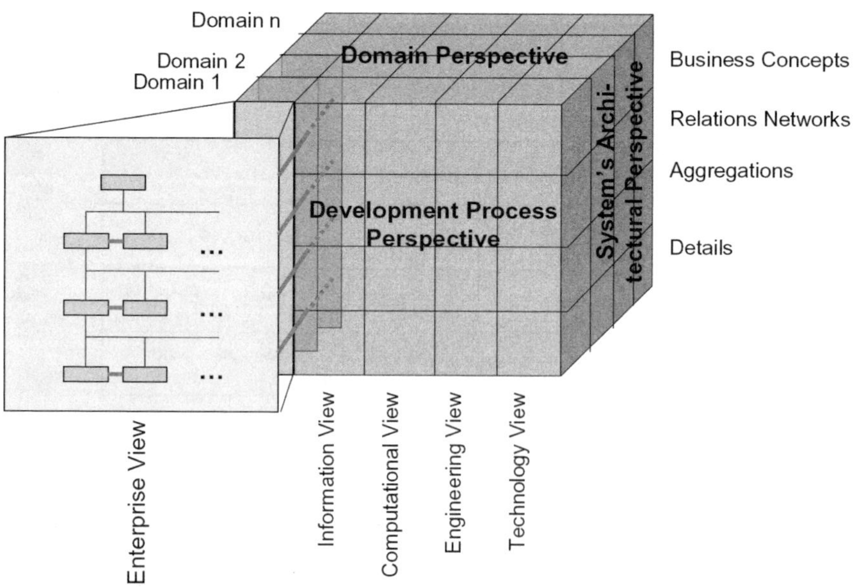

Figure 1. The Generic Component Model

Any instance of a highly dynamic pHealth system which follows a comprehensive architecture framework for open, flexible, scalable, interoperable, service oriented, formally specified, model driven, user accepted and trustworthy solutions as described should meet **just the required complexity level** regarding the level of component aggregation and domain inclusion as well as the resulting interoperability.

Based on the General Component Model (GCM) architectural framework refined to be used as standards taxonomy, all aspects of a pHealth solution covering the composition/decomposition perspective, the domain perspective including the domain mapping challenge, and the development process perspective have to be consistently represented and referenced by corresponding international standards, resulting in a gap analysis which can to be used in the standards development process. For all perspectives, methodology standards, domain-specific standards, and instance management standards are needed. It became obvious that the pHealth modeling challenge is first of all a language and knowledge representation challenge.

2. Results

According to the aforementioned architectural approach to an ideal pHealth system design for individualized ubiquitous care, the required pHealth system aspects have been summarized and presented in Table 2. The architectural approach always starts with restricting the aspects modeled in one step. Modeling one domain, the aggregation level important for describing the business goal has to be designed and refined according to the GCM. The appropriate model hierarchy (specialization/generalization by decomposition/composition) has to be provided throughout all viewpoints of the development process. Of course, the starting point for developing a formal system design must be the business case (service orientation), i.e. the computation-independent conceptual model. Here, a multi-facet approach like the Zachman scheme is recommended [9]. While the representation of the platform-independent as well as platform-specific ICT-models is rather simple due to the very restricted ICT ontology (see Figure 1), the representation of the different domains has to manage highly specialized and very different domain ontologies.

To interconnect the components of different and each other constraining domains at the different granularity level, ontology coordination has to be mastered. This is the real challenge of multidisciplinary systems. For meeting the presented challenges, tool support is inevitable. The outcome is the first level of a taxonomy to architecturally evaluate approaches to multidisciplinary systems in the requirements analysis, the design or the implementation phase. The description of the related aspects is the matter of publicly available specifications (PAS) and – more mature – standards, so that the scheme represents a standards taxonomy. Refining the parameters mentioned in Table 2, this taxonomy has been successfully used in the context of different international projects, e.g. [10].

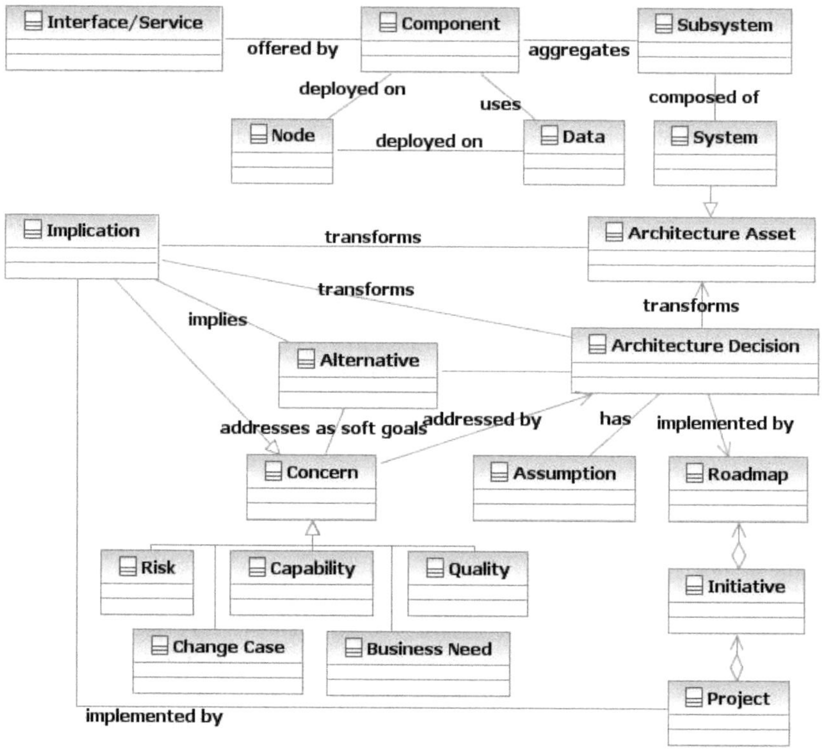

Figure 2. Basic ontology for the GCM system development process perspective (after [11], changed)

Table 2. pHealth system aspects [12]

Architectural Dimension	Architectural Aspect
Architectural composition / decomposition	Aggregations level
	Model Hierarchy
	Reference model based representation
	Constraint / profiling mechanism
	Service orientation
	Ontology based representation
Domain specialization	Clinical
	Biomedical
	Legal / regulatory
	Technology
	Others
Development process	Tool supported
	Presented views
Overall characteristics	Presentation style and means

Among others such as, e.g., technology specifications, a pHealth related health informatics standards taxonomy has to consider specifications defining requirements, architecture, modeling and methodology, communications, interoperability services, infrastructure services including security, safety, privacy and quality, policies, token and ID management but also the way how the concepts are represented. Practically implementable specifications require formal representations based on standardized meta-languages. Verbal narrative specifications like many provided even today in the health informatics domain have just educational, but no practical value. The specifications roughly classified above are provided by different accredited and non-accredited Standards Development Organizations (SDOs) such as ISO, IEEE, IEC, CEN, ETSI, HL7, DICOM, OASIS, W3C, OMG, etc. Table 3 shows a set of arbitrarily selected specifications, standards and norms established with relevance for pHealth environments, thereby exemplifying the use of the taxonomy.

Table 3. Taxonomy of selected standards (Legend: Y-yes, N-no, P-partially, n-narrative, f-formal, E-Enterprise View, I-Information View, C-Computational View, En-Engineering View, T-Technology View, all-All RM-ODP Views)

Architectural Dimension / Standard	Architectural Composition/ Decomposition						Domain-Specialization					Development Process		
	Aggregations level	Model hierarchy	RM based representation	Constraint/ profiling mech.	Service orientation	Ontology based repress.	Clinical	Biomedical	Legal/regulatory	Technology	Others	Present. style and means	Tool supported	Presented views
Requirements & Analysis														
ISO 10781[2]	Y	N	N	N	Y	N	Y	P	Y	P	P	n	N	E
ISO 22857:2004	N	N	N	N	Y	N	N	N	Y	P		n	N	E
ISO TR 20514:2005	N	N	N	N	P	P	N	N	N	N		n	N	E
ISO TS 18308:2004	N	N	N	N	P	P	N	N	N	N		n	N	E
HL7 DAMs	N	N	P	Y	Y	N	Y	Y	Y	N		f	P	EI
Architecture														
ISO EN 12967	P	P	N	N	Y	N	P	N	P	N		f	N	EIC
ISO EN 13606-2	N	N	P	Y	N	P	Y	N	N	N		f	N	I
ISO EN 13606-4	N	N	N	N	N	N	N	N	P	N		n	N	E
Modeling&Methodology														
ISO HL7 27932	Y	Y	Y	N	N	N	Y	Y	Y	N		f	Y	I
ISO IEC 10181	N	N	Y	N	Y	N	N	N	Y	Y		n	N	EI
ISO IEC 27000	N	N	N	N	Y	N	N	N	Y	Y		n	N	E
ISO 10746	N	N	N	Y	P	N	N	N	N	Y	Y	f	Y	all
Communications														
ISO 21090	Y	Y	Y	Y	N	N	P	N	N	N	Y	f	N	I
CEN EN 14822	Y	Y	Y	Y	N	N	Y	N	N	N	Y	f	N	IC
Infrastructure														
OMG EIS	Y	P	N	Y	Y	N	N	N	N	N	Y	f	N	EIC
Terminology&Ontology														
…														

[2] The current HL7 EHR-S Service Functional Model overcomes some of the limitations. The most critical deficiency is the lack of formalization.

As the assessment reflects qualities of the considered specification, there might be different view depending on contextual conditions, skills, experiences and intentions of the evaluator.

3. Using the Results for Evaluating HL7's Approach to pHealth Interoperability

HL7 claims to offer a messaging standard for enabling over the time advancing levels of interoperability. Starting with an EDI protocol providing structural interoperability in its earliest versions, HL7 grew up to syntactic interoperability in the later 2.x versions offering agreed terminology and low level clinical documents. With the advent of HL7's model-based approach of version 3 and the definition of the HL7 development framework, semantic interoperability could be defined at specification level, also including application roles and implementation guides. Because of the lack of an ontological basis (despite the vocabulary efforts), shared understanding of communicated information as well as appropriate behavior of interconnected applications and their offered services could not be guaranteed. The focus on the messaging paradigm resulted in the agnosticism about the behavior of communicating applications defining practical interoperability.

The inclusion of services in the scope of HL7, but even older HL7 specifications such as CCOW or the functional EHR/PHR models introduced the move of HL7 beyond the messaging paradigm, despite the lack of formalization in the latter case. But also for comparing and interconnecting the different HL7 artifacts as well as for providing quality of services definitions, the next level of consideration is inevitable to solve these problems which are "environmental" from a messaging paradigm perspective.

Based on the long term work on architectural frameworks including active engagement in the specification of the predecessor of ISO/IEC 10746 and many OMG standards, in 2007, the International Representatives to HL7's T3F (Technology Transition Taskforce) group brought the urgent need for an architectural framework to consistently and sustainable managing HL7's and other SDO's artifacts on the table.

As a result, the Service Aware Enterprise Architecture Framework (SAEAF) project has been launched [13]. It practically reuses most of the definitions, specifications and principles including formal description techniques of ISO/IEC 10746 for the specification of an open distributed processing systems architecture, nevertheless in some part remaining clearly behind this standard. ISO 10746 defines object modeling, viewpoint specifications, distribution transparency, and conformance. In that context, basic modeling concepts (objects, interfaces and interaction points, behavior and state), specification concepts (composition/decomposition, behavioral, type and class, templates, roles, base classes and derived classes), and structuring concepts (groups and domains, naming, contract, liaison and binding) have in major parts been introduced in the predecessor model of ISO 10746 – the German Generic Component Model – in 1994, and completed in the ISO ODP-RM in 1996 already. More details regarding the evaluation of HL7 specifications can be easily derived from the general discussion provided in the following section.

4. Using the Results for Evaluating Different Interoperability Paradigms

The shortest, but really pregnant definition for interoperability is the ability of two actors to meet a common business objective. For assessing the collaboration realized, the entire information cycle has to be considered. Depending on the environmental and contextual conditions, i.e., the perceptive abilities for managing the data and the cognitive abilities (knowledge) for interpreting them as well as both competence and capability for taking the right action, different interoperability levels summarized in Table 1 are sufficient for performing comprehensive collaboration.

The different phases of the information cycle and their reflection in related interoperability levels correspond to different interoperability paradigms: EDI paradigm, message paradigm, and service paradigm. These paradigms will be shortly discussed using the GCM.

The service paradigm reflects the business domain in question represented by the application regarding structure, function, and behavior within an architecture-centric approach. It corresponds to the GCM dimensions development process and component system architecture within one domain represented by the application ontology, which is derived from the related domain ontology.

The message paradigm (including documents) reflects the business domain informationally and is usually application agnostic. Therefore, just parts of the GCM development process dimension are considered, while all other aspects are completely ignored. Concepts are represented by an ICT ontology informationally reflecting the application environment.

The EDI paradigm reflects the information view of a system solely from an ICT perspective. Therefore, it is represented by ICT ontology, just focusing on technical issues and completely ignoring the business domain.

As clearly shown, the different paradigms are served by different ontologies, in the most challenging case of service paradigm even requesting ontology transformation. As more challenging the ontology is as more insufficient the offered specification follows the GCM requirements. This is also manifested in the standards evaluation sheet of Table 2, following the taxonomy derived from the GCM.

5. Conclusion

As pHealth requires intelligent, flexible and comprehensively interoperable solutions based on a multi-disciplinary architectural approach according to an advanced architectural framework such as the Generic Component Model, the specification and standards guiding analysis, design, specification, and deployment of such solutions have to comply with the aforementioned framework as well. Modeling such multi-disciplinary systems using open system sciences, which have a long tradition in system theory and system engineering as well as the broad fields of domain-related cybernetics (biocybernetics, economic cybernetics, societal cybernetics, etc.) is inevitable.

Different from other domains, there is neither a specification nor a specification set which comprehensively reflects the GCM framework in health informatics. Despite the limited scope regarding the RM-ODP views considered, the more informational or even technical specifications (i.e. the platform-independent or even platform-specific ones) come closer to the offered taxonomy parameters than the business domain related specifications (i.e. the computation independent ones). This is caused by the complexity level of the underlying ontologies, which also relates to the level of formalization realized in standards so far. Particularly for the business domain – and here especially for the domain of life sciences – a hierarchy of ontologies much more complex than the ICT ontology has to be considered. Another challenge is the multi-disciplinary approach of the GCM – clearly reflecting the real world of pHealth – which is represented by different ontologies, which have to be coordinated for managing the real system in question.

Acknowledgements

The authors are indebted to Stefan Schulz (University of Freiburg) and their colleagues from IFOMIS (University of Saarland) for kind cooperation as well as to IBM and OMG for supporting R&D in the paper's domain.

References

[1] European Commission, Directorate-General for Informatics, DIGIT/01 - European eGovernment services (IDABC). Final European Interoperability Framework - November 2004 (EN)
[2] Blobel B. Analysis, design and implementation of secure and interoperable distributed health information system. Amsterdam: IOS Press; 2002. (Stud Health Technol Inform; vol 89).
[3] Object Management Group, Inc. [Online]. Available from: URL: http://www.omg.org (last access: 1 March 2010).
[4] Blobel BGME, Pharow P, Norgall T. How to Enhance Integrated Care towards the Personal Health Paradigm? In: Kuhn KA, Warren JR, Leong T-Z, editors. MEDINFO 2007. Amsterdam, Berlin, Oxford, Tokyo, Washington (DC): IOS Press; 2007. p. 172-76.
[5] Blobel B. Application of the Component Paradigm for Analysis and Design of Advanced Health System Architectures. Int J Med Inf 2000;60(3):281-301.
[6] Blobel B, Pharow P. Analysis and Evaluation of EHR Approaches. Methods Inf Med 2009;48(2):162-9.
[7] Kamareddine F, Laan T, Nederpelt R. A Modern Perspective on Type Theory. New York: Kluwer Academic Publishers; 2004.
[8] Bloe R, Kamareddine F, Nederpelt R. The Barendregt Cube with Definitions and Generalized Reduction. Information and Computation 1996;126(2):123-43.
[9] Zachman J. A framework for information systems architecture. IBM Syst. J. 1999;38(2-3):454-71.
[10] BioHealth Consortium. Security and Identity Management Standards in eHealth including Biometrics-Specific Requirements having an Impact on the European Society and on Standardisation. [Online]. Available from: URL: www.bio-health.eu (last access: 1 March 2010).
[11] Akerman A, Tyree J. Using ontology to support development of software architectures. IBM Systems Journal 2006;45(4):813-26.
[12] Blobel B. Architectural approach to eHealth for enabling paradigm changes in health. Methods Inf Med 2010;49(2):123-34.
[13]HL7 International, Inc. [Online]. Available from: URL: http://www.hl7.org/ (last access: 1 March 2010).

Medical and Care Compunetics 6
L. Bos et al. (Eds.)
IOS Press, 2010

doi:10.3233/978-1-60750-565-5-13

Using Collective Intelligence to Fine-Tune Public Health Policy

Andy MARSH[a,1] Denis CARROLL[a] and Richard FOGGIE[b]
[a] *University of Westminster, London, UK*
[b] *Dept. For BIS, UK government, London, UK*

Abstract. The European Union Future Internet Assembly, the roadmap for the Web heading towards semantic interoperability and building on the UK's adoption of the Internet and social media are accelerating the development of Web 3.0. A number of health portals are opening, some with facilities for the capture of Patient Based Records. Collective Intelligence will be generated that, applied to health, has potential to support Public Health policy. By using the Internet, millions of people in the course of their daily activities contribute to uncertified data stores, some explicitly collaborating to create collective knowledge bases, some contributing implicitly through the patterns of their choices and actions. An application of soft computing, called Collective Health Intelligence, that reasons uncertified and certified data could enhance the social pool of existing health knowledge available to the public health agencies. Collective Health Intelligence could be used to complement national programmes by employing innovative sampling techniques, cost-effectively generating anonymous data trends that would quantify policy, indicate epidemiological effects and supply metrics to test policy efficacy.

Keywords. Soft Computing, Fuzzy logic, Collective Intelligence

1. Introduction

By using the Internet two new forms of information stores are being created in real time by thousands of people in the course of their daily activities, some explicitly collaborating to create collective knowledge bases like the Wikipedia and Freebase, some contributing implicitly through the patterns of their choices and actions. Explicit knowledge bases, such as wiki's refine knowledge through the contributions of thousands of authors; implicit data stores allow the discovery of entirely new knowledge by capturing trillions of key clicks and decisions as people use the network in the course of their everyday lives.

The Internet plays a central role in providing health information. Increasingly, consumers are relying on the Internet for help with their health care decisions. According to Pew Internet [1], some 75 to 80 percent of Americans have used the Internet to find health information. As of January 2008, as reported by iCrossing [2], the Internet rivalled physicians as the leading source for health information. Using Web 2.0 tools, the Internet is becoming a platform for convening social networks and when patients managing the same chronic condition share observations with each other, their

[1] Corresponding Author. Visiting professor at University of Westminster and Director of HoIP CIC, The old stable, Coombe Farm, Coombe Lane, Awbridge, Hampshire SO51 0HN, UK. Email: am@hoip.eu

collective wisdom can yield clinical insights well beyond the understanding of any single patient or physician. The knowledge embedded and recorded within these societies or large groups of individuals is a form of **Collective Intelligence** [3].

Discovering and harnessing the tacit intelligence that results from the data generated by the activities of many people over time —revealed through analyses of patterns, correlations, and flows—is enabling ever more accurate predictions about people's preferences and behaviours, and helping researchers and everyday users understand and map relationships, and gauge the relative significance of ideas and events. Examples of uses for this type of intelligence already exist in industry. Google's PageRank system [4], which assigns value to a Web page based on the number of other pages that link to it, user patterns discovered in hundreds of millions of links to determine which Web pages are most likely to be relevant in a list of search results. Amazon.com examines patterns in hundreds of buyer variables to recommend purchases that you might like based on your previous purchases, those of your friends, and other people who may have similar tastes or preferences.

2. Collective Health Intelligence

As the Internet has developed, so has the concept of Collective intelligence as a shared public forum. Web 2.0 has enabled interactivity and thus, users are able to generate their own content. Collective intelligence is a shared or group intelligence that emerges from the collaboration and competition of many individuals. The global accessibility and availability of the Internet has allowed more people than ever to contribute their ideas and to access these collaborative intelligence spaces [5].

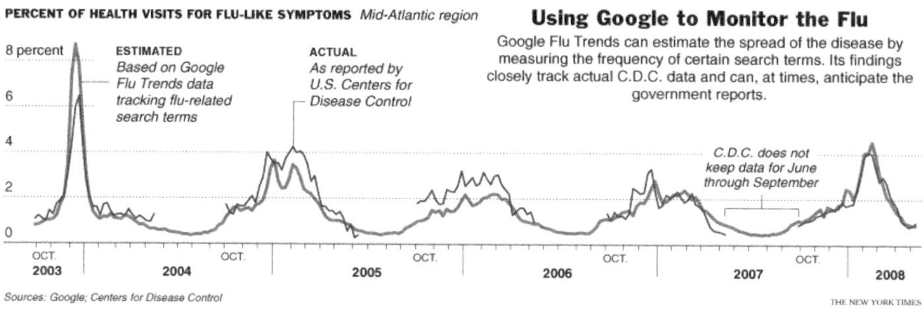

In moving further into the age of machine intelligence and automated reasoning the Web and especially search engines, such as Google, have reached a point where systems have a high machine IQ (MIQ) [6] or in the context of the Web, Web IQ (WIQ) [7]. The data collected by search engines is particularly powerful, because the keywords and phrases that people type into them represent their most immediate intentions. Analysis of the sheer volumes of information available and the ability to differentiate signal trends from the 'background noise' of the Internet has significant potential. Tests of the new Web tool from Google.org suggest that it may be able to detect regional outbreaks of the flu, for the US, a week to 10 days before they are reported by the Centers for Disease Control (C.D.C) [8]. It turns out that a lot of ailing Americans enter phrases like "flu symptoms" into Google and other search engines before they call their doctors. To develop the service, Google's engineers devised a basket of keywords and phrases related to the flu, including thermometer, flu symptoms, muscle aches and chest congestion. Google then dug into its database, extracted five years of data on those queries and mapped it onto the C.D.C.'s reports of influenza like illness. Google found a strong correlation between its data and the reports. Google Flu Trends avoids privacy pitfalls by relying only on aggregated data that cannot be traced to individual searchers. Its Google Flu Trends service [9] analyzes those searches as they come in, creating graphs and maps of the country that, ideally, show where the flu is spreading. The C.D.C. reports are slower because they rely on data collected and compiled from thousands of health care providers, labs and other sources. The premise behind Google Flu Trends —a fruitful marriage of mob behavior and medicine, a form of "collective intelligence" — has been validated by an unrelated study indicating that the data collected by Yahoo, can also help with early detection of the flu.

Existing search engines have many remarkable capabilities. However, what is not among them is a deduction capability—the capability to answer a query by a synthesis of information which resides in various parts of the knowledge base. A question-answering system is by definition a system that has this capability. One of the principal goals of Web intelligence is that of upgrading search engines to question-answering systems [10]. Many modern machine learning, or automated reasoning, methods such as the Semantic Web, Cyc, OWL [11,12,13] and other ontology-centered systems, such as Open Clinical [14], are based on objectivist Bayesian principles—bivalent logic and bivalent-logic based probability theory [15].

One of the crucial features of the Bayesian view is that a probability can be assigned to a hypothesis where a hypothesis can only be rejected or not rejected. One leading example of the application of Bayesian inference is by Autonomy Corporation PLC [16], an enterprise software company with joint headquarters in Cambridge, United Kingdom, and San Francisco, USA. It has developed a variety of enterprise search and knowledge management applications using adaptive pattern recognition techniques centered on Bayesian inference [17] (statistical inference in which evidence or observations are used to update or to newly infer the probability that a hypothesis may be true) in conjunction with traditional methods, such as information theory [18].

Bivalent-logic-based methods of knowledge representation and deduction are of limited effectiveness in dealing with information that is imprecise or partially true [19]. Much of the information that resides in the Web—and especially in the domain of world knowledge—is imprecise, uncertain and partially true [20, 21]. This information can be subdivided into *measurement-based* which can be represented numerically (e.g. It is 35°C, Eva is 28, Tandy is three years older than Dana) or *perception-based* which can be represented linguistically (e.g. It is very warm, Eva is young, Tandy is a few years older than Dana, It is cloudy, Traffic is heavy). More specifically, perceptions are f-granular in the sense that (a) the boundaries of perceived classes are unsharp; and (b) the values of perceived attributes are granular, with a granule being a clump of values drawn together by indistinguishability, similarity, proximity or functionality [22].

For example, designing an expert system to mimic the diagnostic powers of a physician, one of the major tasks to codify is the physician's decision-making process. The physician's view of the world, despite their dependence upon precise, scientific tests and measurements, incorporates evaluations of symptoms, and relationships between them, in a "fuzzy," intuitive manner: deciding how much of a particular medication to administer will have as much to do with the physician's sense of the relative "strength" of the patient's symptoms as it will their height/weight ratio. While some of the decisions and calculations could be done using Bayesian inference an alternative is fuzzy logic. Fuzzy logic is an extension of boolean logic dealing with the concept of *partial truth*. It is related to fuzzy sets and possibility theory and was introduced in 1965 by Dr. Lotfi Zadeh of Berkeley [23]. Whereas classical logic holds that everything can be expressed in binary terms (0 or 1, black or white, yes or no), fuzzy logic replaces boolean truth values with degrees of truth. Bart Kosko [24] has shown that probability is a subtheory of fuzzy logic, as probability only handles one kind of uncertainty.

Fuzzy logic is best applied to perception-based information, whereas Bayesian inference, or probabilistic reasoning, is best applied to measurement-based information. In many cases, especially in health, the available information is a mixture of both and can be interpreted most effectively by using a combination of fuzzy logic and probabilistic reasoning subsuming belief networks, evolutionary computing including DNA computing, chaos theory and parts of learning theory. Referred to as *approximate reasoning*, this hybrid system can also be supported by *search & optimization* techniques, including neural networks, machine learning and evolutionary algorithms. Collectively, these represent the main components of Soft Computing [25] and when applied to health, termed *Collective Health Intelligence,* can be used to enhance the social pool of existing health knowledge available to public health agencies.

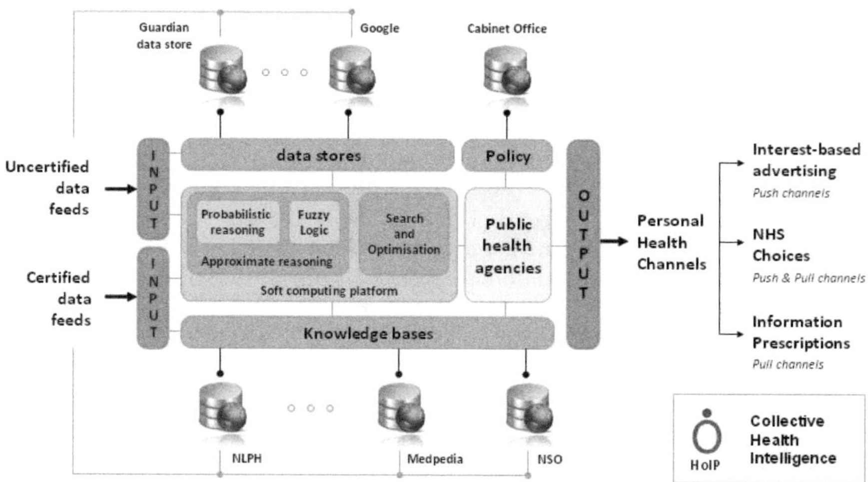

Within a soft computing platform approximate reasoning can be combined with search and optimization techniques to analyze uncertified and certified data feeds in conjunction with their respective stores. Uncertified data originates from the thousands of people using the Internet in the course of their daily activities, some explicitly collaborating to create collective knowledge bases, some contributing implicitly through the patterns of their choices and actions. Certified data feeds represent *measurement-based* information and include Evidence-based reviews, Specialist Libraries, Guidelines, Research publications, information from the Association of Public Health Observatories, APHO [33] and knowledge in the National Library for Public Health, NLPH [34]. Resulting collective intelligence can be used by public health agencies to support public health policy and disseminated over personal health channels.

3. Conclusions

Data is the most basic building block of any modern health information infrastructure. Addressing the *surveillance development and data analysis* theme of the HPA research and development strategy [26] and in accordance with government policy [27,28] one key challenge is to establish a task force to assess the accessibility and interoperability of inter-agency data, information and knowledge that when used by Collective Health Intelligence can directly or indirectly influence public health policy.

By using the Internet two new forms of information stores are being created in real time by thousands of people in the course of their daily activities, some explicitly collaborating to create collective knowledge bases, some contributing implicitly through the patterns of their choices and actions. A key challenge is to develop an open platform in accordance with government policy: Open Source, Open Standards and Re-Use: Government Action Plan [29], for Collective Health Intelligence, with effective surveillance and reasoning capabilities, to conduct complex analyses of these voluminous information stores and assess their impact on public health policy.

One aim of the Department of Health (DH) national information and intelligence strategy called 'Informing healthier choices' [30] is to improve the availability, timeliness and quality of health information across England. A key challenge for Collective Health Intelligence, equal to the NHS information prescription project [31], is to utilise unified communications and social media technologies to promote personalised health channels that will deliver intelligence at the right time ensuring that information is tailored around the specific needs of users when they come into contact with service providers, in the most appropriate way ensuring that information is provided through a range of channels and is accessible and convenient, in the most appropriate format working to develop a range of formats to maximize the inclusiveness of the Information Prescription process, helping to make sure that information is accessible and useable for all and be available at the right place ensuring information is made available from a range of access points, situated at locations convenient for the service user.

The success of Collective Health Intelligence depends on the use of technologies that provide timely and accurate measurement-based and perception-based information. There must be an infrastructure for information collection, exchange and analysis with interoperability that facilitates information sharing between organizations, regions, and agencies. A key challenge for Collective Health Intelligence would be to demonstrate its effectiveness and potential impact on public health policy by addressing one of the six overarching priorities in the public health white paper Choosing Health [32] such as reducing obesity and more specifically childhood obesity.

Acknowledgments

The authors would like to acknowledge the Public Health, Research and Development Department of Health and the i4i Programme of the National Institutes for Health Research in the UK for financially supporting the research scoping study and background material for this chapter.

References*

[1] [Online]. Available from: URL: http://www.pewinternet.org/Reports/2008/The-Engaged-Epatient-Population.aspx.
[2] [Online]. Available from: URL: http://www.icrossing.com/research/how-america-searches-health-and-wellness.php.
[3] [Online]. Available from: URL: http://en.wikipedia.org/wiki/Collective_Intelligence.
[4] [Online]. Available from: URL: http://www.google.com/corporate/tech.html.
[5] Flew, T. New Media: An Introduction. 3rd ed. Melbourne: Oxford University Press. 2008.
[6] Zadeh LA. Fuzzy logic, neural networks, and soft computing. Comm. of the ACM—AI 1994;37:77–84.
[7] [Online]. Available from: URL: http://www-bisc.cs.berkeley.edu/zadeh/papers/A Note on Web Intelligence, World Knowledge and Fuzzy Logic-2004.pdf.
[8] [Online]. Available from: URL: http://www.nature.com/nature/journal/v457/n7232/pdf/nature07634.pdf.
[9] [Online]. Available from: URL: http://www.google.org/flutrends/.
[10] Arjona J, Corchuelo R, Pena J, Ruiz D. Coping with web knowledge. In: Advances in Web Intelligence. Berlin, Heidelberg: Springer-Verlag; 2003. p. 165–78.
[11] [Online]. Available from: URL: http://www.w3.org/2001/sw/.
[12] [Online]. Available from: URL: http://www.opencyc.org/.
[13] [Online]. Available from: URL: http://www.w3.org/TR/owl-guide/.
[14] [Online]. Available from: URL: http://www.openclinical.org/ontologies.html.
[15] Bishop CM. Pattern Recognition and Machine Learning. Springer; 2007.
[16] [Online]. Available from: URL: http://www.autonomy.com/.
[17] [Online]. Available from: URL: http://en.wikipedia.org/wiki/Bayesian_inference.
[18] [Online]. Available from: URL: http://en.wikipedia.org/wiki/Information_theory.
[19] [Online]. Available from: URL: http://www-bisc.cs.berkeley.edu/zadeh/papers/A Note on Web Intelligence, World Knowledge and Fuzzy Logic-2004.pdf.
[20] Novak V, Perfilieva I, editors. Discovering the World with Fuzzy Logic. Studies in Fuzziness and Soft Computing. New York, Heidelberg: Physica-Verlag; 2000.
[21] Zadeh LA. From computing with numbers to computing with words from manipulation of measurements to manipulation of perceptions. IEEE Transactions on Circuits and Systems 1999;45(1):105–19.
[22] Bargiela A, Pedrycz W. Granular Computing—An Introduction. Boston, Dordrecht, London: Kluwer Academic Publishers; 2003.
[23] [Online]. Available from: URL: http://www.bigpedia.com/encyclopedia/Lotfi_Zadeh.
[24] [Online]. Available from: URL: http://sipi.usc.edu/~kosko/.
[25] [Online]. Available from: URL: http://modo.ugr.es/en/soft_computing.
[26] [Online]. Available from: URL: http://www.hpa.org.uk/web/HPAweb&HPAwebStandard/HPAweb_C/1203064747700.
[27] Data Retention (EC Directive) Regulations 2009. [Online]. Available from: URL: http://www.opsi.gov.uk/si/si2009/draft/ukdsi_9780111473894_en_1.
[28] Communications Data Bill. [Online]. Available from: URL: http://www.commonsleader.gov.uk/output/page2667.asp.
[29] [Online]. Available from: URL: http://www.cabinetoffice.gov.uk/cio/transformational_government/open_source.aspx.
[30] [Online]. Available from: URL: http://www.dh.gov.uk/en/Consultations/Closedconsultations/DH_4135308.
[31] [Online]. Available from: URL: http://www.informationprescription.info/index.html.
[32] [Online]. Available from: URL: http://www.dh.gov.uk/PublicationsAndStatistics/Publications/PublicationsPolicyAndGuiance/PublicationsPolicyAndGuidanceArticle/fs/en?CONTENT_ID=4094550&chk=aN5Cor.
[33] [Online]. Available from: URL: http://www.apho.org.uk.
[34] [Online]. Available from: URL: http://www.library.nhs.uk/publichealth/.

System Design and Evaluation

Medical and Care Compunetics 6
L. Bos et al. (Eds.)
IOS Press, 2010

doi:10.3233/978-1-60750-565-5-21

Quality Evaluation of Health Information System's Architectures Developed Using the HIS-DF Methodology

Diego M. LÓPEZ [a,b1] Bernd BLOBEL[a] and Carolina GONZALEZ[c]
[a] *eHealth Competence Center, University Hospital Regensburg, Germany*
[b] *Telematics Engineering Research Group, University of Cauca, Colombia*
[c] *Software Engineering Research Group, University of Cauca, Colombia*

Abstract. Requirement analysis, design, implementation, evaluation, use, and maintenance of semantically interoperable Health Information Systems (HIS) have to be based on eHealth standards. HIS-DF is a comprehensive approach for HIS architectural development based on standard information models and vocabulary. The empirical validity of HIS-DF has not been demonstrated so far. Through an empirical experiment, the paper demonstrates that using HIS-DF and HL7 information models, semantic quality of HIS architecture can be improved, compared to architectures developed using traditional RUP process. Semantic quality of the architecture has been measured in terms of model's completeness and validity metrics. The experimental results demonstrated an increased completeness of 14.38% and an increased validity of 16.63% when using the HIS-DF and HL7 information models in a sample HIS development project. Quality assurance of the system architecture in earlier stages of HIS development presumes an increased quality of final HIS systems, which supposes an indirect impact on patient care.

Keywords: Information Systems, Architecture, Quality Evaluation, Semantic Interoperability, Standards, HIS-DF, RUP, HL7

Introduction

Characterizing a system by its inherent technical, environmental, or policy conditions, collaboration between different actors in any health-related process requires open, flexible, scalable, service-oriented, intelligent, semantically interoperable, and trustworthy information systems. Requirement analysis, design, implementation, evaluation, use, and maintenance of such complex systems have to follow an agreed development process [1]. Furthermore, analysis and design of health information systems architecture, especially their underlying business and information models describing basic concepts, business and relation networks have to be based on e-Health standards [2]. Unfortunately, most health information system (HIS) development projects, including national e-health programs, still need to focus on the practical adoption of generic models and common clinical concept representation [3].

[1] Corresponding Author: Diego M. Lopez, PhD, Associate Professor; Telematics Department, Universidad del Cauca; Calle 5 Número 4-70, Popayán, Colombia; Phone: +57-2-8209800 ext 2117. Fax: +49-2-8209810. Email: dmlopez@unicauca.edu.co; http://www.unicauca.edu.co

HIS-DF (Health Information System Development Framework) [1] is a comprehensive development process consisting of a set of principles and guidelines as well as methodologies and techniques for designing and implementing the architecture of semantically interoperable components and applications based on existing e-Health standards.

HIS-DF offers an architecture framework in a standard way, documenting tasks, responsible persons, artifacts, products, guidance, phases, and workflows as no other methodology does. Particularly important is the personalization of formal software processes engineering methods such as the Rational Unified Process (RUP) framework, ISO 10746 Information Technology – Reference Model Open Distributed Processing standard (RM-ODP) and the HL7 Development Framework, as well as of architectural approaches such as Model Driven and Service-Oriented Architecture [1].

For reusing e-Health standards, HIS-DF defines a development Guideline called "Standards Harmonization". The method is based on UML extensibility mechanisms by defining UML profiles for e-Health standard information models [2]. This new approach allows to "annotate" the system models with Domain Reference Models and Vocabulary (e.g. HL7 RIM, D-MIM, vocabulary), enriching its semantic quality. UML and OCL have limitations for modeling knowledge such us for example its lack of strict semantically control, many times causing ambiguities [4][5], but this is the standard language used in the software industry and in many eHealth standards. Moreover, the annotation process proposed based on UML profiles provides other advantages such as model transformations, exchangeability, extensibility, automatic code generation, etc.

HIS-DF has been so far evaluated in the analysis, design, and implementation of a prototype architecture for the Integrated National Health Information System in Colombia. The prototype implementation is based on a Model Driven Development (MDD) process, transforming a HIS-DF-designed platform-independent architecture into Enterprise JavaBeans [6]. Moreover, this work is currently supporting the design of a reference architecture for EHR systems integration in Colombia, provided by the newly created Colombian HL7 committee on EHR [7]. The adoption of the methodology in large scale projects is however a long-term process with the necessity to perform several adjustments and configurations of the methodology. In the meantime, is possible to take advantage of empirical methods to formally evaluate the main aspects of the methodology.

The objective of this paper is to provide an empirical demonstration of the quality improvement of HIS architectures developed with HIS-DF. Being HIS-DF-designed architectures expressed as a set of UML models, the increased quality of the architecture have to be measured in terms of the increased quality of the created UML models (e.g., Classes Diagrams, Use Cases, Sequence Diagrams, etc) when they are profiled with healthcare standards (Domain Information Models and Vocabulary).

1. Materials and Methods

Quality evaluation of architectures is an open research topic in health informatics and software engineering disciplines. In the health informatics arena, evaluation has been specially focused on health information system's impact as well as organizational and social aspects [8]. However, it has been recognized that evaluation is valuable from early stages of the system's design. In software engineering, several methods for evaluating software architectures have been proposed, commonly addressing multiple quality attributes such as performance, maintainability, testability, and portability [9]. Semantic quality evaluation is an important quality attribute especially for semantically interoperable systems. Unfortunately, there is no clear definition of quantitative indicators to formally evaluate semantic quality of models. Research on quality measures for semantic quality is an important step towards the design of high quality HIS architectures as prerequisites for realizing an increased quality of final HIS.

Considering that the experimental objects in this study are software artifacts (architectural models derived from HIS-DF), the validity of HIS-DF would be better demonstrated using empirical methods for evaluating software artifacts commonly used in software engineering. In the discipline of software engineering, three empirical methods are well known: formal experiments, case studies and surveys [10]. The selection of the right technique is part of the design activity in any empirical study. In this study, surveys are discarded because they are more suitable for long-term projects. Several guidelines help to decide whether to perform a case study or an experiment, but the central factor for having chosen the design of a formal experiment was its flexibility to control the different variables influencing (confounding factors) an HIS development project.

In the next subsection, a brief review of approaches for evaluating the semantic quality of models is presented. Following, the design of the formal experiment for evaluating the semantic quality of HIS-DF architectures is explained.

1.1. Semantic Quality Evaluation of System Models

HIS-DF supports the design of UML Business Analysis, Requirements, Analysis and Design Models. Those models are different in nature and scope. The principal model in HIS-DF is the Analysis model (particularly the Harmonized Domain Analysis Models –HDAM). HDAM is foremost important in HIS-DF because it is the result of applying the "Harmonize Information Models" Task. It is intended to improve the semantic quality of Analysis Models by creating "semantic annotations" using the HL7 Information Models and Vocabulary. If an increased quality of HDAM is demonstrated, it can be inferred that it was principally influenced by the process of harmonization of healthcare standards.

HDAM is considered a sort of conceptual model. Conceptual modeling is a software engineering discipline as such offering several frameworks for evaluating the quality of conceptual models. As an example of a very well used framework is the Lindland framework [11] which defines three levels of conceptual models quality:

- *Syntactic quality*: Defines how a given model adheres to the syntax of the modeling language.
- *Semantic quality*: Defines the quality of a model in terms of how the model describes the domain. It considers not only syntax, but also relations among statements and their meaning. Semantic quality is commonly described in terms of validity and completeness attributes. Validity implies that all statements in the model are correct and relevant to the problem domain. Completeness implies that the model contains all statements about the problem domain that are correct and relevant.
- *Pragmatic quality*: This category addresses the comprehension aspect of the model from the stakeholders' perspective. The comprehension goal specifies

that all audience members (or interpreters) completely understand the statements in the model that are relevant to them.

Evaluation of syntactic quality in UML models is in theory not complex, because it relies on the correct use of the UML syntaxes, which is commonly supported by UML modeling tools. Pragmatic quality assessment is manageable, as it relies only on user's perception. However, semantic quality is very difficult to evaluate as it is hard to perceive the reality, to represent this knowledge and finally to reach a common agreement through UML models [12].

Restricted to completeness and validity metrics for semantic quality in UML models as defined by Lindland, diverse and overlapping metrics were identified. Unhelkar [13] defines quality metrics for semantic correctness. Correspondingly, Bolloju and Leung [14] identify and classify the most typical set of errors frequently committed by novice systems analysts designing UML Use Case, Class, And Sequence diagrams; thereby discussing how those errors affect the quality of models. Despite referring to semantic quality as defined in the Lindland framework, quantifiable metrics for completeness and validity are not defined. Shanks [15] defines metrics to compute completeness as defined by Lindland, but centered on data models (Entity–Relationship Models). Evaluation of completeness is based on the number of major and minor errors found in the data models compared to a "correct" data model. Major errors include missing entities or relationships. The algorithm proposed by Shanks for completeness is:

$$\text{Completeness} = (N\text{-}E1 - 0.3E2)/N * 100 \quad (1)$$

where N is the number of constructs (entities and relationships) in the "correct" model, E1 is the number of major errors for each construct and E2 is the number of minor errors.

1.2. Experimental Design

Considering that HIS-DF architectures are expressed as a set of UML models, the increased quality of the architectural models have to be measured in terms of the increased quality of UML models compared with models created with a baseline architectural development framework. The baseline used for the evaluation is the Rational Unified Process (RUP), the most widely used development process in software engineering. In RUP, the system architecture is created using the Architectural Development method. Figure 1 briefly describes the experiment.

In the Architectural Development method of RUP, the DAM corresponds to the Analysis Class Artifact which is the main output artifact of the Use Case Analysis Task. In HIS-DF, the Domain Analysis Model (DAM) is first developed following the same RUP process. Following, this DAM is further refined into an HDAM using the HIS-DF "Harmonize Information Models" Task [1]. In consequence, for the sake of evaluation it is possible to compare the quality of the HIS-DF HDAM and the RUP DAM because both are represented as UML Class Diagrams.

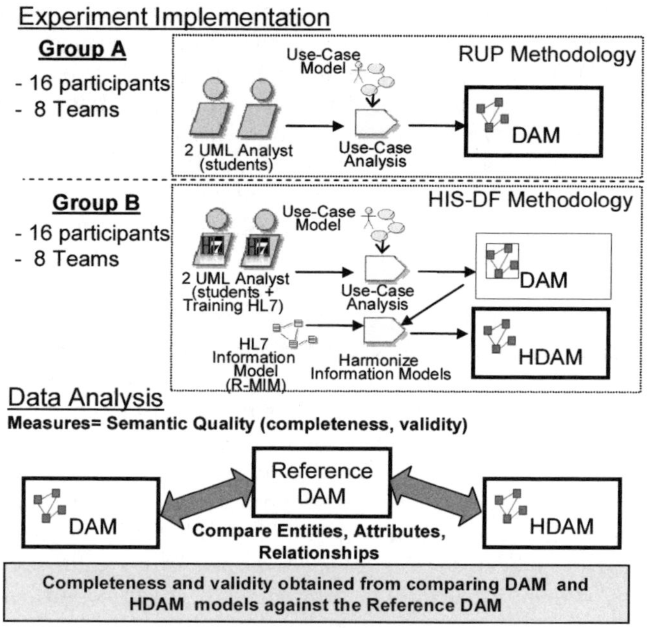

Figure 1. Experimental Design

The experiment's design elements are described in the following subsections.

Hypothesis: The following hypothesis has been defined and proven: "Semantic quality of HIS Analysis Models (HDAM artifact) created using HIS-DF is higher than semantic quality of HIS Analysis Models (DAM artifact) created using the RUP guidelines for the Software Architecture development"

Experimental Subjects: Being an Architecture development project, experimental subjects are HIS System Analysts. The Experiment was performed using 32 undergraduate students in Telecommunications Engineering at the University of Cauca in Colombia. The students have all already taken three software engineering courses (180 hours in total), having in average similar training and experience in RUP and UML design. All subjects are randomly assigned to two groups: Group A and Group B. Group A is the control group (they perform the design of the RUP DAM for a HIS scenario). Group B is the group receiving the treatment (performs the design of the HDAM for the same scenario using the HIS-DF methodology). To make use of the advantages of pair programming and design, each role (system analyst) is performed by a software development team of two students.

Experimental objects. The experimental objects are two types of HIS Analysis Models:

- Harmonized Domain Analysis Model (HDAM)
- Domain Analysis Model (DAM)

Both models are UML Class Diagrams with the difference that the HDAM is an Analysis Model which has been "annotated" with the semantics of a HL7 Domain Information Model, also conforming to the HL7 Vocabulary. Using HIS-DF implies using an HL7 Domain Information Model as Reference. The HL7 model used in the scenario is a UML Profiled Model based on the HL7 Notifiable Condition Report R-MIM (PORR_RM100001UV01). The model has been already described in [1]. This model was translated into Spanish, to improve understandability by the participants.

Treatment and Control Treatment: The control treatment (Group A) consists in the design of a DAM for the Public Health Surveillance in Colombia. The students receive a Use Case Model describing the system requirements. They have to follow RUP guidelines for DAM design (Use Case Analysis Task). No additional training on RUP and UML is required. The treatment consists in the use of HIS-DF methodology in the design of the Harmonized Domain Analysis Model (HDAM) for the same scenario. The students participating in Group B received additional training on HIS-DF (4 hours). The total time available to complete the design tasks is 4 hours for both groups.

In order to calculate the validity and completeness variables, a reference DAM needs to be used. To assure quality of the reference model, the model was taken from the official documentation of the national Public Health Surveillance in Colombia. This reference model has been previously created by experts in the problem domain (this is verifiable because it was designed in a real project by experts responsible of designing the public health system at the public health authority in the country). Also, being a national project, the resources invested (time, personnel) were higher, therefore the quality of the reference model needs to be higher than the quality of the models in the experiment (control and experimentation groups) which had only 4 hours in total of work in the models, and were created by students with-out experience in the domain. The Reference DAM model doesn't consider the use of e-Health standards, so if an increased quality is demonstrated after using HIS-DF, it can be attributable to the use of eHealth standards.. The reference model has 24 Entities, 106 Attributes and 22 Relationships.

2. Results

The first step in the study was to define quantifiable metrics for semantic quality. Subsequently, the experiment was completed.

2.1. Semantic Quality Metrics

Semantic quality metrics include the definition of completeness and validity. Completeness is measured as the percentage of correct and relevant statements (constructs) of the Reference DAM which are included in each of the models under evaluation (DAM and HDAM). If all statements are captured in those models, the completeness is 100%. Statements in UML models are represented as UML Classes, Attributes and Relationships. The overall completeness is obtained by averaging the completeness for each modeling:

$$\text{Completeness} = (\text{CEntities} + \text{CAttributes} + \text{CRelation ships})/3 \quad (2)$$

where:

$$\text{CEntities} = (\text{NEr} - \text{NEmm} - 0.3\text{NEaAm})/\text{NEr} \times 100 \quad (3)$$

NEr is the total number of Entities in the Reference DAM, NEmm is the number of Entities of the Reference DAM missing in the model under evaluation (missing either as entity or attribute), and NEaAm is the number Entities of Reference DAM found as Attributes.

$$\text{CAttributes} = (\text{NAr} - \text{NAmm} - 0.3\text{NAaEm})/\text{NAr} \times 100 \quad (4)$$

NAr is the total number of Attributes in the Reference DAM, NAmm is the number of missing Attributes of Reference DAM in the model under evaluation (missing either as attribute or entity), and NAaEm is the number Attributes of the Reference DAM found as Entities.

$$\text{CRelationships} = (\text{NRr} - \text{NRmm})/\text{NRr} \times 100 \quad (5)$$

NRr is the total number of Relationships in the Reference DAM, NRmm is the number of missing Relationships of the Reference DAM not found in the model under evaluation.

In a similar way, Validity is measured as the percentage of correct and relevant statements in the models under evaluation (DAM or HDAM) which are part of the Reference DAM. If all Attributes, Classes and Relationships the DAM or HDAM are defined in the Reference DAM, validity is 100%. The overall Validity is obtained by averaging the validity for each modeling construct (UML Classes, Attributes and Relationships):

$$\text{Validity} = \text{VEntities} + \text{VAtributes} + \text{VRelationships}/3 \quad (6)$$

where:

$$\text{VEntities} = (\text{NEm} - \text{NiEmmr})/\text{NEm} \times 100 \quad (7)$$

NEm is the total number of correct and relevant entities in the model under evaluation; NiEmr is the number of (invalid) entities of model not present in Reference DAM.

$$\text{VAttributes} = (\text{NAm} - \text{NiAmr})/\text{NAm} \times 100 \quad (8)$$

Nam is the total number of Attributes in the model, and NiAmr is the total number of (invalid) attributes of model not found in the Reference DAM.

$$\text{VRelationships} = (\text{NRm} - \text{NRmr})/\text{NRm} \times 100 \quad (9)$$

NRm is the total number of Relationships in the model, NRmr is the number of Relationships of the model not found in the Reference DAM.

2.2. Completeness and Validity Results

After performing the experiment, 16 UML models were obtained: 8 DAM developed by Group A, and 8 HDAM developed by group B. For each model, the completeness and validity variables presented in equations (2)–(9) were calculated. Following, the overall completeness and validity was calculated for Groups A and B, averaging the results obtained from the 8 models in each group. The overall completeness and validity metrics for Groups A and B are presented in Table 1 and Figure 2. The table also presents the standard derivation, and probability for each variable.

Table 1. Completeness and Validity results

	Completeness				
	Group A		Group B		Probability*
	%	SD	%	SD	
Entities	59,06	10,46	68,75	7,88	0,055
Attributes	45,81	14,01	54,85	5,90	0,115
Relationships	18,18	19,74	42,61	15,35	0,015
Overall	41,02		55,40		

*t-test for mean comparisons

	Validity				
	Group A		Group B		Probability*
	%	SD	%	SD	
Entities	82,84	9,11	93,95	8,64	0,118
Attributes	82,10	21,03	86,59	12,64	0,428
Relationships	46,57	21,03	80,85	10,74	0,001
Overall	70,50		87,13		

*t-test for mean comparisons

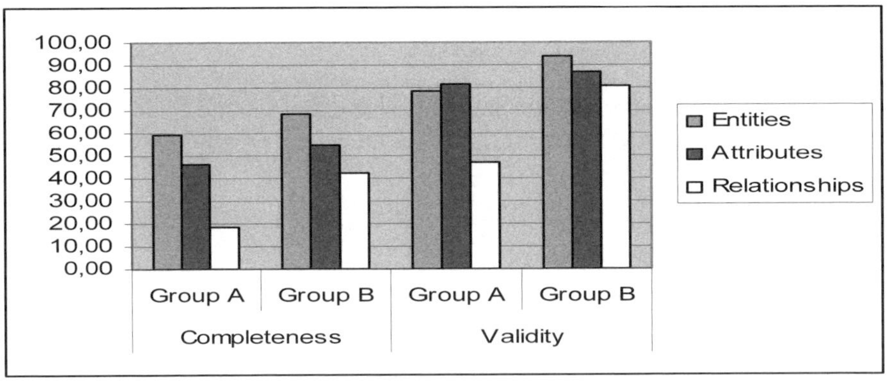

Figure 2. Completeness and Validity Results

3. Discussion

An assessment of semantic quality of HIS architectures developed using HIS-DF compared with architectures developed using traditional RUP Architectural Development has been presented. Semantic quality has been measured in terms of completeness and validity variables. From the results of Table 1, some statements can be formulated:

Overall Completeness of the architecture is increased by 14.38% due to the use of HIS-DF instead of the RUP Architecture Development method. The increased Completeness of Entities, Attributes, and Relationships in group B are respectively: 9.68 %, 9.03 % and 24.43 %. The significance of the results was statistically analyzed using a t-test calculation for mean comparison. The increased Completeness of Relationships was found strongly significant ($\rho = 0{,}015$), the increased Completeness of Entities was found nearly significant ($\rho = 0{,}055$), and Completeness of Attributes was found not significant ($\rho = 0{,}115$).

The increased completeness obtained is explained because the HL7 reference model (Notifiable Condition Report R-MIM) used by Group B provides a lot of common elements as defined in the reference DAM, therefore helping the Analyst to discover new Entities, Attributes and Relationships. The higher contribution of relationships completeness (24.43 %) could be especially due to large and detailed number of Relationships defined in HL7 models. Low Relationships Completeness in Group A might be explained due to the fact that the requirements provided to the analyst (students) included only static information about the surveillance scenario, therefore, ambiguities in behavioral aspects of information caused several errors in Relationships representation. Summarizing, it can be concluded that HIS-DF is useful for discovering new Entities, Attributes and Relationships, but only statistically significantly for discovering new Entities and Relationships.

Overall Validity is increased by 16.63% due to the use of HIS-DF instead of the RUP Architecture Development method. Increased validity of Entities, Attributes, and Relationships is respectively: 11.11%, 4.69%, and 34.27 %. The significance of the results was statistically analyzed using a t-test calculation for mean comparison. The increased Validity of Relationships was found strongly significant ($\rho = 0{,}01$), but the increased Completeness of Entities and Attributes was found not significant.

The validity of Attributes and Entities in the control group is high (82,4% and 82,1%) , therefore is difficult to demonstrate a significant increasing of the validity caused by HIS-DF. This result is reasonable because validity is measured with respect to the model itself (validity of entities present in the model). A model with only two entities can be 100% valid; despite it doesn't completely describe the problem domain. The more entities are present in the model, the more validation errors can occur. Validity of Attributes is also high (82.1% and 86.59 % in Groups A and B, respectively). However, the contribution of using HIS-DF is relatively low (4.49%). An explanation could be that the attributes presented in the HL7 R-MIM model (provided by HIS-DF) are so difficult to understand (specially due to the presence of HL7 data types) that system analyst prefer not to use them as reference. Summarizing, it can be concluded that HIS-DF is especially useful for describing valid Entities and Relationships, but only significant for identifying valid Relationships.

The analysis of results clearly demonstrates a significant improvement of completeness and validity of HIS architectures using HIS-DF. Many other analyses can be performed based on the collected data, specially the co-relationships between completeness and validity variables, as well as co-relationships between Entities, Attributes and Relationships. Also the contributions of using HL7 information models, attributes and data types in the HIS design process, as well the impact of using of UML profiles can be evaluated. This analysis is however, out of the scope of the paper.

The use of students to assume the role of HIS Analyst, as well as the limited training in HL7 standards offered to the participants could be a limitation of the study. However, according to [12], using students instead of practitioners allows easier control of human factors. Moreover the experimental tasks performed don't require high levels of industrial experience. It is also recommendable to increase the sample size in new experiments in order to improve the significance of the results.

4. Conclusion

Through an empirical experiment, it has been demonstrated that using HIS-DF for HIS architectural design, increases the architecture's semantic quality, compared to traditional RUP architecture development process. The increased quality of the architecture presumes an increased quality of final HIS systems and an indirect impact on patient care. Semantic quality has been measured in terms of completeness and validity attributes of UML Domain Analysis models (DAM). Validity implies that all statements in the model are correct and relevant to the problem domain (healthcare scenario). Completeness implies that the model contain all statements about the problem domain that are correct and relevant. The experiment demonstrated increased completeness of 14.38%, and an increased validity of 16.63% when using the HIS-DF combined with HL7 information models in a sample HIS development project.

Acknowledgments

The authors are indebted to thank their partners from HL7, OMG and other organizations for collegial collaboration. This work was founded by the German Academic Exchange Service DAAD and, projects SALUS (Qualidade em Sites na Área da Saúde 508RT0361) and MD-HELF (ID 2550) at the University of Cauca.

References

[1] Lopez DM, Blobel BG. A development framework for semantically interoperable health information systems. Int J Med Inform 2009 Feb;78(2):83-103.
[2] Lopez DM, Blobel B. Enhanced semantic interoperability by profiling health informatics standards. Methods Inf Med 2009;48(2):170-7.
[3] European Commission, Semantic Interoperability for Better Health and Safer Healthcare. Deployment and Research Roadmap for Europe,SemanticHEALTH Report. European Commission. Information Society and Media. 2009
[4] Lopez DM. Semantic Interoperability between Clinical and Public Health Information System for Improving Public Health Services. Stud Health Technol Inform 2007;256– 67.
[5] Lano K.. A compositional semantics of UML-RSDS. Software and System Modeling 2009;8(1):85-116.
[6] Lopez DM, Blobel B. Architectural Approaches for HL7-Based Health Information Systems Implementation. Methods Inf Med 2009 (submitted).
[7] HL7 Colombia. [Online]. Available from: URL: http://www.hl7.org.co (Accessed 15 Sep 2009)
[8] Anderson JG, Aydin CE. Evaluating the Organizational Impact of Health Care Information Systems. 2th ed. New York: Springer; 2005.
[9] Mårtensson F. Software Architecture Quality Evaluation. PhD Thesis, Blekinge Institute of Technology. 2006.
[10] Wohlin C et al. Experimentation in Software Engineering. An Introduction. Boston: Kluwer Academic Press; 2000.
[11] Lindland O, Sindre G, Sølvberg A. Understanding Quality in Conceptual Modeling. IEEE Software 1994;11(2),42-9.
[12] Maes A, Poels G. Evaluating Quality of conceptual modelling scripts based on user perceptions. Data & Knowledge Engineering 2007;63(3):701-24.

[13] Unhelkar B. Verification and Validation for Quality of UML 2.0 Models.New Jersey: John Wiley & Sons; 2005.
[14] Bolloju N, Leung SK. Assisting Novice Analysts in Developing Quality Conceptual Models with UML. Communications of the ACM 2006;49(7):108-12.
[15] Shanks G. Conceptual Data Modelling: An Empirical Study of Expert and Novice Data Modellers. Australian Journal of Information Systems 4(2):63-73.

Medical and Care Compunetics 6
L. Bos et al. (Eds.)
IOS Press, 2010

doi:10.3233/978-1-60750-565-5-32

Setting Core Standards: Privacy, Identity & Interoperability

B. Manning[1] and S. Benton[2]
[1] *Department of Informatics, University of Westminster*
[2] *The Business Psychology Centre, University of Westminster, 309 Regent Street, London W1B 2UW*

Abstract. This position paper focuses on strategic developments and underlying concepts emerging out of the standards and associated domains. It addresses the issue of personal privacy in the wider context of interoperability across an ever-growing range of e-health and social care support systems and processes. These will increasingly be driven by major growth in the elderly segment of national populations where unambiguous identification of both patients and care staff both in hospitals and the community will become significant issues. This is particularly so where remote patient monitoring and access control to personal data is concerned, and is further complicated where racial, cultural and linguistic barriers are prevalent.

Keywords. Privacy, Identity Management, Interoperability, Semantics

Introduction

The advent of evermore sophisticated and pervasive computing combined with micro-miniaturized monitoring devices is increasingly putting personal privacy at risk. At the same time the standards and regulatory communities' interests are beginning to overlap in terms of processes and procedures and of interoperability and interaction, especially where personally identifiable information is concerned.

As a result the fundamental issue of invasion of personal privacy is beginning to be considered in terms of degrees of intrusion involving a delicate balance between risk and benefits to the person concerned, as well as to the wider community. However it is equally important to ensure that they are correctly identified before significant harm occurs – especially where clinical interventions are concerned.

Privacy

To date most effort has so far been focused on Data Protection in terms of unauthorised access to personally identifiable information, either in transit or storage. However increased use of remote monitoring will impinge on the more fundament privacy rights surrounding personal behaviour and activities [1]. Moreover this will extend the need for protective measures out into ethical governance and public policy.

The ethical dimension has long been deeply embedded in clinical practice, especially in the context of surgical interventions, typically through the use of Informed

Consent procedures. By contrast the diverse nature of public policy is highly variable in its application and compliance both within and between legislative bodies, and with its service providers.

The forecasted doubling in the proportion of the elderly toward 35% of population of many nations [2] is likely to radically increase the use of Smart Home/Environment and Telemedicine/care support services out in the community [3]. Inevitably this will involve a variety of intrusions into personal privacy through the use a variety of physiological/location based monitoring and interactive support systems.

Dependent on the degree of support needed this will require an equivalent form of Informed Consent that enables the individual concerned to assess and balance the relative risks and benefits involved. However in this instance the decision process is far more complex as it affects ongoing quality of life across its whole spectrum.

Paradoxically most people are likely to take such significant decisions at an almost superficial motivational level, one influenced by personal expediency, without much consideration of other more subtle factors [4]. This essentially places a greater responsibility on professionals not only to back their recommendations with solid evidence, but also to ensure the individual concerned considers all the factors involved.

Behind the purely motivational judgment level lays the long-term worth of trading degrees of privacy for potential benefits in on-going quality of life. This in turn has to be set against exposure to unforeseen risks/issues, which will depend on the degree of trust and confidence that can be placed on service providers [Fig.1].

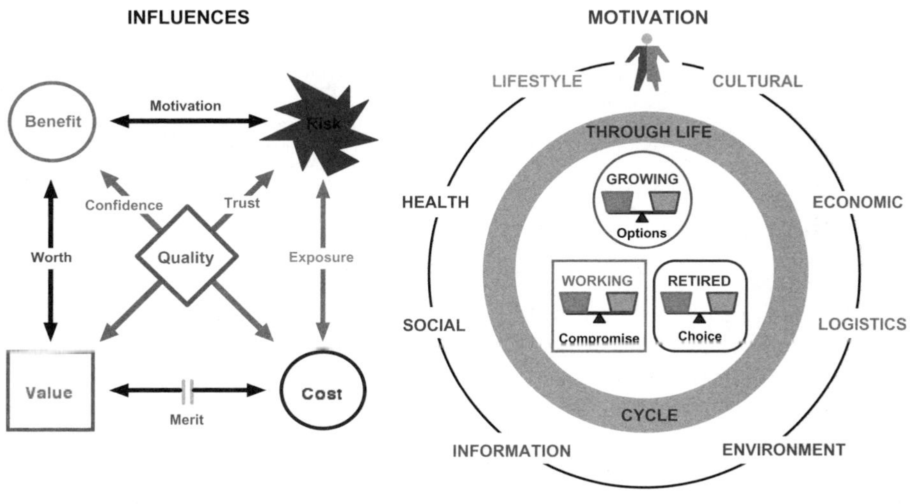

Fig.1 Behavioural Factors

Unfortunately continuity and quality of service provision are difficult, if not impossible to guarantee over any reasonable period due to the vagaries of life, public policy and funding availability. This is especially so as service merit is not generally equated in terms of any shared or reliable cost-to-value criteria. Further downside exposure comes from the lack of effective interoperability and coordination between support service providers, regardless of whether they operate on an insurance or governmental basis.

Identity Validation

In these circumstances confirmation of the identities of those concerned, from both the perspectives of the intruded upon as well as the authorized intruder, is of major importance. However obvious and simple it sounds, this is a highly complex and politicized problem, with a host of cultural, perceptual and logistical influences lurking behind them.

Although biometrics can be a key component in the identification process, their use entirely depends on there being an effective reference link to the formal identity of an individual currently registered under the relevant national jurisdiction [Fig.2]. Whilst this would seem a relatively simple task, it is bedeviled not only by the complexity and variability within and between national registry systems from birth onwards, but also by migration, marital relationships, dual nationality and many other issues.

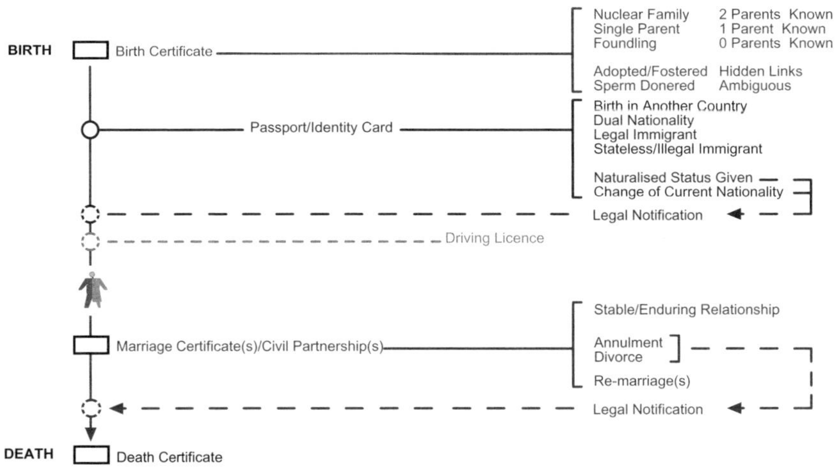

Fig.2...Identity Registration Life Cycle

Ideally the issue of a Death Certificate should conclude the registration life history of individual – thus preventing many identity thefts. Unfortunately this is not generally possible due to the slow, incremental process of developing interoperable centralised electronic registries, as well as the idiosyncratic and increasingly peripatetic nature of the life cycle followed by many individuals.

Despite this key dependence a task group of International Standards Organisation Technical Committee [ISO] TC215 – Health Informatics has been investigating how advances in "lab-on-a-chip" rapid DNA swab processing and string-selection methods could be used as a global health reference biometric identifier. Its ultimate aim would be to replace local/national numbering systems with one that would give secure world-wide access to relevant clinical information needed for emergency treatment.

A further aim of this approach will be to link this identification information with the DNA allergy markers that are beginning to emerge from current clinical research, as the preface to the electronic health record [EHR]. Prompts that highlight allergic susceptibilities to clinicians on entry to the EHR should help in reducing the risk of triggering analeptic shock and loss of life through inappropriate interventions.

Whilst the potential benefits that this approach offers patients are significant, their introduction would need to counter the innate suspicion that the collection of physiological biometric data – and in particular DNA - is destined to be misused by the authorities and turned against the best interests of the individual.

Interoperability

The key to rapid world-wide access in emergencies to EHR data centers on strictly controlled secure access via the internet to its source in the patient's home country. Whilst a laudable and achievable objective, it is beset by a number of practical problems, commencing with fundamental political and linguistic issues.

This is best illustrated by efforts within the European Union to establish a framework for effective interoperability between its member states. This identifies five basic levels [5] at which major harmonization and alignment must take place[Fig.3].

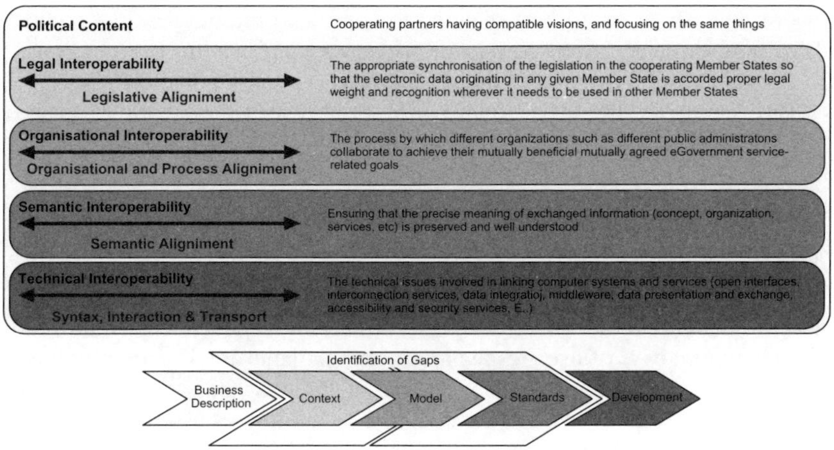

Fig.3 European Interoperability Framework

This neatly illustrates the contextual structure within which all good systems design should take place. However all too frequently technology inspired and led ventures make the fatal error of launching into major programs without carefully considering - or even in some instances discounting - the many legal, socio-political, socio-economic and psycho-social factors on which success ultimately rests.

The key lesson is that the role of technology is ultimately to be the supporting enabler of many improvements in services across a vast span of human endeavors - not "the be all and end all" focus of scientific interests! It has invariably to be set in the context of the needs and aspirations of society, ranging from the highly personal through a variety of organizational circumstances out into the wider community.

This is especially true in the health and social care domain. Whilst the primary interaction is between clinical/care staff and patients, systems and technology have an equally important interactive role to play in the care delivery process. Indeed the former are not only an integral part of the systems "loop" - but are unfortunately the source of significant ambiguity, variability and instability within it.

Interoperability is thus the "glue" without which most operational processes all too easily can and do fall apart - often disastrously!

As if this is not difficult enough to deal with successfully, increasingly multi-cultural and multi-lingual societies add a further layer of complexity. Systems - technological and organizational alike - have to take account of the sensibilities and perceptions that arise cross these divides in terms of both semantic and cross-cultural interoperability.

A parallel study on e-health interoperability [6] has surveyed the current progress and future projections from a broad policy perspective, taking account of stakeholder perspectives from both clinical and technical viewpoints. However this valuable body of knowledge needs to be seen in the context of the wider socio-political perspective on which its delivery will largely depend.

From this perspective the key issue is to identify the major gaps, disparities and disconnects that need to be resolved. Central to this is the establishment of a clear understanding of the end-goals and their context; the strategic service delivery model; the standards needed to ensure performance consistency and quality; and finally the basis for its successful implementation, development and governance. Moreover the past focus on records needs to be expanded to cope with the burgeoning expansion in demand for both the elderly and low-level primary mental health care monitoring and interactive well-being support out in the community.

As ever, standards are there to provide a reference framework to ensure best practice is followed appropriately and in context – especially where cross-compatibility between enabling technology and operational infrastructures will be at a premium.

The five tier European Union concept of interoperability spans what are all too frequently separate jealously guarded "silos" to link citizens (patients), businesses (clinical services) and administrations (Departments of Health, Local Authorities and other agencies) across traditional and national boundaries. Secure access and information transfer should ideally operate transparently between multiple-linked portals for maximum ease of use – especially where patients are directly involved.

A critical success factor centers on this need for trust and confidence in service quality and speed of response where the enabling technology is essentially invisible yet all pervasive. However as ever success in this field will come down to the human element and the preparedness to compromise to achieve worthwhile benefits both professionally and for the good of patients.

Semantics

The multiplicity and diversity of source systems involved underline the need for a federated approach to locating and consolidating specific cross agency content to meet a potentially vast range of highly focused user needs [7]. Moreover the quality of the source content should be maximized since it will be maintained by its local stakeholders/originators.

The size and geographic spread of sources and involved parties within national borders almost certainly require registries – such as the "Spine" system within the UK. These in turn will need to be consolidated at a supra-national level servicing the interoperability needs in the EU which are a collation of sets of information from individual states plus that of the EU itself. For the federated approach to operate effectively across multi-lingual, multi-cultural and multiple administrative structures a key requirement is to enable semantic interoperability across these complex domains, as outlined below [Fig.4]. The solution to these two problems lies in the addition of two further registries.

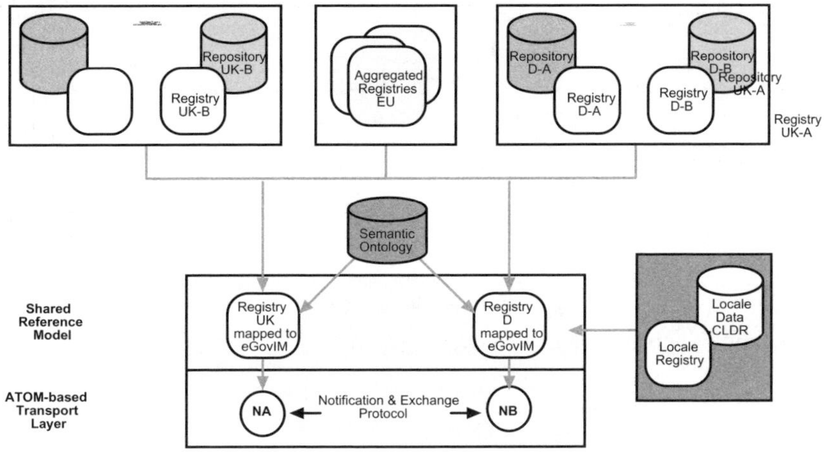

Fig. 4 Networked e-Government Services

The first is based on the creation of a semantic ontology system that acts as a terminological reference registry. This holds a linguistic cross-index of synonyms and "semi-synonyms", where the latter are sub-indexed as instances of "is equivalent to". The second will collate, compare and draw attention to cultural sensitivities in different areas as Cultural Locale Data Registries [CLDR].

The use of resource federation between parties who have agreed to share or exchange information allows users to search concurrently in multiple distributed repositories, rather than along the lines of distributed searching. This process enables the 'harvesting' of relevant information from 'open' areas from other collaborating repositories to be consolidated back into that of a particular interested party. Whilst this can then be browsed using their own search facilities as required, it can also provide further 'harvesting' access to others.

The underlying technology is designed to manage terms and their semantic relationships, as shown below [Fig.5] and will operate to:

1. Deal with information contained in documents that needs to be processed by applications, as opposed to situations where the content only needs to be presented to humans.
2. Explicitly represent the meaning of terms in vocabularies and the relationships between those terms.
3. Has more facilities for expressing meaning and semantics than XML, RDF, and RDF-S, and thus goes beyond these languages in its ability to represent machine interpretable content on the Web

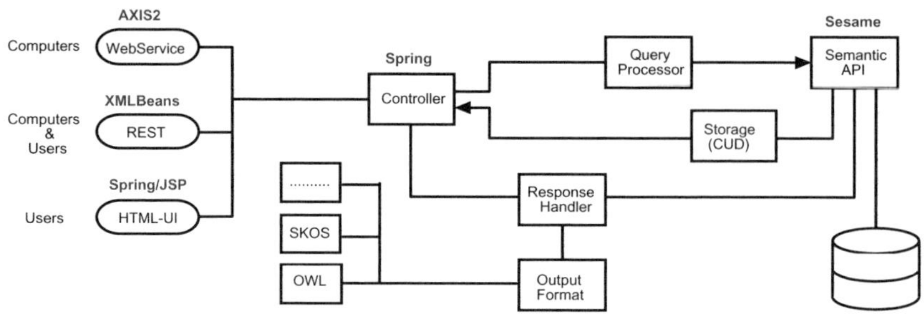

Fig. 5 Semantic Interoperability System

This type of approach has the advantages that:

It can express:
- Terms (text)
- The natural language of a term
- A relationship to other terms

From a user perspective their use of the system is limited to asking the TRN for a specific term and for its relationships to other terms

It is interesting to note that the development and proof of this concept has been carried out under the auspices of the Centre European de Normalisation [CEN] as an exploratory exercise as the prelude to the creation of a new standard based on this suitably funded research.

Conclusions

The three topics of privacy, identity and interoperability are delicately intertwined not only in the hospital and GP domains, but also increasingly in community care support settings. Whilst advances in biometric techniques can radically enhance identification accuracy to address patient safety and privacy concerns, these must be reference linked to an individual's formal identity records. This in turn would be dependent on secure and effective interoperability for identity validation at all levels. However the greatest significance of interoperability lies in radically improving evolutionary change in health and social care practice - bridging the gaps between human and technology domains - that should be the core of objective of Compunetics.

References

[1] ISO/TMB TFP Internal Report of the 1st Meeting of the ISO Technology Management Board Task Force on Privacy, DIN Berlin; 2008 Dec 10-11.

[2] Commission of the European Communities. e-Health – making healthcare better for European citizens: An action plan for a European Health Area. COM (2004); 356

[3] Manning BRM, McCann J, Benton S, Bougourd J. Active Ageing: Independence through Technology Assisted Optimisation. In: Bos L, Blobel B, Marsh A, Carroll D, editors. Medical and Care Compunetics 5. 2008 Jun. Amsterdam: IOSPress; 2008. p. 257-261. (Stud Health Technol Inform; vol 137)

[4] Bauman S. The Individualist Society. Polity Press. 2001 Jan 8. ISBN 0-7456-2507-X

[5] Commission of the European Communities: Draft Pan-European Interoperability Framework.

[6] Editorial Project Team CEN/CENELEC/ETSI: e-Health-Interop Report Phase 1. EU Mandate/403. 2007
[7] CEN/ISSS Workshop Agreement – CWA 15971:2009 parts 1 - 6 "e-Gov-share" Discovery of and Access to e-Government Resources

Medical and Care Compunetics 6
L. Bos et al. (Eds.)
IOS Press, 2010

doi:10.3233/978-1-60750-565-5-40

An Improved Method of Measurement of ECG Parameters for Online Medical Diagnosis

H.R SINGH [a,1], Rahul SHARMA [b], Nitin SAHGAL [c], Poonam SETHI [a], Rahul KUSHWAH [d] and Pranav KACHHAWA [b]

[a]*Biomedical Measurements and Standards Group, National Physical Laboratory New Delhi -110012, India*

[b]*B.Tech student BITS Pilani Goa Campus, Goa -403004, India*

[c]*B.Tech student RV College of Engineering, Bangalore- 560059, India*

[d]*M.Tech student NIT Kurukshetra-136119, Haryana, India*

Abstract. The accuracy in the online measurement of ECG parameters has a decisive role in the better diagnosis and effective treatment of the diseases. The present paper describes a Lab-VIEW based programming using Pan Tompkins method to extract out QRS complex whereas QT interval measurements were carried out using Mat-lab based math-script module. Hilbert transform has been applied on the ECG signal to convert it into an analytical signal for better peak detection. Peak detection and other parameters like RR interval, HR and several time domain measures of heart rate variability such as RR mean and standard deviations, HR mean and standard deviations, RMSSSD, NN50 count, pNN50 etc were calculated for several other clinical applications apart from online disease diagnosis.

Keywords. Biomedical measurements, Biomedical computing, ECG parameters extraction, ECG wave analysis

Introduction

A healthcare delivery system, with precision measurements becomes a more reliable diagnostic tool for an effective treatment of a disease. From a clinical point of view, the disease diagnosis is characterized by proper observations and accurate measurements of concerned parameters. Thus, proper evaluation of a signal, in the present context say ECG signal, helps clinicians in quick treatment decision for better healthcare [1]. The real time biomedical signal acquisition with online time interval measurements has always been in demand and is required to be taken up on priority for an early diagnosis in an automatic manner, mainly in case of elderly patients monitoring [2], [3] living in remote areas. A number of researchers and academicians have put their viewpoints on the need of automation [4], [5], [6] of ECG parameters over the manual detection. New technological developments and the use of information technology to support the delivery of quality healthcare offer promising prospective towards the precise

[1] Corresponding Author: H.R Singh, Biomedical Measurements and Standards Group, National Physical Laboratory, New Delhi-110012, India

parameter measurements and ultimately online diagnostic success. Such systems and technologies could be employed in the detection and time measurements of several waves such as P wave, T wave, QRS and QT and interpretation of abnormalities arise out due to variations in shape, size and occurrence of these waves in the ECG stream. On screen e-calipers and precisely calibrated simple calipers have been quite common for use in biomedical measurements to obtain various parameters like QRS, QT, PR and QT_c and their mean deviations etc. for clinical applications.

The present paper outlines a Lab-VIEW based method for the automatic evaluation of ECG and other such biomedical signals for an appropriate diagnosis and their correlation to the cardiac abnormalities of the patients.

1. Methodology

Pan Tompkins algorithm and Hilbert transform have undoubtedly been the most accepted solutions to extract out the parameters from the raw ECG signals. In the present application QRS and QT detection were performed using Pan Tompkins while most of the other parameters such as RR interval, BPM, Peaks, RR measurements and several other statistical and geometric measures were detected using Hilbert transform. In order to isolate the QRS energy predominant portion, the raw signal after acquisition is pre- processed [7] by proper signal conditioning and removing base line wandering. These parameters after extracting out from the enhanced ECG signal have been significantly used in diagnostic applications with accuracy acceptable to provide higher order of care to the patient.

1.1. QRS detection

A Lab-VIEW based program was developed to detect QRS complex using Pan Tompkins method [8]. The program takes on the characteristics features of slope, width and amplitude of the signal. The ECG signal is passed through a band pass filter with upper and lower cut-off frequencies at 12 and 5 Hz respectively to reduce the influence of muscle and 60 Hz interferences and baseline wandering etc. using low thresholds to increase the sensitivity of detection. The filtered signal is differentiated in order to provide better QRS complex slope information followed by point by point squaring of the derivatives emphasizing higher frequencies (ECG frequencies). In addition to the slope of R wave, the wave form feature information is obtained by inserting moving window integration as shown in the following equation

$$y(nT) = 1/N\sum_{n=1}^{n=N} X(nt-(N-1)T) \quad (1)$$

Where, N is the number of samples in the width of integration window. The width of this window should be approximately the same as the widest possible QRS complex. For our sample rate of 125 samples/second the window is 18 samples wide (144 ms). Since there was no VI available in Lab-view to implement moving window integration the math script module in Mat-lab was used to generate the relevant code. The QRS corresponds to the rising edge of the integration waveform. The time duration of rising edge is equal to the width of the QRS complex and is finally computed by differentiating the signal and checking for how long is the derivative positive. A block diagram implementing the above stated stages in Lab-VIEW program is shown in Figure 1 for QRS detection. The results evaluated on samples from MITBIH database [9] show sensitivity of high order.

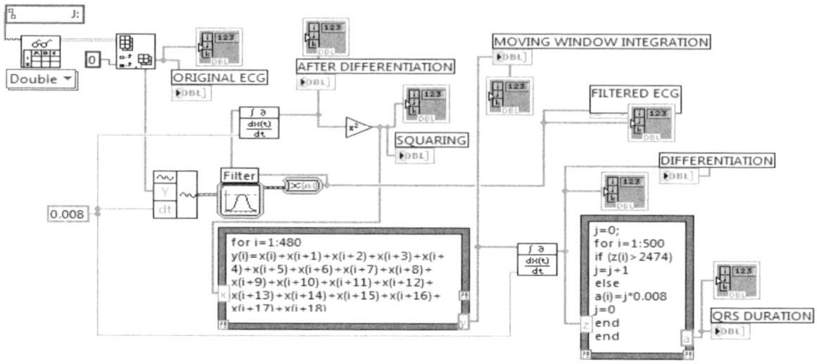

Figure 1. Block diagram of QRS detection

Figure 2 displays the corresponding waveforms after executing every stage of the above VI on a normal sinus rhythm as input.

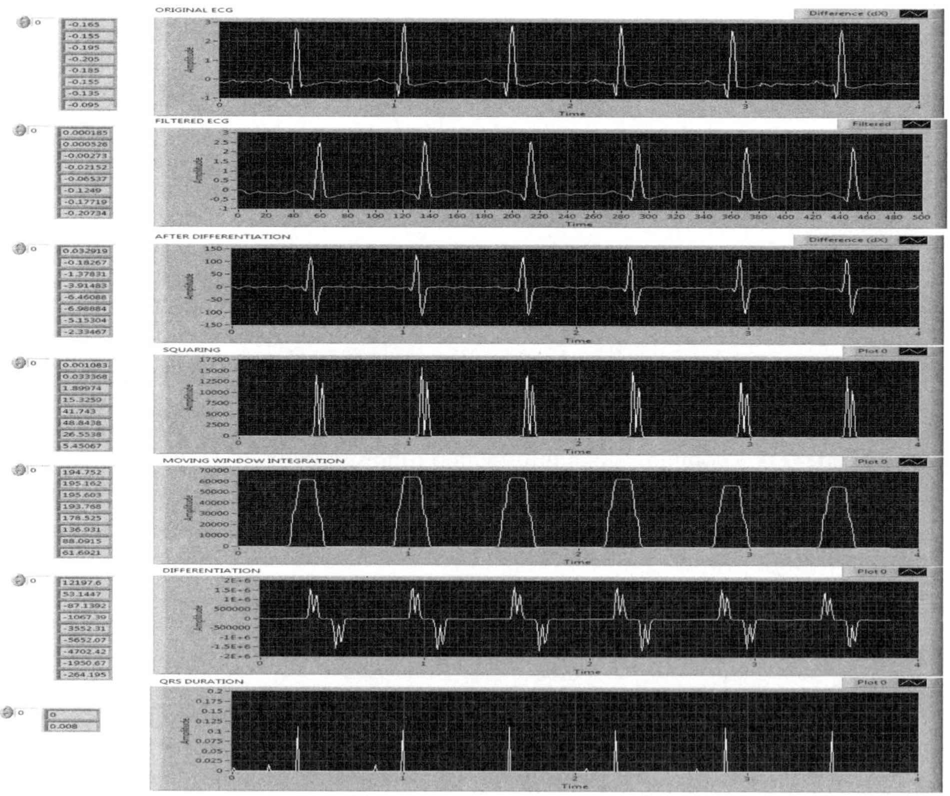

Figure 2. Input/Output waveforms of a Normal Sinus Rhythm

1.2. QT detection

Another highly informative and diagnostic element complex in ECG wave analysis is QT interval measurement, which needs to be calculated online for the safety assessment of the new drug during its developmental stage, in order to avoid any clinical implications. This automation in QT interval helps professionals to make a quick assessment of the prolongation of even a few ms in QTc timing and to study the spontaneous variability in QT interval. The gap interval between Q $_{onset}$ and T $_{offset}$ values is calculated on a signal as acquired and processed in the previous section of QRS complex determination. The block diagram developed for the detection of QT interval and Q point and T point time measurements is shown in Figure 3.

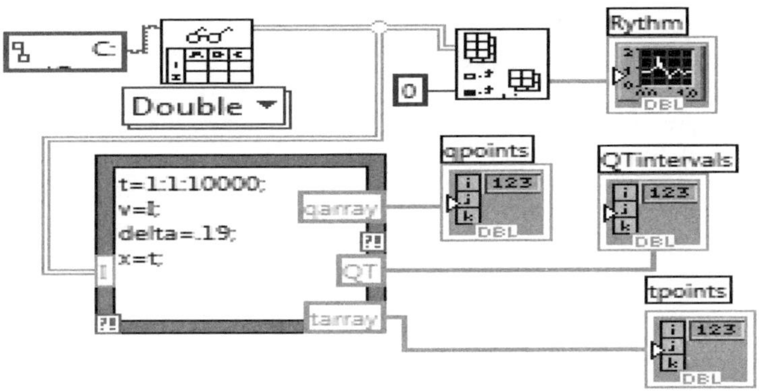

Figure 3. Block Diagram for detection of QT interval

The corresponding QT interval measurement displaying the QT $_{off}$ and QT $_{on}$ values separately along with the signal acquired is shown in Figure 4.

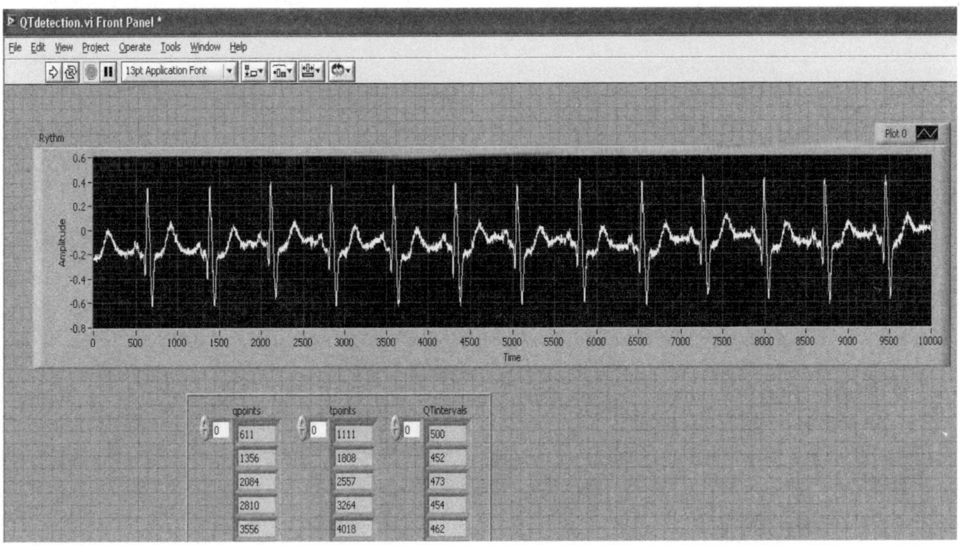

Figure 4. Front panel of QT detection

1.3. RR interval and Time domain Heart rate Variability Analysis

The derivative of the signal acquired after filtering and base line wandering elimination using median filter is taken on which Hilbert transform is performed. The reason Hilbert transform is used for these measurements is to turn the ECG signal to an analytic signal, which gives a better peak to detect. This process will give an enhanced ECG signal as compared to raw ECG signal first obtained. Peakdetection.vi algorithm is developed to find all the peaks and their locations by setting appropriate threshold parameters. The RR intervals are extracted by measuring the time interval between two consecutive peaks. The heart rate is calculated as follows:

Sampling rate*60/ RR interval (ms)

The most common method of heart rate variability analysis is time domain analysis where only the temporal RR interval signals are used to extract out a few statistical and geometric measures. These measures are mean and standard deviation (RR mean) of all RR intervals and heart rate (HR), RMSSD (square root of mean of sum of square of differences between adjacent RR intervals), NN50count (Number of pairs of adjacent RR intervals differing by more than 50 ms) and HRV triangular indcx (total no. of all RR intervals divided by height of the histogram of all RR intervals) etc. The process of acquiring various signal parameters as stated above is shown in Figure 5.

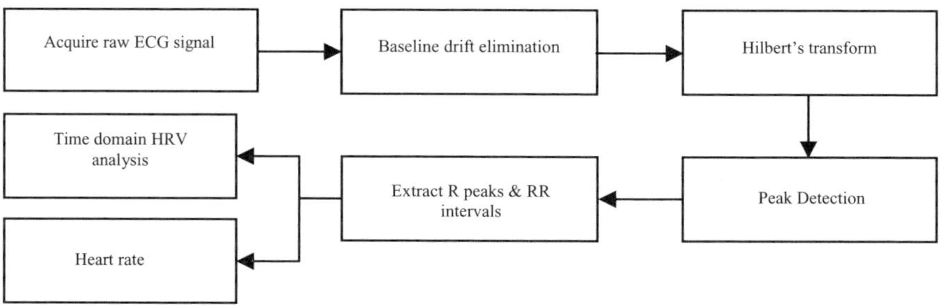

Figure 5. Process of acquiring signal parameters

The block diagram of the time domain HRV analysis in lab-view is shown in Figure 6.

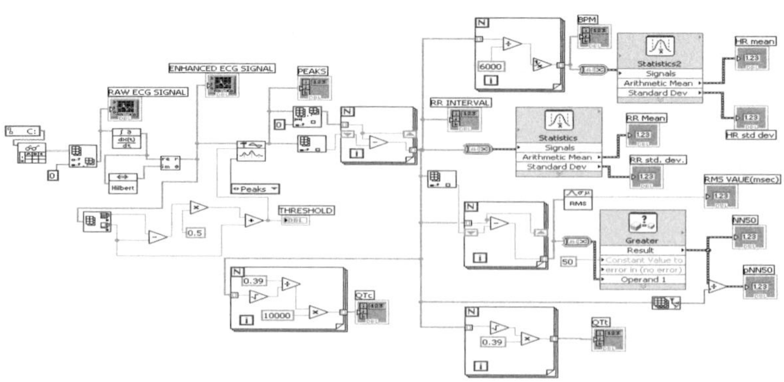

Figure 6. Block diagram of Time domain HRV analysis

The execution of above VI in lab-view yields the following time domain statistical and geometric measures (Fig. 7) from the original RR interval.

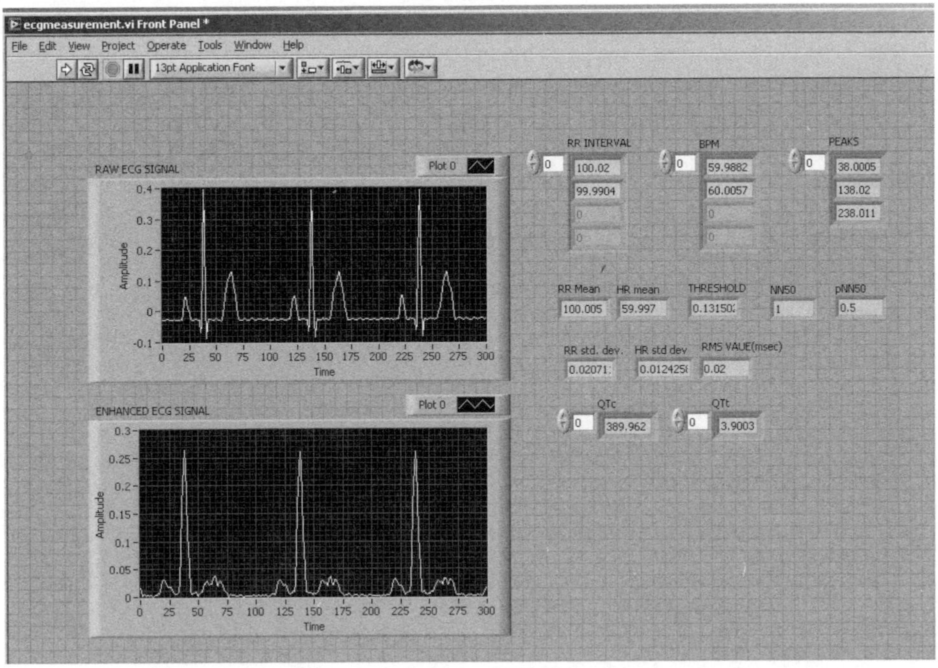

Figure 7. RR interval, Peak detection and HRV parameters of ECG Signal

A few of the parameters measured as above are extremely helpful in clinical applications for specialists to arrive at a quick and decision making opinion about the disease whereas the others are highly informative R&D elements to show the interdependencies of parameters with each other.

Conclusion

VI's for the determination of QRS duration using Pan Tompkins algorithm is developed and stepwise execution of every stage is displayed in the front panel diagram. For QT interval measurement, math-script tool in mat-lab is used and the corresponding QT intervals along with their Q point and T point time measurements are displayed in the respective front panel diagram. QT interval measurements are highly desirable in the safety assessment of new drugs before it is actually put on trial on patients. A single window VI for the measurement of all time domain statistical and geometric measures such as RR interval, HR, HRV time variant analysis, RR and HR mean and standard deviations, RMSSSD, NN50 count is also developed and results are displayed. These results and their interdependencies on each other are highly desirable to study the spontaneous variability in their time intervals in order to avoid any spurious confusion among the patients.

Acknowledgement

Authors are grateful to the Director National Physical Laboratory, New Delhi, India for the encouragement received during the work. We are also thankful to Dr. P. Banerjee for his help and encouragement. The extensive discussion with Prof. V.R Singh, Advisor AICTE and his help is highly acknowledged.

References

[1] Forker-Dunn J. Internet based Patient self care: The next generation of Health care Delivery. J Med Internet Res 2003;5(2):e8.

[2] Alwan M, Dalal S, Kell S, Turner B, Leachtenauer J, Felder R. Impact of monitoring Technology in assisied living: outcome Pilot. IEEE Trans on info Tech in Bio-med 2006;10(1):192-8.

[3] Singh HR, Singh M. Design and development of Knowledge driven web based ECG monitoring and diagnostic tool in Lab-view. In: Bos L, Blobel B, Marsh A, Carroll D, editors. Medical and Care Compunetics 5. IOS press; 2008. p. 170-80.

[4] Murray A, Mclaughlin NB, Campbell RB. Measuring QT dispersion man Vs machine Heart. 1997;77(6):529-42.

[5] Langley P, Murray A. Comparison of Manual and automatic QT dispersion measurement in clinical groups. Computer Cardiol 2001;28:1645.

[6] Madias J. Manual based Vs Automation based measurements of the amplitude of QRS complexes and T wave in patients with edematous states – clinical implications. J. of Electrocardiography 2008;41(1):13-8.

[7] Daskalov I. Electrocardiogram signal preprocessing for automatic detection of QRS boundaries. Medical Engineering and Physics 1999;21(1):37-44.

[8] Pan WJ, Tompkins J. A Real time QRS detection Algorithm. IEEE Trans Bio-med Eng., 1985;BM1232: 230-6.

[9] MIT-BIH Arrhythmia database. [Online]. Available from: URL: www.physionet.org

Medical and Care Compunetics 6
L. Bos et al. (Eds.)
IOS Press, 2010

doi:10.3233/978-1-60750-565-5-47

Evaluation of Response Time Delay of a Pen-Tablet System in Thin-Client Computing Environments: Implications for Usability

Kei TERAMOTO [a,c,1], Shigeki KUWATA [a], Andre W. KUSHNIRUK [b], Elizabeth M. BORYCKI [b], Maki NOMURA [c] and Hiroshi KONDOH [a]
[a] *Medical Informatics Division, Tottori University Hospital, Tottori, Japan*
[b] *School of Health Information Science, University of Victoria, Victoria, Canada*
[c] *Graduate School of Medical Science, Tottori University, Tottori, Japan*

Abstract. Changeover from the traditional paper-based patient records to the computerized patient records has been spreading rapidly in medical facilities. Since ordinary input devices such as a keyboard and mouse are often thought insufficient for the needs of medical workers using electronic patient records (EPR) compared with traditional pens and paper-based patient records, a pen-tablet system (PTS) as a digital pen interface tends to be used instead. On the other hand, with the growing adoption of thin-client computing (TCC) in medical facilities, the usability of PTS with TCC has come to be a concern because of possible reduction of the usability due to delays of response time occurring in TCC environments. To analyze the factors that influence the usability of PTS with TCC, the authors focused on the relationship between length and its scattering of the response time delay. The results indicated that the delay scattering could be a more influencing factor than the delay length itself and that values of the scattering should be within approximately 35 milliseconds for the best usability. This study would provide useful indicators for evaluating the usability of PTS in incorporating it into the EPR system with TCC environments.

Keywords. Electronic Patient Record, Pen-Tablet System, Thin-Client Computing, Usability

1. Introduction

Thin-Client Computing (TCC) is computer system architecture in which applications, usually running on end-user's PCs in the traditional system, are centralized and executed in the server-side system. A low cost machine with inexpensive hardware, e.g. diskless thin client, can therefore be adopted in TCC. The innovative architecture has been utilized not only in common business settings but also in the hospital information system (HIS) in term of its superiority with regard to cost reduction and privacy protection. An example clarifying the effectiveness of TCC was illustrated in a hospital with about 700 beds and 1,100 thin client PCs [1] [2]. TCC was also used as an infrastructure for cross-reference system of Electronic Patient Records (EPR) between a central hospital and its surrounding hospitals in a rural district [3]. On the other hand,

[1] Corresponding Author: Kei Teramoto, MHSc., Medical Informatics Division, Tottori University Hospital, 36-1 Nishi-cho, Yonago, Tottori, 683-8504, Japan; E-mail: kei-tera@umin.net

it was pointed out that adoption of EPR with TCC architecture might address some issues on the usability of pen-tablet systems (PTS), frequently used with EPR by medical workers, because of delays of screen updating due to response time prolongation being intrinsic to TCC environments [4]. With the increase of adoption of TCC in medical facilities, it would be much more needed to evaluate the usability of PTS as an input device of EPR.

1.1. Using Pen-Tablet System on Electronic Patient Record

Preceding studies found that existing technologies of EPR for documentation and data entry comparing with traditional paper-based health record were problematic [5] [6]. The major reason was that computer requires use of a keyboard and mouse, poorly suited to editing on EPR. PTS, a substitutive man-machine interface for a mouse, was frequently utilized by medical workers for writing signatures, drawing graphics, pointing at a portion of PC screen and annotating radiology graphics on EPR (**Figure 1**) [7] [8]. Moreover, PTS was also applicable to the man-machine interface for patients to input their signatures in the case of informed consent or to respond to medical check-up questionnaires preceding doctor's consultation.

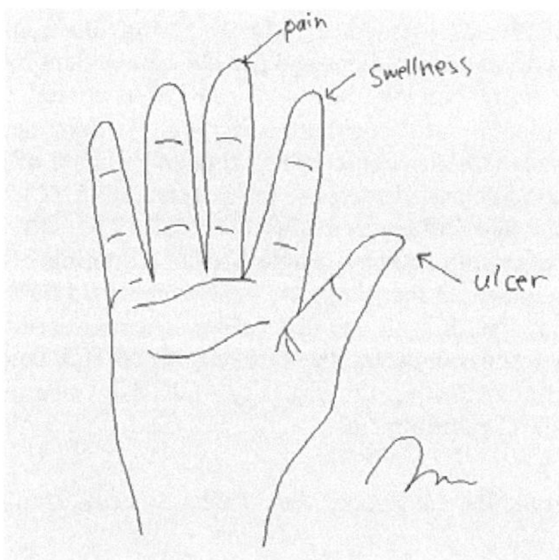

Figure 1. A sample graphic drawn by a nurse using a pen-tablet system

1.2. Characteristic of Thin-Client Computing

TCC architecture makes it possible to centralize all application functions to remote servers and provide virtual desktop information created and sent by remote servers with the end-user's machine. Typically TCC software installed in the remote server communicates with the thin clients via TCP/CP network. Common mechanisms of the TCC applications are as follows: (a) The end user's machine sends the information of input commands of mouse, keyboard and PTS to the remote server over the network, (b) The remote server receives the command to process application by oneself, and (c) The remote server responds to the commands. Since each process completes in a short moment, end-users feel as if the client PC were handling all application processes. Various TCC applications with different mechanisms were developed to realize the virtualization by many vendors; the difference due to TCC applications usually lay in the last process (c). The TCC applications used in this study were GO-Global (GG) by GraphOn [9], Citrix Presentation Server (Citrix) by Citrix [10] and Windows Terminal Service (WTS) by Microsoft [11]. Citrix adopted the Independent Computing Architecture Protocol as an advanced version of WTS to implement considerable compression and optimization to render the application. GG adopted the Rapid-X protocol to send only drawing API commands to clients. Since the processes from (a) to (c) were executed over the network, delays of screen updating at the client PC were frequently prolonged as compared with standalone PC.

2. Purpose

The aim of this study is to measure the limiting factor on the delay of screen updating for implementing PTS to EPR, under the hypothesis that the delay influenced compatibility between TCC and PTS [4] [12]. The results of this study would be one of indices in developing the EPR system with a usable PTS on TCC architecture as well as on cloud computing in which response time delays would become inevitable cause of reducing the usability.

3. Methods

This study was composed of experiments including two scenarios. The first scenario as a preliminary experiment was conducted to obtain fundamental data for the second scenario. The method included three steps: Step 1) measurement of velocity of writing signatures (referred to as 'signatures' for simplicity) and drawing graphics ('graphics') on PTS, Step 2) measurement of the delay length when using PTS and Step 3) usability questionnaires of PTS. The second scenario as a main experiment aimed at specifying limiting range of the delay in response time by an observation of the usability under the controlled delays varied within a possible range of practical use of PTS.

3.1. Preliminary experiment

3.1.1. Step 1: Measurement of writing velocities of signatures and graphics

Writing velocities of signatures and graphics were measured for five subjects including three medical workers and two system engineers of a hospital who had over ten years experience of computer operation. Age of the subjects ranged from 28 to 41. The subjects were asked to write signatures and draw graphics three times respectively using PTS on the screen of Mc5, an application to measure the writing velocity developed by FAREND Technology Inc. [10]. The movement of mouse-cursor synchronized with the operation on PTS that was recognized as a mouse device by operation system. Mc5 stored the data of moving distance and time calculated by the position of mouse-cursor on coordinates at intervals of 1/100 second. The subjects practiced typical operations of PTS before the experiment so that they were able to use PTS just like traditional pens on the paper and that they could memorize sample graphic images that they would asked to draw in the following experiment not to stop their PTS operation during the experiment.

3.1.2. Step 2: Measurement of delay length

Mc5 was installed in the remote server to recognize mouse-events of the user. It has a user interface that allows users to draw arbitrary objects as Microsoft Paint does. The delay length was measured using five lines drawn with three different velocities (Low, Middle and High) on Mc5 for three major TCC applications (GG, Citrix and WTS). The authors supposed that the difference of the usability between signature and graphics would be caused by the nature of delay length that originated from the difference of velocities between them. The average velocities of moving mouse-cursor were set to Low: 320.7, Middle: 600.1 and High: 1628 (in pixels/sec) as typical velocities that were decided according to the results in Step 1, to make their influence on delay length distinguishable.

3.1.3. Step 3: Evaluation by questionnaires

The subjects who participated in the Step1 experiment were asked to answer five-grade usability questionnaires on difference between TCC and standalone PC. The evaluation was categorized as follows: 5: no difference, 4: partly inferior but no influence on work, 3: inferior but no influence on work, 2: inferior but usable under some limitation, and 1: completely inferior and not usable on work. The order of evaluating the TCC applications was changed for each subject and a product name of the TCC applications was hidden to exclude a bias that could influence the results of the questionnaires.

3.2. Main experiment

In the preliminary experiment, the authors found that the delay length could be a possible index of the usability and that the degree of its fluctuation was also considered of importance (*cf. 4.1 Results of preliminary experiment*). The purpose of this experiment is to scrutinize the relationship between the length and fluctuation of the response time prolongation and the usability of PTS to obtain limiting factors for implementing PTS to EPR systems on TCC environments. The experiment was conducted for five subjects at the age ranging from 27 to 40 who operated PCs during daily work and experienced use of PTS. The subjects were asked to write signatures using PTS with various settings of the delay on drawing application (described below). Subsequently, they were asked to answer three-grade questionnaires on the usability, focusing on the differences from the ordinary stand-alone environment with no delays. The options for the answers were: (a) no difference (score 5), (b) a little inferior but no problem for business use (score 3) and (c) obviously inferior and not usable for business use (score 1).

3.2.1. Devices used in the experiment

The devices used in the experiment included a laptop PC (Lenovo, ThinkPad X61 8930-96J), PTS (WACOM, Intuos3), and a drawing application (FAREND Technologies Corporation, Mc6). Mc6 provides a drawing tool like Microsoft Paint and produces an artificial delay by inserting a deliberate pause into system responses. The length and standard deviation of the delay, represented as average and standard deviation respectively, were controlled by MC6 to the values ranging from 0 to 120 milliseconds (msec) with 20 msec intervals and from 28 to 110 msec with approximately 3 msec intervals, respectively. These values were determined according to the results from the preliminary experiment suggesting that the substantial change of usability scores would occur within those conditions.

4. Results

4.1. Results of preliminary experiment

4.1.1. Results of measurements of writing velocities (Step 1)

Figure 2 shows the results of the measurement in Step1. The averages of velocities of signatures and graphics were 288 and 121 respectively (in pixels per second). For each subject, the velocity of signatures was 1.75–3.6 times higher than that of graphics. It was confirmed that signatures tended to be written with higher velocities than graphics.

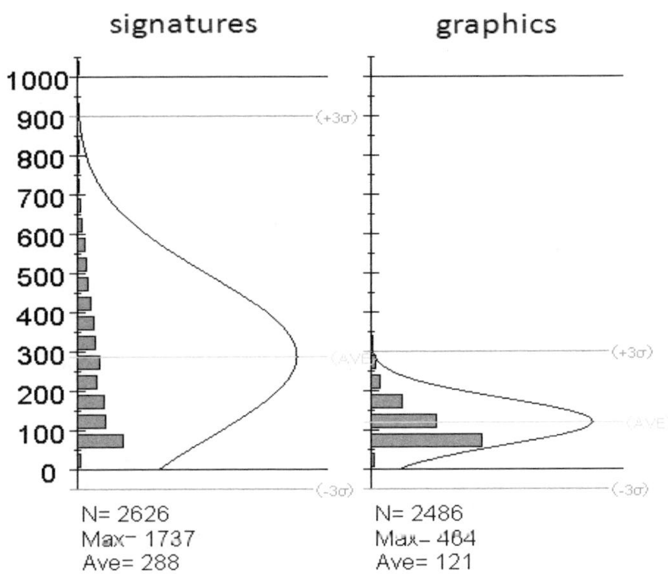

Figure 2. Histogram of velocities of signatures and graphics (Vertical units are pixels per second)

4.1.2. Results of measurement of delay length (Step 2)

Variances of delay length for each TCC application were compared using the statistical method of Bartlett test. Values of the delay length of GG, Citrix and WTS for each velocity range were Low: 46.4 ± 28.7, 16.9 ± 17.7 and 5.7 ± 5.7, Middle: 51.4 ± 30, 41.4 ± 34.3 and 34.5 ± 20.5 and High: 124.8 ± 56.5, 110.3 ± 67.0 and 98.1 ± 77.1 (Mean ± SD in pixels per second) respectively (**Figure 3**). For all TCC applications the values tended to increase with velocity, and their averages were found as WTS < Citrix < GG.

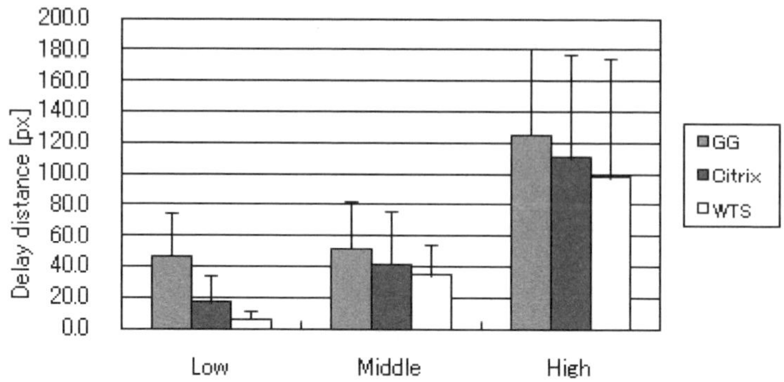

Figure 3. Distribution of delay length for three TCC applications for three different velocities (Units are pixels described as px; Bars represent Mean and lines represent SD)

On the other hand, regarding the scattering (standard deviation) of the delay length, in spite of the result as WTS < Citrix < GG for Low velocity, the relationship of the delay length among three TCC applications was reversed for High velocity, and the scattering of the delay length increased for Citrix and WTS when writing velocity increased. In particular, scattering of the delay length had significant difference ($p<0.01$) between GG and WTS (**Figure 4**). Consequently, 1) for higher velocities the delay length tended to be greater than for lower velocities for all TCC applications, 2) Citrix and WTS were more sensitive to the velocity than GG resulting in greater scattering of the delay length as the velocity increased.

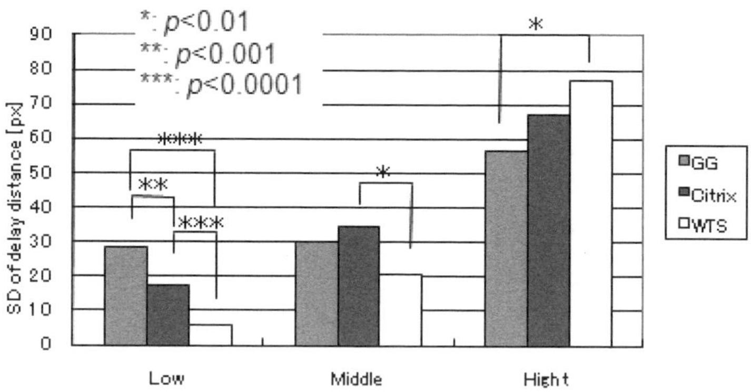

Figure 4. Comparison of standard deviation of delay length for three TCC applications for three different velocities (Units are pixels described as px; probabilities were calculated using Bartlett test)

4.1.3. Results of usability questionnaires (Step 3)

Table 1 shows the results of questionnaires for signatures and graphics evaluated by the subjects. The best usability was obtained for GG followed by Citrix and WTS for both signatures and graphics. The scores for signatures were overall lower than those for graphics. All subjects marked the best scores for GG, which represented that GG had the almost same usability as standalone PCs, particularly for graphics. The results coincided with those from Step1 and 2 in that the usability was reduced as the delay length increased and that it was also sensitive to the growing delay scattering as the writing velocity increased.

Table 1. Results of questionnaires for signatures and graphics for different TCC applications

signatures

	subject A	subject B	subject C	subject D	subject E	average
GG	5	5	3	5	4	4.4
Citrix	4	4	3	4	3	3.6
WTS	1	3	1	2	1	1.6

graphics

	subject A	subject B	subject C	subject D	subject E	average
GG	5	5	5	5	5	5.0
Citrix	5	4	5	4	4	4.4
WTS	3	4	2	2	5	3.2

4.2. Results of main experiment

Figure 5 shows the distribution of the average scores obtained from the subjects. The vertical axis indicates the delay length and the horizontal axis does the scattering. Deep blue color represents the best scores of the usability, which means that all the subjects answered 'no difference' under the conditions as the axes indicated, where deep red color does the worst score. For the scattering of delay length less than approximately 35 msec, the usability was equal to or above the average regardless of the values of delay length, while for more than approximately 45 msec it was less than the average no matter how small the delay length was, which meant that use of PTS was inappropriate under those conditions. In short, it was of great importance to remain the scattering within the threshold value to obtain the best quality of the usability of PTS on TCC environments.

Figure 6 shows the delay length and its scattering obtained from the preliminary study (Step 2). The result indicated that all plots for GG except three fell within 35 msec of the delay scattering, which coincided with that fact that GG obtained the best usability in the experiment of Step 2.

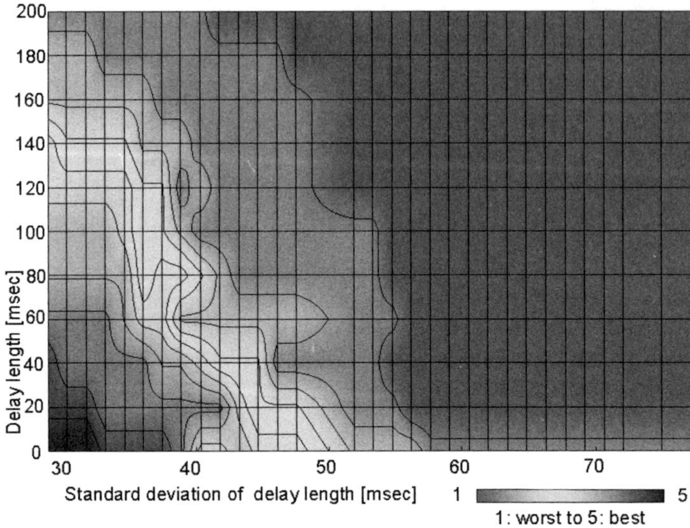

Figure 5. Distribution of the usability questionnaire by the subjects under controlled delays. Deep blue color means the best quality (Score 5) and deep red color does the worst (Score 1). Scores were averaged for each subject. Units are milliseconds for both axes.

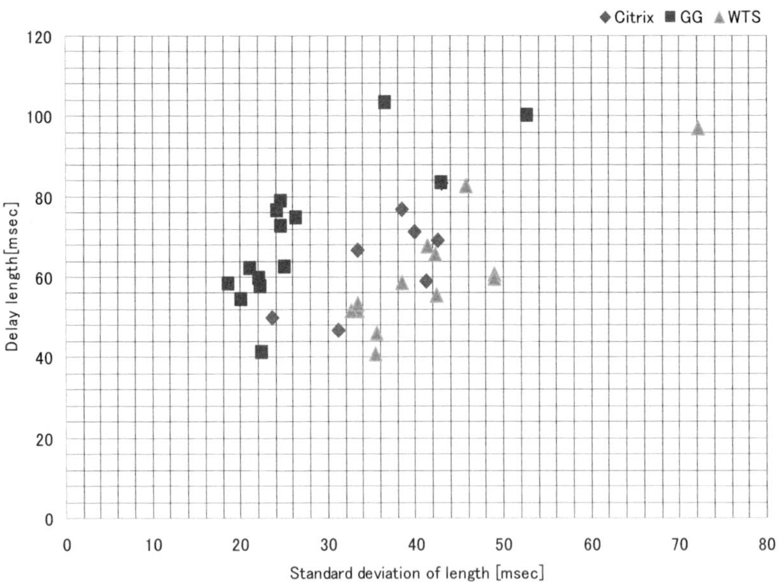

Figure 6. Plots of delay length and its standard deviation for three TCC applications for three different velocities, obtained from the preliminary study.

5. Discussion

Delays in response time necessarily occur when using EPR over the network. To make the impact on the usability by the delay less serious, some TCC applications deliberately crop some part of the response information to shorten the delay. The technique would be effective within a certain range of the delay, but it might make the users confused with unnatural system behavior by excessive cropping when the transmission rate is very low: Cropping with increase of the fluctuation would ruin the usability. From the finding of our study, it would be important to limit the delay scattering within a given range to obtain the best usability, specifically approximately 35 msec in our experimental settings, even letting the delay last for some periods.

How the delay scatters generally depends on how TCC applications crop screen-updating information when responding to the PC client. The manner of the cropping would be optimized for various purposes with various settings; therefore it should be noted that the results of the study would not discuss the superiority of any TCC application, since three TCC applications in this study were used with their default settings, without allowing for the optimization.

PTS on EPR is often used in drawing graphics as well as writing signatures, but in the main experiment the usability only for writing signature was considered. This is because the preliminary study presented that pen movement by users tended to be much slower in drawing graphics than in writing signature. With that drawing velocity, no significant delay of response time was found on TCC environment.

This study included the relatively small subjects in the experiments. It is possible that large number of the subjects with different backgrounds may yield the different results of the usability. The limitation would be reexamined in further studies.

6. Conclusion

To analyze the factors that influence the usability of PTS on TCC architecture, the authors focused on the relationship between length and its scattering of response time delays produced by the architecture. The results from the experiments of this study, it could be concluded that the delay scattering could be a more influencing factor than the delay length itself and that values of the scattering should be within approximately 35 msec to obtain the good usability for practical use. This study would provide useful indicators for evaluating the usability of PTS in incorporating it into the EPR system with TCC environments.

References

[1] Kuwata S, Teramoto K, et al. Effective Solutions in Introducing Server-Based Computing into Hospital Information System. Stud Health Technol Inform 2009;143:435-40.

[2] Teramoto K, Shigeki K, et al. Development of a design model of Hospital Information System based on Server-Based Computing. Japan Journal of Medical Informatics 2007;27 (suppl.):666-8.

[3] Kimura H, Nakahara K, et al. The operative experience of five years of the regional medicine cooperation system (Ajisai net). Japan Journal of Medical Informatics 2009;29(suppl.):530-1.

[4] Teramoto K, Kuwata S, et al. Evaluation of the Usability of a Pen Tablet System Using Server-Based Computing. Proceedings of Asia Pacific Association for Medical Informatics 2009. 2009;182-6.

[5] Yen P, Gorman PN. Usability Testing of a Digital Pen and Paper System in Nursing Documentation. AMIA Annu Symp Proc 2005;844-8
[6] Nakazawa K, Ashihara T, et al. A Comprehensive Computer Interface for Electronic Medical Recording Systems Supporting Hand-writing Inputs by Pen Device. Japan Journal of Medical Informatics 2002;22 (suppl.):364-5.
[7] Main DS, Quintela J, et al. Exploring Patient Reactions to Pen-Tablet Computers. Ann Fam Med 2004;2(5):421-4.
[8] Kieffer S, Gouze S, et al. Towards Standardized Pen-Based Annotation of Breast Cancer Findings, Human-Computer Interaction. In: Interacting in Various Application Domains. Heidelberg, Berlin: Springer; 2009. p. 524-33
[9] GraphOn Corporation. [Online]. Available from: URL: http:// www.graphon.com/.
[10] Citrix Systems Inc. [Online]. Available from: URL: http://citrix.com/lang/English/ home. asp.
[11] Microsoft Corporation. [Online]. Available from: URL: http://msdn.microsoft.com/ja-jp/library/bb521701.aspx.
[12] Teramoto K, Kuwata S, et al. Issues on Evaluation of the Usability of a Pen Tablet System using Server-Based Computing. Stud Health Technol Inform 2009;150:415.
[13] FAREND Technologies Corporation. [Online]. Available from: URL: http://www.farend.co.jp/.

Medical and Care Compunetics 6
L. Bos et al. (Eds.)
IOS Press, 2010

doi:10.3233/978-1-60750-565-5-57

Development of an Alarm Management System to Manage those alarms occurred during the Illness Prevention and Management inside and outside the Hospital Environment

Fátima RODRÍGUEZ[a1], Alejandro LAMELO[a], Francisco ARNAL[b], Camino REMÓN[c], Rosa VILLANUEVA[d] and Guillermo VÁZQUEZ[a]
[a] *INIBIC-ATIS[2], IT Department, A Coruña University Hospital, Spain*
[b] *Pathological Anatomy Department, A Coruña University Hospital, Spain*
[c] *Clinical Analyses Department, A Coruña University Hospital, Spain*
[d] *Microbiology Department, A Coruña University Hospital, Spain*

Abstract. A great amount of information is available to be exploited thanks to the use of information technologies. However, the systems that analyze this data lack the ability to alert the right clinical staff to important events, having some of the latest developments centered on the possibility of sending events from specific areas. The following system tries to solve these dependencies and offers a unique system capable of analyzing any data source and communicates the alarms through different means in an effective way.

Keywords. Alarm system, rules engine, efficient care.

Introduction

A great amount of information is available to be exploited thanks to the use of information technologies. In view of this fact, several information systems have been developed with the capability of dealing with this data and showing it in a clear and simple way to the users.

However, most of these systems are specific area directed, without bearing in mind other areas where patient data could be stored, which makes it far harder to obtain complete knowledge about the patient's state. For example, a hospital may have three different information systems for the departments of Radiology, Pathological Anatomy and Laboratory.

The solution was to find a new information system able to bring together all the data from these different data sources on demand by the user. In this way, the user could analyze every piece of information as a whole. The problem with these new

---

[1] Corresponding author. Fatima.Rodriguez.Calvo@sergas.es
[2] INIBIC - ATIS: Biomedical Research Institute of A Coruña – Advances in Telemedicine and Health Information Technologies

information systems is that they lack proactivity, that is, the information is only displayed on demand, which can make the information not as productive as at the moment it took place.

The system presented here tries to offer a unique point of analysis of the information produced in different areas. In addition, it gives the necessary proactivity by means of the analysis of the data produced in the different systems and sending the information that is considered to be important. Three central areas were chosen to be our initial data sources: Clinical Analyses, Microbiology and Pathological Anatomy.

Nowadays, the system, after meeting the requirements of the Galician Health Service (Servizo Galego de Saúde), is used in our hospital, which has 1400 beds. The Galician Health Service is the entity that governs the health field in our autonomous community.

1. Objectives

The main objective is to develop a unique system capable of managing any type of data received from any kind of external or internal data sources. In order to do so, it has to achieve several points:

- Independence: although the developers will have to make a specific development for each new data source, it should be minimal.
- Standardization: the use of communication standards will simplify the previous task.
- Scalability: with a modular system, it would only be necessary to add a specific module for each new data source.
- High availability: no malfunction is acceptable when the life of patients is at stake.
- Operate with proactive and monitored applications: the system will have the option to be waiting for the information sent by a proactive application or to monitor periodically the non-proactive applications.

From another point of view, the system needs to be able to analyze the data received and to know in advance which set of data will trigger an alarm. One of the options is the integration of a rule engine in the system, using a rule repository to store the rules that can be activated by the received data.

The system must be able to raise complex rules with different data sources involved, enabling the use of all the information concerning the patient and not just the one referred to a specific hospital area.

Furthermore, the system to be developed must have the possibility to send the detected alarms to the proper addressee, including patients. This should be possible in different ways, such as e-mail, SMS or an electronic warning through an information system.

2. Materials and Methods

The used methodology was divided into two large sections. On the one hand, the first section is used to identify the relevant events that could happen in the specified areas and, on the other hand, the methodology for the computer development.

2.1. Identifying the Relevant Events

Our current system was modeled to know with accuracy the possible ways by which the samples travel in the departments previously mentioned. Also, we wanted to know when events capable of being considered alarms could take place. For this task, the ARIS® [1] Toolset software developed by IDS Scheer was chosen, because of its ability to generate Event-driven Process Chains (EPCs) [2]. These EPCs allow the designing of models of easy comprehension for real processes by means of the use of functions (shown in green in the figure) and events (shown in pink). While functions represent actions to do, events are their possible results. Figure 1 shows an example of the arrival of the samples to the Clinical Analyses Department.

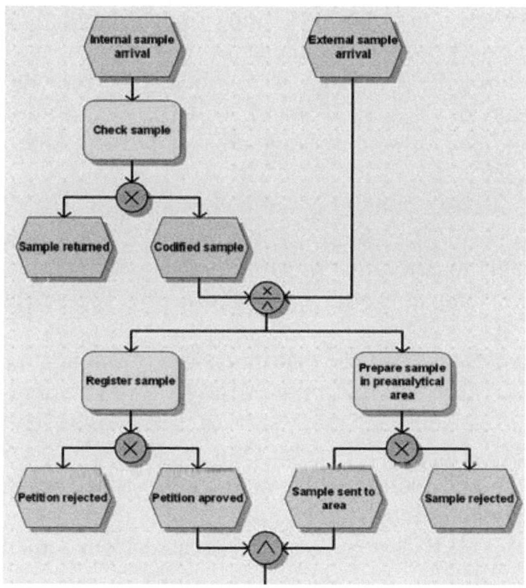

Figure 1. EPC example.

2.2. Software Development

For the software development, we used the methodology of the Technological Architectures Commission of the Health Ministry (Comisión de Arquitecturas Tecnológicas da Consellería de Sanidade). This methodology establishes an iterative process of development where the most significant stages are these: Functional Analysis, Definition of the Technical Architecture of the System, Technical Design, System Development, Implementation and System Acceptance.

The obtained system, known as SION, has been developed using the J2EE platform (Java 2 Platform, Enterprise Edition) with EJB 2.1 and has been tested with

IBM Websphere Application Server 6.1 cluster configured. It is a complex system that has been split into subsystems minimizing the coupling among them. The message queues of Websphere, which follow the JMS standard (Java Message Service), help in the task of diminishing the dependence among the parts of the system.

The rules engine is one of the most important components. It allows the storing of the business logic related to the detection of information events susceptible of generating alarms and to make decisions about each one of the alarms detected in the form of business rules. The rules engine that belongs to the Jboss's business logic integration platform called Drools 5.0 [3] is the one that has been used.

The database server which has been chosen both for the rules repository and for the final system's database is MS SQL Server 2005.

2.3. How to Build a Rule

Inside Drools you can find Guvnor, which is a Business Rules Management System that is also used as a centralized rules repository. With it, business rules can be managed and created in a simple way. To illustrate this, we will next show how a rule is built to alert the correct staff of a patient with high amylase values.

In our case, we are interested in defining rules using natural language so that any type of user, clinical or not, can understand and modify the business logic of the application. Therefore, the first step is to obtain the rule in natural language; for example: "when Amylase is greater than 250 IU/L, send a message to the caregiver". Once the rule is defined in natural language, we have to split it into its elements in order to analyze them.

Like any rule, it has a condition and a consequence. The condition is of the type *parameter operator value*, that is to say, we have to compare the value of a parameter with a reference value to determine if it fulfills the condition. If this rule is transformed into a more generic one, it would be like this: "If {parameter} is {operator} than {value}".

As for the consequence, we see that it consists of sending an alarm to an addressee and, generalizing it: "Then send alarm with {text} to {addressee}".

In Drools, two elements are necessary to create rules made of natural language sentences: the DSL (Domain Specific Language) and the DSLR (Drools Specific Language Rules). A DSL consists of a set of key - value pairs, where the key is the sentence written in natural language and the value is its translation to the DRL (Drools Rule Language). A DSLR is a set of rules created from sentences defined in one or more DSLs.

The DSL for the amylase would look like this:

```
[when] If {parameter:ENUM:Parameter.name} is
{operator:ENUM:Operator.operation} than {referenceValue:([0-9])+\.?([0-9])*}
IU/L =  p: MDTO (codMet == {parameter}, paramResult: result, paramResult
matches "([0-9])+\.?([0-9])*", idPatRes: idPatient)
PatientClassificationVO(idPat:idSion, historicalRecordNum == idPatRes)
eval(UtilRules.{operator}( paramResult,"{referenceValue}"))

[then] Alarm detected with message = AlarmVO alarm = new AlarmVO(idPat,
UtilRules.trim(idPatRes), Calendar.getInstance(),
UtilRulesServolab.formatTxtAlarmOrigin (p.idPeticion,p.fecPetition,p.numLab));
```

[then] - clinician > {cause} has been detected = alarm.setMessageCli(new AlarmMessageVO("{cause}"));

[then] Send alarm to be processed = alarms.add(alarm);

In this example, MDTO is an object that is received from the laboratory application with the information necessary to evaluate the condition.

Guvnor contains an editor for DSLs and another one for rules; the last one allows the creation of rules with a friendlier interface than a simple text editor. For example, the elements that appear between curly brackets are drop-down lists that allow the choice of different options for the same type of rule. In this rule, we can choose from a list of parameters.

Once the DSL is completed, we can begin to make new rules. The rule for the amylase would look like this:

WHEN
If Amylase is GREATER than 250 IU/L
THEN
Alarm detected with message:
    - clinician > "High Amylase" has been detected
Send alarm to be processed

3. Results

3.1. Types of Rules

There are five different types of rules in the rules repository:

- Classification rules: used to know if the information received of a monitored application generates an alarm.
- Reclassification rules: similar to the previous type, but used for proactive applications.
- Action rules: they define what the system should do when an alarm is generated.
- Escalation rules: they specify what to do if an alarm is not acknowledged.
- Subscription rules: they allow users to subscribe to events that are not considered to be alarms, but that have some importance for the user.

The alarms have been ranked depending on their importance, which also defines the maximum response time during which every addressee has to acknowledge the reception of the alarm. In case the system does not receive this acknowledgment, the alarm would be scaled up to an addressee of higher rank in the hierarchy. Four levels of alarm have been defined, being the level 1 the highest one and the level 4 the lowest one and their maximum response time varies between 1 hour and 3 days. In addition, it has been created another level for the events of subscription previously mentioned, as well as a special level for certain events of immediate response, such as the ending of a report of an intraoperatory biopsy, have been created.

The reception of the data by the system is performed in two different ways, depending on the ability that the data source has to send data or if it is necessary to request it. In the case of a proactive application, the system has a message queue ready to receive these events, whereas in the case of the monitored ones there are timer objects that will manage the request process occurring periodically.

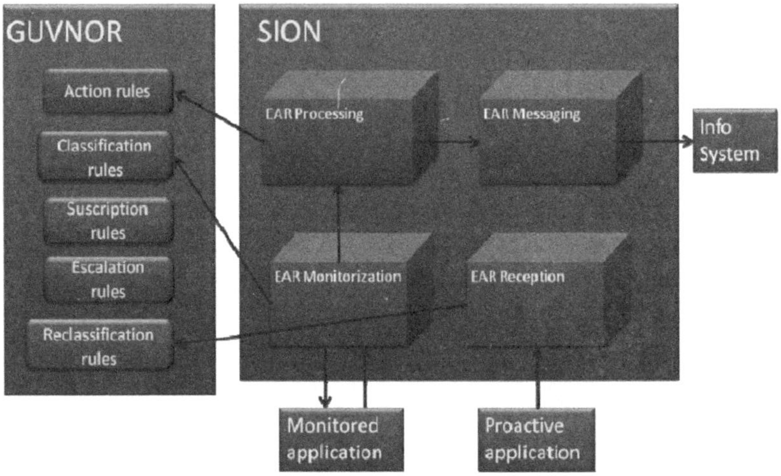

Figure 2. Alarm processing.

Once the data has been obtained, it is analyzed by means of its matching with the existing classification or reclassification rules in the rules repository. When a rule is activated, an alarm is generated and the related data as well as its source is sent to the processing subsystem. This subsystem is in charge of evaluating the information received with the action rules that can be found in the repository. The consequences of the action rules are sent to the messaging subsystem, which is the manager of the process that sends the alarms to their primary addressees.

In order to define those who must be the addressees of each alarm, three different hierarchies have been established: one for clinicians, another for nurses and the final one for people who should be informed about the event. These hierarchies can be seen in table 1. The reason to split the addressees into hierarchies is to allow the system to make different actions to different types of addressees at the same time. In addition, specific groups exist for certain alarms, like the multi-resistant microorganism control which evaluates the alarms generated by microorganisms with high number of resistances to antibiotics.

Table 1. General addresses hierarchies.

Scaled grade	Clinical	Nursing	Informative
4	Clinical staff in charge of the patient	General nurses	Petitioner General practitioner Subscriber
3	Department Head	Supervisor	
2	On duty bleeper	General supervisor	
1	On duty Head	Nursing management	
0	Clinical management		

3.2. Some Examples of Rules

The system currently has more than 200 rules defined. The next ones exemplify different types of them:

- Result operator value: similar to the one shown in the previous example (Amylase > 250 IU/L).
- Existence: looking for a certain event (Bottle without sample in Microbiology).
- Voluntary: the event is not always going to be considered an alarm, only if the clinician who validates the results decides so (Yeast in sterile sample Report in Mycology).
- Text search: the rules look for a certain character string inside the results (Positive hemocultive report ("...has been isolated")).
- Results of a specific sample type: the system sends the alarm only if the event has taken place in a certain area (Positive S. pneumoniae antigen report in cerebrospinal fluid).
- Multi-resistant microorganism control: special case for finding microorganism resistant to certain antibiotics (Pseudomonas aeruginosa resistant to all the antibiotics).
- Historic: rules that take into account what has happened before the current events. There are several types (First haemoglobin < 9 g/dL., Positive cultive report with negative staining in Micobacterium area) and are used to find Hospital-acquired infections, where you have to look for a microorganism with the same resistances infecting different patients in the same area.

At present, the system is in the final testing phase and is waiting for the approval to be put into production environment. Because of this, the alarms are only being sent to staff that have accepted to cooperate in this phase. Two monitoring modules have been developed for the connection with the external applications, which are at this moment: Servolab® Laboratory Information System (Siemens), where the reports of the Clinical Analyses and Microbiology departments are stored, and EOS® (Servizo Galego de Saúde), where the reports of the Pathological Anatomy department are stored. For example, between the 1st and 11th of January 2010, more than 1300 alarms were sent while analyzing more than 43,000 results.

4. Discussion

During the first interviews with the health staff users of the project, they have shown their general satisfaction with the use of the system in the hospital. On the one hand, the health staff of the central departments think that the using of this product will allow them to improve their efficiency, because of not having to be searching for the right people to give them the information that they have just obtained about the patient.

On the other hand, the health staff of the peripheral departments of the hospital believe that this system offers them the safety of knowing the relevant facts of the patient at the moment they take place, which will lead to a more effective treatment of the conditions of the patient. This advantage will be more relevant with the incorporation of the Primary care staff to the reception of alarms, since they sometimes feel distanced from the specialized care and this system could bring them closer.

So far, we have only spoken of how SION changes the health process from the point of view of the monitoring of hospital information and the execution of actions that only involves the clinical staff. Although this functionality of the system is in an initial phase, the patient is just a new type of addressee to whom relevant information is sent. Nevertheless, the patient empowerment in this case must be supervised closely, since a lot of the information obtained by SION cannot be seen by them before the clinician has evaluated it.

But a chronic patient being able to anticipate the exacerbations of his condition is a reality. By means of the use of applications for home follow-up, which can send the information about the patient to our system, SION can react to it. Among the tests that are being carried out, with patients suffering rheumatologic, cardiac and neumologic chronic conditions included, their respective systems send the most recent information which is evaluated by our system, and then launch an alarm to the patient and order them to do several different actions.

5. Conclusion

The proactivity that SION incorporates allows that the evaluative process of the patient will be made in the minimal time bearing all the available information in mind about him at the moment in which it is validated, giving better patient care and, possibly, a cost reduction.

The system to create rules is simple enough so any type of user may create them and flexible enough to implement complex rules that make use of data from several data sources.

In addition, different types of addressees important to the health process have been taking into account and, by means of the use of scaled hierarchies, the most effective patient care is guaranteed.

Acknowledgment

This work is a part of a project funded by the Health Research Fund (Fondo de Investigación Sanitaria) of the Carlos III Health Institute (Instituto de Salud Carlos III) with the PI 061430 code.

References

[1] ARIS Platform. [Online]. Available from: URL: http://www.ids-scheer.com/en/ARIS_ARIS_Platform/3730.html. (Last access: 18/12/2009)
[2] Event-driven Process Chains. [Online]. Available from: URL: http://www.ids-scheer.com/en/ARIS/ARIS_Modeling_Standards /EPC/79740.html?mod_srch[result_link]=1. (Last access: 18/12/2009)
[3] JBoss Drools. [Online]. Available from: URL: http://www.jboss.org/drools/. (Last access: 30/12/2009)

Medical and Care Compunetics 6
L. Bos et al. (Eds.)
IOS Press, 2010

doi:10.3233/978-1-60750-565-5-65

Metaboli-Net: Online Groupware System Providing Counseling Guidance for Patients with Metabolic Syndrome

Shigeki KUWATA [a1], Shin-ichi TANIGUCHI [b], Atsuko KATO [c], Kazuoki INOUE [b], Naoya YAMAMOTO [b], Tsuyoshi OHKURA [b], Kei TERAMOTO [a], Chiaki SHIGEMASA[b] and Hiroshi KONDOH [a]
[a] *Division of Medical Informatics, Tottori University Hospital, Yonago, Tottori, Japan*
[b] *Tottori University Faculty of Medicine, Yonago, Tottori, Japan*
[c] *Kofu Municipal Office, Kofu, Tottori, Japan*

Abstract. This study presented a newly developed online groupware system, Metaboli-Net, to yield counseling guidance on diet and exercise to patients with metabolic syndrome. A distinctive feature adopted in the system to maintain the retention rate of patients was the social network service (SNS) that enables the patients to share their dietary and relevant health information with other participants in the same group on the network. A pilot study was conducted to prove the effectiveness of the system in improving the patient's lifestyle and dietary health awareness. SNS also contributed to the participant's adherence to intervention programs.

Keywords. Dietary program, intervention, patient education, computer-assisted online system and social network service

1. Introduction

Since the fiscal year of 2008, as a part of medical system reforms, the Japanese government has enforced regulations for healthcare insurers aiming at the implementation of health checkups and counseling guidance focused on metabolic syndrome [1]. Accordingly the insurers in Japan are preparing for dietary and physical activity programs to establish the effective and efficient implementation of checkup and guidance. The authors formerly developed a web-based system, Metaboli-Net, to assist nutrition and exercise education for prospective patients and conducted a pilot study [2] that formed a part of the Tottori-Kofu Study, a long-term clinical trial focused on diabetes in rural districts of Japan [3]. The system was developed for both dietitians and patients to facilitate communication with each other, and particularly to assist middle-aged people who had little time to receive counseling guidance from specialists and also had a high probability of lifestyle-related diseases in the future. Subsequent to the pilot study, in 2009, the authors improved the system to release a new version of Metaboli-Net, in response to the need for practical solutions for the computer-assisted online counseling guidance.

[1] Corresponding author. shig@med.tottori-u.ac.jp

The effectiveness of computer-based patient education programs was widely accepted. Revere and Dunbar [4] reviewed that over 90% of the computer-based health behavior interventions that they had investigated were found to be either statistically significant or improved outcomes, though no theoretical basis was established for their tailoring protocols. The Internet-based assistance was also required and expected particularly in the application to diabetes, referred to as telediabetes, as presented by a systematic review conducted by Dalton [5]. A typical large-scale study was exemplified in a web-based nutrition education program conducted by Boston University Medical Center [6], in which 12-month programs were provided via the Internet without in-person meeting and found to be associated with significant weight loss, blood pressure lowering, and dietary improvements.

Such eHealth programs provided on the Internet, however, frequently brought up issues on how continued usage could be encouraged [7]–[9]. Woodall et al. [7] found that iterative messaging by email promoted in use of their web-based programs, though its effect was valid for a short-term period. Kroeze et al. [10] supported those findings by presenting that web-based interventions had shorter-term effects compared with print-delivered interventions in a computer-tailored nutrition education program.

Thus, the Internet-based education systems appear promising in its short-term effect, while new strategies for enhancing the participant's retention are needed to provide a longer-term effect as much as traditional in-person programs do.

2. Objectives of the Study

This study was conducted to confirm the effectiveness of the system with newly implemented features by examining the results of a pilot study in participation with 10 subjects and a dietitian.

3. Methods

3.1. Overview of system design

In the previous version of the system, the authors elucidated the necessity of countermeasures against possible participant dropouts; distinctive tactics were required to maintain a certain level of patient retention. In an attempt to keep the participants motivated, the following user interfaces were adopted (**Figure 1**): (a) visualization of the participant's progress in the program, (b) visualization of the outcome evaluated by the dietitians or exercise instructors as an avatar's face with five grades ranging from "sad (bad)" to "smiley (good)", (c) a function that enables the participants to view other participant's data on diet in the same team and its relevant health information, which was derived from a concept of Social Network Service (SNS) .

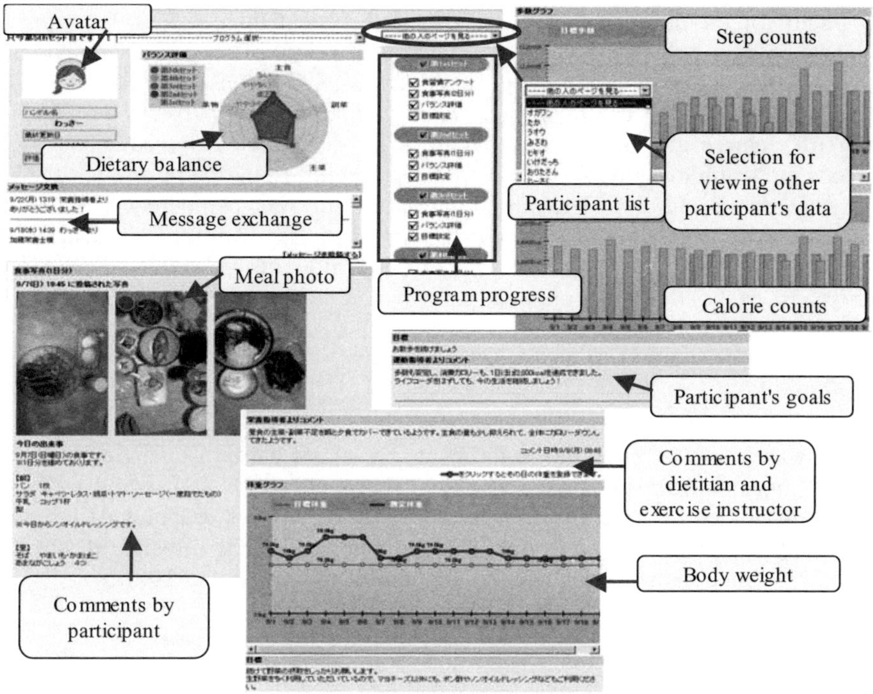

Figure 1. Features in user interfaces were illustrated in a screen example of Metaboli-Net

3.2. Dietary and exercise program and its work flow

It was possible to simultaneously execute multiple dietary and exercise programs in the system. A typical dietary program and its workflow were represented as follows: First, the dietitian sent the registered participants a questionnaire on their dietary habits. The action by the dietitian was executed online and required an email message be sent to the participants. Secondly, the participants received the email, including the URL of the web site of the questionnaire and followed the link to respond to it. Subsequently, they sent photos of their meals of the day taken by a digital camera on their mobile phones to the designated address given upon registration for three consecutive days. Also, they were required to login to the system to register their body weight of the day or add comments on their daily activities at their own discretion. Thirdly, the dietitian viewed the submitted data to evaluate the dietary balance and to set several goals for the participants, occasionally responding to the comments or asking additional questions of them. The procedures described above were defined as a set. Completing multiple sets assigned by the dietitian, the participants answered the final questionnaire to finish the program.

3.3. Design of pilot study

The pilot study to evaluate the newly developed system was conducted for 10 subjects including 6 men and 4 women, with the average age of 34.4±6.8 and the average BMI of 20.7±3.7. The subjects followed the protocol requiring them to: (a) answer an initial questionnaire followed by meal photos of the day for three consecutive days, (b) email meal photos of the day once a week for the subsequent three weeks, (c) input their comments on their daily life and register their body weight of the day and data obtained from a portable activity monitor device (Suzuken, LIFECORDER EX) that counts steps and calculates the calories, intensity and duration of a person's activities, and finally (d) answer a closing questionnaire. The questionnaires were comprised of questions on health awareness with five grades ranging from "not aware (Score 1)" to "highly aware (Score 5)." The initial questionnaire was compared with the final questionnaire to highlight differences in health awareness. Additional questions were included in the final questionnaire on the perception of life-style change and the effectiveness of the SNS function.

4. Results

Dietary awareness was improved significantly ($P<0.05$; paired t-test) from 1.9 ± 0.9 at the initial questionnaire as compared with 2.7 ± 1.2 (Mean $\pm$ SD), while no obvious difference was found for exercise. The majority of the subjects responded by reporting that use of the system had led to quality improvement of their life-style (8 out of 10) and the SNS function had contributed to the improvement (6 out of 10).

5. Discussion

5.1. Adherence to intervention programs

The more the number of patients with life-style related diseases increases, the more a need for patient education tools of nutrition and exercise grows. Computer-based online systems were considered efficient and effective in the intervention in that they were able to simultaneously yield instant and tailored information to the large number of patients at a low cost [11] [12]. However, it was also pointed out that engagement and retention were important challenges [8] and retention-enhancing strategies were needed [9] in computer-based interventions.

Metaboli-Net had a distinctive attribute derived partly from the generic SNS to retain the participant's motives for health awareness by sharing information with others on the computer network. The design model was developed in response to the findings from the preceding studies that stressed the importance of the existence of community and social supportiveness [13]–[15]. This study was an innovative challenge because few studies have examined the effectiveness of computer-assisted social network systems on patient education. Our results showed that the feature was promising for raising the retention rate usually falling into the range of approximately 20–30% [16][17].

5.2. Issues on Social Network Service

Originally, SNS aimed at building online communities of people who have the same goals or interests, enabling the participants to achieve their goals or fathom the understanding of their interests. With its rapid prevalence these days, SNS has begun to draw the attention of researchers in terms of its social impact and effectiveness as a social good. Some critical issues on SNS, however, have been reported with regard to privacy infringement and vulnerability to disturbances by malicious use or innocent misuse. Hence it is highly expected that the various optimal use-case models for different objectives should be developed in the near future. On the other hand, Metaboli-Net was designed to use the SNS functions only in viewing other participant's data on diet and relevant health information. As a result, the problematic issues stated above were successfully evitable due to a lack of direct communication among the participants. It is proposed that detailed scrutiny be executed in terms of its effectiveness in the viewpoint of patient education, since broader range of the SNS functions might be adopted in the future, in response to the need to improve the participant's usability.

5.3. Effectiveness on health awareness

In spite of the improvement of dietary awareness, no significant changes were found in exercise awareness. The reasons for the difference were considered as follows: a sequence of meal photos of the day with the dietitian's comments would intuitively evoke awareness of diet and practical actions for the dietary improvement that would be readily executable for the participants, e.g., eating more vegetables. On the other hand, measures for increasing exercise would need attentive and tailored instructions, which would not be always feasible given the limited knowledge obtained from online messaging on the life-styles of the participants.

5.4. Limitations and further studies

The results of the study presented that online counseling was effective in improving dietary awareness, while an online dietary advice program had no significant difference from an exercise-only program in reducing body weight [16]. The authors did not confirm the effect in reducing body weight, since the period of the study was not long enough to produce distinguishable difference in body weight. As stated in the introduction, recent studies have focused on the effect in a longer-term period, therefore, further studies are needed to prove that the system can yield objective outcomes by its feature that produces the participant's stronger adherence to education programs.

The system needs scalability that is competent to work with a number of groups and their constituents on the assumption that the system would be utilized in social organizations with considerable numbers of departments or divisions. This stems from environments in Japan that business enterprises own healthcare insurance organization for their employees, thus the scalability would matter if the enterprise insurers would adopt the system to reduce the healthcare risk of the employees. Metaboli-net is to be extended and used as SaaS (Software as a Service) on the Internet for a large number of users after the preliminary study. Similar web-based services are provided in a commercial base, however, it would be better to incorporate dietary specialists and structured programs into the system like Metaboli-net as Gold et al. presented that a specialist-led structured program had greater effects than a self-help commercial program [18].

6. Conclusion

The newly developed online groupware system for prevention of lifestyle-related diseases was effective for the participants in improving their lifestyles as well as to raise their health awareness concerning their diet. SNS features that were adopted in the system also contributed to maintain the participant's adherence to the intervention program.

References

[1] Ministry of Health, Labour and Welfare (Japan). Measures against Lifestyle related Diseases through "Health Japan 21" and Promotion of "Shokuiku (food and nutrition education)". In: Annual Health, Labour and Welfare Report 2007-2008, 2009 [updated 2009 June 27]. Available from: URL: http://www.mhlw.go.jp/english/wp/wp-hw2/index.html.

[2] Kato A, Takechi M, Taniguchi S, et al. Development of a IT tool, Metaboli-net, to assist dietary education (The 6th report on Tottori-Kofu Study). The 51st Annual Meeting of the Japan Diabetes Society, Tokyo; 2008:S-315.

[3] Ohkura T, Taniguchi S, Inoue K, et al. Screening Criteria of Diabetes Mellitus and Impaired Glucose Tolerance of the Japanese Population in a Rural Area of Japan: The Tottori-Kofu Study, Yonago Acta medica 2009;52:105-14.

[4] Revere D, Dunbar PJ. Review of computer-generated outpatient health behavior interventions: clinical encounters "in absentia". J Am Med Inform Assoc 2001;8(1);62-79.

[5] Dalton JE. Web-based care for adults with type 2 diabetes. Can J Diet Pract Res 2008;69(4):185-91.

[6] Moore TJ, Alsabeeh N, Apovian CM, et al. Weight, blood pressure, and dietary benefits after 12 months of a Web-based Nutrition Education Program (DASH for health): longitudinal observational study. J Med Internet Res 2008;10(4):e52.

[7] Woodall WG, Buller DB, Saba L, et al. Effect of emailed messages on return use of a nutrition education website and subsequent changes in dietary behavior. J Med Internet Res 2007;9(3):e27.

[8] Spittaels H, Bourdeaudhuij ID, Vandelanotte C. Evaluation of a website-delivered computer-tailored intervention for increasing physical activity in the general population. Prev Med 2007;44(3):209-17.

[9] Weinert C, Cudney S, Hill W. Retention in a computer-based outreach intervention for chronically ill rural women. Appl Nurs Res 2008;21(1):23-9.

[10] Kroeze W, Oenema A, Campbell M, Brug J. The efficacy of Web-based and print-delivered computer-tailored interventions to reduce fat intake: results of a randomized, controlled trial. J Nutr Educ Behav 2008;40(4):226-36.

[11] Cousineau T, Houle B, Bromberg J. et al. A pilot study of an online workplace nutrition program: the value of participant input in program development. J Nutr Educ Behav 2008;40(3):160-7.

[12] Brug J, Campbell M, Assema P. The application and impact of acomputer-generated personalized nutrition education: a review of the literature. Patient Educ Couns 1999;36:145-56.

[13] Burns D, Soward AC, Skelly AH, et al. Effective recruitment and retention strategies for older members of rural minorities. Diabetes Educ 2008;34(6):1045-52.

[14] Medina DP, D'Antonio AM, Smith SM, et al. Successful recruitment and retention strategies for a randomized weight management trial for people with diabetes living in rural, medically underserved counties of South Carolina: the POWER study. J Am Diet Assoc 2004;104(1):70-5.

[15] Fortune T, Wright E, Juzang I, Bull S. Recruitment, enrollment and retention of young black men for HIV prevention research: Experiences from The 411 for Safe Text project. Contemp Clin Trials 2010;31(2):151-6

[16] Booth AO, Nowson CA, Matters H. Evaluation of an interactive, Internet-based weight loss program: a pilot study. Health Educ Res 2008;23(3):371-81.

[17] Douketis JD, Macie C, Thabane L, Williamson DF. Systematic review of long-term weight loss studies in obese adults: clinical significance and applicability to clinical practice. Int J Obes (Lond). 2005;29(10):1153-67.

[18] Gold BC, Burke S, Pintauro S, et al. Weight loss on the web: A pilot study comparing a structured behavioral intervention to a commercial program. Obesity (Silver Spring) 2007;15(1):155-64.

Medical and Care Compunetics 6
L. Bos et al. (Eds.)
IOS Press, 2010

doi:10.3233/978-1-60750-565-5-71

The Potential of RFID Technology in Blood Center Processes

V. KEBO[a], P. KLEMENT[a], Z. ČERMÁKOVÁ[b], J. GOTTFRIED[a], M. SOMMEROVÁ[a], A. PALEČEK[a]
[a]*VŠB-Technical University of Ostrava*
[b]*University Hospital Ostrava*

Abstract. Current RFID technology deployment is limited by safety, procedural and physical limitations in healthcare field. It is important to define and ensure safe operation of technologies without actual deployment in real operation. Potential problems could arise due to the consequences of technical and physical characteristics of RFID technology and its improper location. This article deals with manipulation of blood products and the definition of suitable places for radio identification. Each suitable place must undergo laboratory experiments and tests. The results can provide a convenient base for defining efficient and safe deployment of RFID technology in Blood Centers with substantial financial savings for Czech healthcare.

Keywords. safety, efficiency, RFID potential, blood and blood products

Introduction

RFID - Radio Frequency Identification represents modern identification technology of objects by radio waves, which can provide large amounts of real-time information related to certain objects.

The information is electronically saved to small storages (tags) from which it can be read and rewritten multiple times with the use of radio waves. The RFID technology is called "a successor" to bar codes, though not intended to be a full replacement. Use of barcodes will dominate some areas of the marketplace and in others a combination of bar codes and RFID technology may predominate, for example Smart Label Tags. Similarly to the bar codes, the data are written into the data storage (tag), which is fastened onto the traced object. The tag includes a small chip with antenna and memory. RFID tags represent a basic element for collection and transfer of information through the electro-magnetic waves. The present reading devices can read, in parallel, hundreds of tags per second. [3]

1. Interference from risks connected with RFID application in health care

RFID application in health care can be very useful in many respects. Many examples are known of efficient application of RFID technology in health care from the global perspective, including identification or location of patients or medical equipment, evidence or identification of drugs, laundry or medical material manipulation, etc. The technology can be (and is) generally used in logistic (supply) chains to simplify and intensify the logistic processes, such as in the distribution of medical material. Our laboratory has conducted practical tests, for example marking of breast implants or intraocular lenses by RFID to simplify identification. [1]

RFID technology application in health care brings many benefits, namely elimination of mistakes connected to patient identification of medical application, speeding and improvement of the main logistic processes in hospitals, economical treatment of blood and blood products by automatic identification of a blood bag with temperature monitoring. On the other hand, there are some RFID technology application hazards, which can restrict the medical applications. The hazards can be classified in a few groups:

1. Physical restrictions: The principle of RF signal propagation is such that certain materials (metal, liquids), interfere with the RF signal, decreasing the quality or disallowing signal propagation. Blood and blood products include, similar to the human body, significant amounts of water that cause unfavorable conditions for RFDI technology application.
2. Interference of the RF signal with medical equipment: A majority of medical apparatus uses electric energy for operation, and is equipped with many smart sensors and actuators that communicate with control units, very frequently based on digital control. All these parts can be negatively influenced by RF signals or by the presence of RFID technology. This is proven by a paper [2] published in JAMA magazine. The results document a total of 123 tests of interaction of RFID tags with medical equipment, where in 34 cases the equipment was influenced by Tag presence.
3. RFID safety – Unauthorized and malicious use: A potential risk caused by RFID technology use in medical care, for example in a blood centre, is the possibility of a malicious change of tag information regarding the blood product. This manipulation can cause fatal problems for the patients.
4. Personal data protection and other ethical considerations of RFID application in medical care – The use of RFID technology can include a risk of unauthorized access to personal patient data (health condition, location, and movements). It is therefore necessary to study the ethical dimension of RFID technology application in medical care. There is a Bureau for personal data protection in the Czech Republic that carefully observes all the handling and operations around the area of personal data to protect against unauthorized use, collection and storage. On one hand this regulation protects patient privacy, but on the other hand this regulation can cause ineffective, limited application of RFID technology and consequently low benefits from the technology.
5. Risks of mistakes generated by integration of RFID with medical IS – This risk is comparatively unimportant. But it must be mentioned that by extension of the current IS by these new modules we do increase the complexity and the potential for mistakes.

2. RFID technology

When making a choice of new technology and its application in health care we should take into account a few basic factors: 1 – physical fundamentals, 2 – applied technology, 3 – human factor.

From the standpoint of physics, the dielectrical properties of each product are very important and similarly the properties of product coverings have different characteristics. The tag location on the marked object influences the tag antenna impedances and therefore the used frequency of a RFID system. There is the reason for different tag-type construction for different areas of application to compensate the RFID system power caused by the presence of materials problematic to radio-frequency in the surroundings.[7] We can classify materials as RF emitter or RF friendly materials, RF nontransparent materials, and materials absorbing radio waves. Definition of materials as RF absorbing or RF nontransparent is very relative, as it depends on the frequency of the radio wave. The power of the RFID system is also influenced by the distance of tag and reader. Very important is the reciprocal orientation and obviously the antenna's dimension in particular system components. The tag size is important in the case where we want to mark the objects regarding the unit level, as a small tag requires a small area on the product. The tag antenna dimension depends on the frequency of RF signal and wave length of the signal. If we do not respect this dependence, the power of the whole RFID system is decreased.[5]

The knowledge of the electrical parameters of the surface of wrapping technologies and knowledge of blood product properties is necessary for the study of radio wave reflection on the blood bag. Fundamental, for radio wave reflection, is the influence of water content on a given volume or on the surface or according to the permittivity. Radio-wave propagation can be effected in multiple ways due to interaction of radio wave with the air and the construction materials used for data storage. It could be caused by unsuitable antenna location or inappropriate marking or storage of blood products. Inducted prostructs or holes in the reading pole can cause a power decrease of the entire RFID system, or even cancel the reading of the information from the tag. [6] This is the reason why it is necessary to carry out a study of RFID technology convenience with respect to operational environment of planned RFID system application.

The key question for the selection of an RFID system is the choice of appropriate system frequency – UHF or HF. The application of UHF or HF RFID technology is very often discussed for use in medical care (patients' observation and identification, use of laundry and hospital equipment, medicals dosing or marking etc.).[3] The RFID technology based on UHF frequency (Ultra High Frequencies 866 – 960 MHz) is most widespread for product marking, but the frequency range is not standardized globally. The world is divided into regions with different frequency ranges for UHF technology. This technology is characterized by power decrease caused by the presence of metals and liquids that could be compensated by useful tags or antenna construction for UHF RFID tags. The big advantage to HF technology is the reading range of up to 10m and the existence of global standards (EPC Electronic product code), similar to bar codes. The second most popular for frequency for RFID technology is HF (High Frequency) working at 13.56 MHz. The typical applications are at access systems, ID cards, marking of drugs in health care, etc. [7] The use of HF technology is suitable for the marking of blood products, as the principle of energy transfer between the reader and tag provides the possibility to acquire higher power when the tag is located on the surface of RF-interfering materials like liquids or metal particles. The reading distance is reduced to tens of centimeters. It is generally valid for all RFID technology that the tag antenna construction always depends on the specific properties of materials where the tag has to be located.

The entire RFID system has to be robust enough from the standpoint of physical, chemical or mechanical influences, but also regarding proper use. The mobile RFID systems should have suitable ergonomic design and a high level of stability and intelligence. The software solutions based on RFID technology can automate many processes to prevent possible mistakes from the human factor. They provide the possibility to share important information among the management and staff, provide the necessary information for strategic production control, reserves stock control, and expediting blood products. The RFID system is as powerful as is the data acquisition system, RFID technology benefits are created in SW components – Middleware and in the level of business control systems.

3. RFID in a Blood Centre

One of the most important features of medical care is reliable identification of all components, and in the case of a blood center it is identification of blood products in all preparation processes. RFID technology provides the possibility to apply new identification methods to improve the blood center processes' safety and quality.

The blood center of the University Hospital Ostrava is a model pattern for the RFID technology application. The main activities of this blood centers are production of transfusion materials for clinical medical institutions in Ostrava city and production of blood plasma for subsequent preparation into blood derivates (for foreign partners). The blood takings, autologous takings, plasma takings, thrombocyte and granulocyte takings are carried out at the blood center. For all the processes identification bar codes are used, applied by self-adhesive labels. RFID technology application will increase the production quality and provide better safety of blood products.

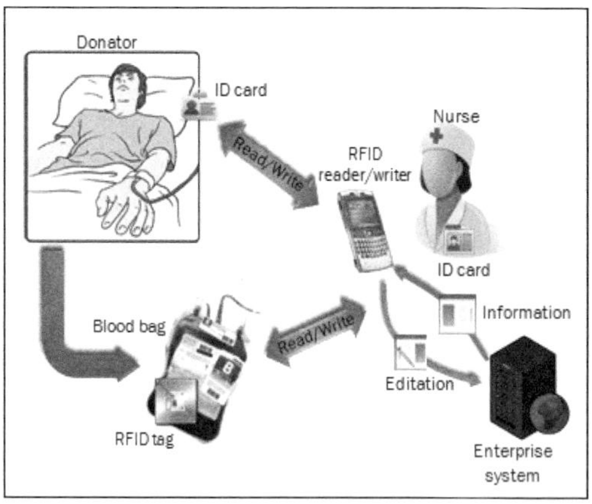

Figure 1. The use of RFID technology at the place of blood taking

RFID technology will be used for blood product manipulation from the very beginning of the blood taking process at the donor, when the whole blood and its components are taken into special blood bags. The blood bags have to be assembled before the blood taking according the type of taking. A large amount of information must be written down before the taking, such as the charge number of blood bags, and other labels according the taking type. The natural taking is identified by bar code with the taking number; nurse ID, taking (capitation) device with its technological parameters (time, weight, temperature, etc…). Then the information is passed into the

IS and to the production. If the RFID tag is integral part of the blood bag it will be advantageous in that it will simplify the transfer of bag information to the IS, and at the same time provide a tool for recording of the taking of information straight into the RFID tag during the taking process. (Figure 1.).

The blood bags are transported in a thermo-box to the production division, where the whole blood is processed onto erythrocyte mass, erythrocytes without leukocytes, plasma and thrombocytes and finally for the human serum. The blood bags with plasma have to be frozen immediately and consequently stored frozen. The information about the blood products should be recorded before the freezing process. RFID technology makes batch reading of the information from the blood bags possible. Plasma intended for the clinical use is stored in quarantine, where it must remain for six months. The blood products with granulocytes and thrombocytes from aferesis are stored in an agitator. All the information regarding the processing and laboratory tests are continuously recorded and eventually automatically stored into IS. Consequently it is necessary to mark the blood bag by label with all important information including the bar code.

In the case of negative results of all the laboratory tests, the transfusion products can be released to the expediting group – or conversely it must be liquidated. The RFID technology application enables the information storage into the tag in the blood bag directly, without necessity of bag label changing. This method ensures the monitoring and control from the donor reception up to expedition or liquidation of the products.

The blood products are, after the release, inserted into special thermo-boxes – containers, warmed or cooled to the temperature satisfying the limits for blood product storage and then passed to the expediting group for the entering into a repository. See the figure 2.

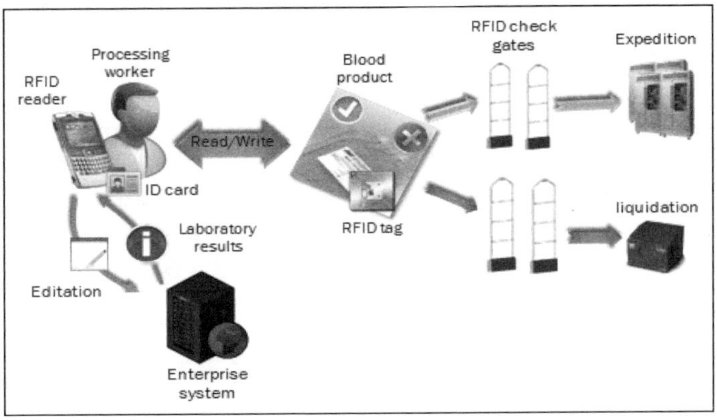

Figure 2. RFID technology at the processing of blood products

There are few possibilities of RFID technology application in the expediting group. The released blood products go through RFID check gates and which products were accepted into the store are recorded in the IS. Subsequently the responsible worker in the expediting group will check the accepted blood products relative to documentation. The entry into storage is implemented according to the type of transfusion product into the freezing, cooling device or agitator.

The blood products are stored onto shelves according the blood group and expiration date, when all the equipment is connected to the electronic system to monitor the inner temperature, times of door openings, etc. The access into this storage spaces is also monitored, and can be ensured by RFID card only for authorized persons.

Blood products are expedited from storage for particular patients according the request, or to other blood banks and hospitals according the orders. The worker will search for the particular products for particular recipients. A product test must be done after the release of the products from storage. The charge numbers at the products for expedition must be read, these numbers are compared with the order for delivery for the blood products. Then the blood products in the special thermo-box are passed to the responsible person. In this process it is possible to use a mobile RFID reader for automatic information recording into the IS when searching for blood products. After the necessary control steps the blood products in the special thermo-box go through the RFID gate to check the correctness of actual blood products (compare to delivery order), Figure 3.

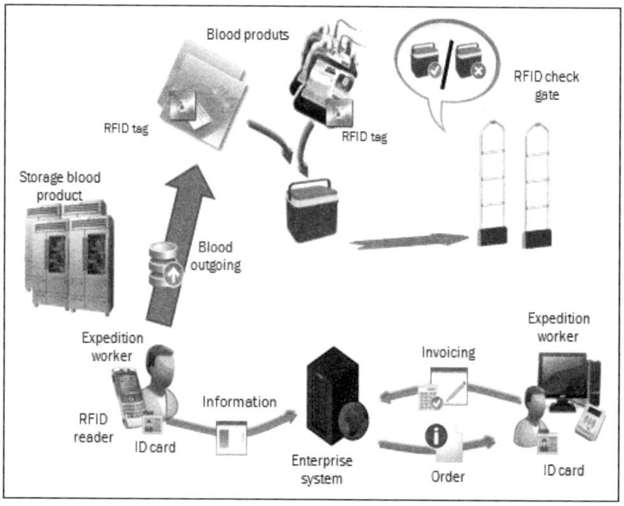

Figure 3. RFID technology at expedition, release of blood products

Further benefit of RFID technology can be gained by the use of an active RFID tag with continuous temperature measurement. This device can guarantee the return storage of unused blood products, as we can declare the security of technological conditions of transportation.

4. Conclusion

Current RFID technology is advanced such that it can monitor the whole life cycle of blood products from the donor identification, through blood taking, blood products processing, product storage, expediting, and finally to product consumption. These technologies do not bring only benefits, but also hazards. The paper at the initial part of the process describes certain risks that can develop in the use of RFID technology in medical care. There are not only technical risks, but also those connected to ethical problems.

There is a large area of RFID use in medical care logistics. The internal memory of tags can store all the important information for each of product life cycle step. The blood bag can be equipped by RFID semi-passive or active tags with sensors of temperature, acceleration or moisture, so we can store and monitor all the information along the product transportation. The stored data can give a proof of technological conditions of transportation and consequently save much used blood products with respect to the safety of patients. This brings improvement of efficiency of blood products economies. The introduction of RFID technology into the blood centers takes place by pilot projects in some countries, for example in Italy, Austria or UK. Parallel to these activities is the effort of blood bags producers to implement RFID tags into their products. The possibility of storing and sharing the blood product tag information induce the necessity of global standards development for blood products labeling and tag data structure. These activities are under development and cooperation with worldwide standard organization GS1 Global, which historically introduced the global standard for use of bar codes.

Acknowledgements: The contribution was prepared under support of Czech Science Foundation project GACR # 105/09/1366.

References

[1] Gottfried J, et al. Final tests report, Internal research report Ilab-RFID. VŠB-TU Ostrava 2010. p. 49
[2] van der Togt R, et al. Electromagnetic Interference From Radio Frequency Identification Inducing Potentially Hazardous Incidents in Critical Care Medical Equipment, J Am Med Assoc 2008;299(24):2884-90.
[3] RFID portal, Základní informace o technologii RFID. Czech Republic. 2010.[Online]. Available from: URL: http://www.rfidportal.cz/index.php?page=rfid_obecne.
[4] Lahiri S, RFID Sourcebook, Pretice Hall PTR. United States; 2005. p. 304. ISBN 0-13-185137-3
[5] Banks J, Pachano M, Thompson L, Hanny D. RFID Applied. John Wiley & Sons, New Jersey, 2007. ISBN 978-0-471-79365-6
[6] Pechač P, Zvánovec S. Základy šíření vln pro plánování pozemních rádiových spojů. Nakladatelství BEN – technická literatura, Prague (Czech Republic). 2007. ISBN 978-80-7300-223-7
[7] Miles SB, Sarma SE, Wiliams JR. RFID Technology and Applications. Massachusetts Institute of Technology, Cambridge University Press, 2008, ISBN-13 978-0-521-88093-0
[8] Jones EC, Chung CA. RFID in LOGISTICS A Practical Introduction. United States: CRC Press; 2008. p. 522. ISBN 978-8493-8526-1

Computer-Assisted Learning

Medical and Care Compunetics 6
L. Bos et al. (Eds.)
IOS Press, 2010

doi:10.3233/978-1-60750-565-5-81

Co-morbidity Analysis And Decision Support on Transplanted Patients using Machine Learning Techniques

G. Iago CORBAL[a1], Mariano J. CABRERO[b], Lino CARRAJO[a], Olaia VÁZQUEZ[a], Loli RIMADA[a] and Guillermo VAZQUEZ[a]

[a] *R&D&I, Information Technology Department, A Coruña University Hospital Complex, Spain*

[b] *Laboratory for Biomedical Applications of Artificial Intelligence, Department of Computer Science, Faculty of Informatics, University of A Coruña, Spain*

Abstract. The A Coruña University Hospital Complex is developing an expert system to improve the decision support for transplanted patients. The system will access the data collected during the monitoring of patients and generate a database of statistics that will aid health professionals in several stages of the transplant process. All historical data will be revised to give an estimation of the patient's parameters evolution depending on his medical record and his actual treatment. We will use two different machine learning techniques to do both clustering and classification.

Keywords. Patient monitoring, User interfaces, Data analysis extraction tools, Surgery.

1. Introduction

The A Coruña University Hospital Complex (CHUAC) is implanting a system called SiMON that simplifies and automates data acquisition during the monitoring of transplanted patients. Each transplant protocol has defined a group of parameters that are taken at the moment of the operation (age, weight, diagnosis, surgical technique, etc.) and another group that will be collected during successive check-ups (laboratory analytical data, pharmacokinetics levels, etc.). A third group of data, called events, will be inserted if the patient incurs in any state defined as important for study in the protocol (exitus, re-transplant, infections, tumors, hospitalizations, etc.). This type of data will go associated with a date, so our system will be capable of drawing survival curves of any defined event. Finally, SiMON will also manage the medication patients take and the variations made by the specialist during every check-up.

SiMON access the different hospital services to import most part of this data, so the user only has to supervise the correctness of the values and add comments if necessary. When it comes to define the treatment, the system will copy the last one prescribed and present it to the user for modifications. This will improve efficiency on

[1] Corresponding author. Gerardo.Iago.Corbal.Ramon@sergas.es

prescription and ensure that the patient doesn't miss any of his medication. The system also contains basic rules to change the treatment dose if the parameters reach certain levels that require action. To achieve this we use a business rule based on a JBoss product called Drools[2]

An immunosuppression plan is also prescribed based on the transplant data inserted using a business rule engine. It is at this point when we find the need for a feedback that allows our system to notice if the rules applied are effective or, on the contrary, are not helping the patient's correct evolution. The system described below will be used to give information to monitoring systems (like SiMON) about possible problems that may arise after giving a determined medication, based on the statistical data collected from previous patients.

Currently, this system is still under early stages of development. We expect to have enough registries on our database by the time it is completed to allow accurate predictions and begin testing.

2. Material and Methods

2.1. Objectives

The system will use the information stored in the database generated by SiMON. This database contains the four basic groups of information described before, and is updated daily by nurses and doctors at the hospital. Our objective here is to parse this information and obtain statistical data which will allow us to:

1. Perform Comorbidity analysis of a transplanted patient or on waiting list. The system will access historical data from other patients with similar characteristics and will make an estimation of possible adverse events that may turn up caused by the transplant.
2. Generate alerts if an unfavorable patient evolution is detected. Parameters collected during transplantation, events and treatment will be taken into account.
3. Propose medication plans that have proved favorable for other patients with similar characteristics.

2.2. Design Aspects

2.2.1. Collected data types

Our system will analyze four kinds of different data for each patient to create a statistical model capable of giving quick responses to the monitoring system:

- **Transplant parameters**: collected before, and a short time after, the operation. This includes different data: basic information about the receptor/donor, pretransplant, surgical, immunosuppression, serology and discharge. The parameters defined for each transplant type will follow international models, whenever existing, so data can be exported to other

[2] More information at http://www.jboss.org/drools/

major databases. This will also make possible the interchange of statistical information between hospitals. So far we have Heart and Lung models implemented following the ISHLT[3] specifications.

- **Visit parameters**: these ones are gathered when the patient comes for a checkup. Most of this data is extracted from other subsystems that deliver patient's result tests. We can group here laboratory analysis (including microbiology and pharmacokinetics), biopsies, hemodynamic or radiology data.
- **Visit Treatments:** treatments are prescribed after every checkup. This involves several phases: first the last medication the patient received is copied, afterwards, the system applies a set of business rules to adjust the doses based on the collected parameters (decision support system), and finally this medication is presented to the specialist to allow a manual adjustment.
- **Events:** Events are registered at anytime through the follow-up of the patient. They usually consist on a patient comorbidity or a success that will affect patient's evolution in some way. Death, re-transplant, infections, hospitalizations, organ rejections, etc. This type of registries will be useful when making studies of the protocol by, for example, drawing survival curves. Most of this data is registered by the Hospital Information System (HIS) and daily updated into our monitoring system.

2.2.2. Learning techniques used

2.2.2.1. Clustering (K-Means)

The clustering techniques or cluster analysis, have the objective of separating a group of observations into subgroups called clusters depending on a predefined property. Clustering is a non-supervised learning method commonly used for statistical data analysis in many fields of knowledge, including machine learning, data mining, pattern recognition, image analysis and bioinformatics. We will be using the K-Means algorithm since it is commonly used for other problems of similar nature and it allows us to specify the number of clusters.

In this kind of clustering (k-means) the Euclidean distance is used by default. We find a problem when defining quantitative distances between the possible values of a qualitative characteristic. For example, if we consider a parameter that represents the presence of cytomegalovirus antibodies (CMV), and we have it defined with 5 different qualitative values: *Cannot be specified*, *Undetermined*, *Negative*, *Not done* and *Positive*. The distance between *Negative* and *Positive* should be big, whereas between *Undetermined* and *Not done* should be 0, since, for our study purpose, it is the same value. Whereas in this parameter it seems easy to define the distances, there are other variables that will require a complex calibration before comparison. To solve this we will need to define distances for each one of the qualitative characteristics used. These distances will be specified by the medical team based on the similarity of the values represented and kept as part of our model.

2.2.2.2. Statistical classification (SVM)

Statistical classification is another learning technique where an observation can be categorized as member of a group based on the quantitative information of one or more of its inherent characteristics. This process will require a previous training of the

[3] The International Society for Heart & Lung Transplantation

system with a population previously labeled. We will be using Support Vector Machines (SVMs) to develop this kind of system, since it is widely used nowadays for classification and it has a strong connection with statistical learning theory. A SVM can be considered an approximate implementation of a structural risk minimization method, where the goal is to minimize the maximum value of generalization before minimizing the training error. This approach makes it a more efficient generalization than other conventional techniques.

2.2.3. Architecture

Due to security issues and performance, our system would follow a multilayered architecture based on J2EE technology:

- The access layer to data and business logic would be implemented using EJB's technology according to the requirement of J2EE 1.4.
- Data is stored in a relational database capable of enduring a high transactional load.

For the server layer we would be using IBM WebSphere Application Server v6.1. In the Database Management System (DBMS) layer we choose IBM Informix Dynamic Server v9.4. These two layers communicate using the Informix JDBC Driver 3.00 JC3. The client access the methods in the server through EJBs, each of these calls will be logged, storing detailed information about what data is being retrieved and which user is responsible for the operation.

We briefly describe the different components needed to carry out the defined tasks. Figure 1 illustrates the processes that will take place to achieve our objectives.

- **Communication manager:** will be in charge of receiving the petitions and organize the information before transmitting it to the rest of the components.
- **Coordinator:** distributes the petitions received and generates the solution with the results obtained.
- **DB controller:** manages the calls to the data base to obtain the structured information contained in the monitoring system tables.
- **Cluster manager:** carries out the tasks of clustering and cluster information maintenance on memory, allowing fast data extraction during statistics generation. Our system will manage two different kinds of clusters, for transplants and visits.
- **SVM classifier:** chooses the correct cluster to which the register given should belong. To do this task the SVM models will be previously trained with the information given by the cluster manager.
- **Statistics manager:** this information will be generated from the data obtained in the cluster and evolution managers. For each transplant cluster, statistics will be calculated based on the events occurred to all the transplants defined on the cluster.
- **Rule extractor:** generalizes the parameters from a determined cluster and extracts the medication plan used to generate a treatment rule.

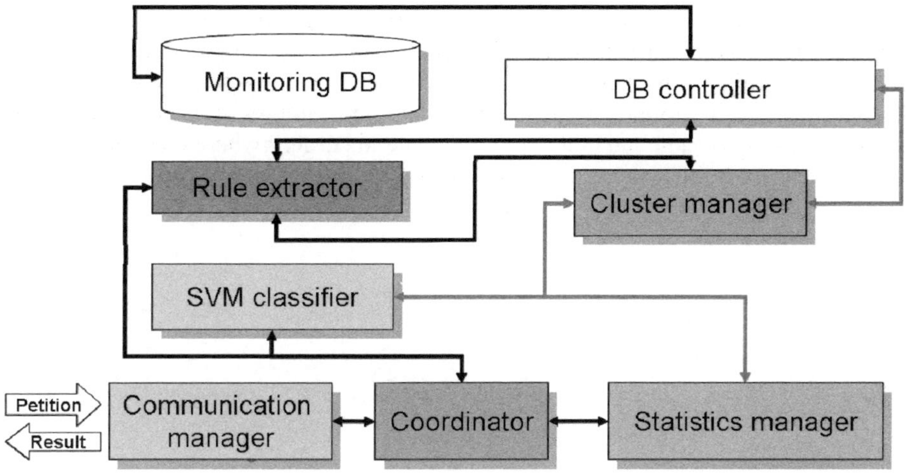

Figure 1: System's architecture

3. Discussion

This task will use two of the techniques already described: clustering and classification. Starting with a set of observations extracted from transplanted patients, and translated to our system as transplant parameters or basal characteristics, a process of clustering is made to obtain patient groups with similar characteristics. As we pointed out before, this requires a previous analysis work for all the variables involved to define the distances between possible values. All these characteristics will also have an associated weight defined by the specialist, creating big groups based on the heaviest variables and subdividing them with the lighter ones. We can see in Figure 1 how the grouping is done based on six basic variables like diagnosis, receptor/donor age and gender, and urgency level. Unfortunately, the set of variables is not always small. We are collecting over 200 variables for some transplant protocols. Defining distances and weights for each one of these variables is a complex task that needs to be done with the help of specialist and through different iterations to test the groups generated.

System validation will be done through different meetings with the experts, generalizing the groups defined by the system and asking the experts to classify a set of transplanted patients they have treated based on those generalizations. When a divergence is found, the case must be studied to find which variable weight must be reconsidered. Once the variable weight is adjusted we will ensure the patient is correctly placed.

The number of variables to consider is always directly proportional to the size of our population. For heart transplant, for example, we deal with no more than 700 cases, which we could group in seven different sets or reference groups. To do this grouping we can use 10 to 20 variables, depending on their type and the way patients are distributed on this multi-dimension space. This situation will change as the population grows, since we will be able to make more specific groups. Our system can do this automatically by selecting a ratio for the population needed to form a group (in our example 1/100). The clustering manager will then split our population in the number of groups given with no need to change our model. So, for renal transplants, where we have more than 2000 cases we find that 20 different groups can be created. This will result in more adjusted statistical information. Once our population has reached the maximum number of possible groups (our variables can only produce a limited number of subsets), each group can grow over the limit imposed, making more precise assumptions. This same method applied to general surgery where there are hundreds of patients being operated each week can render even more accurate results.

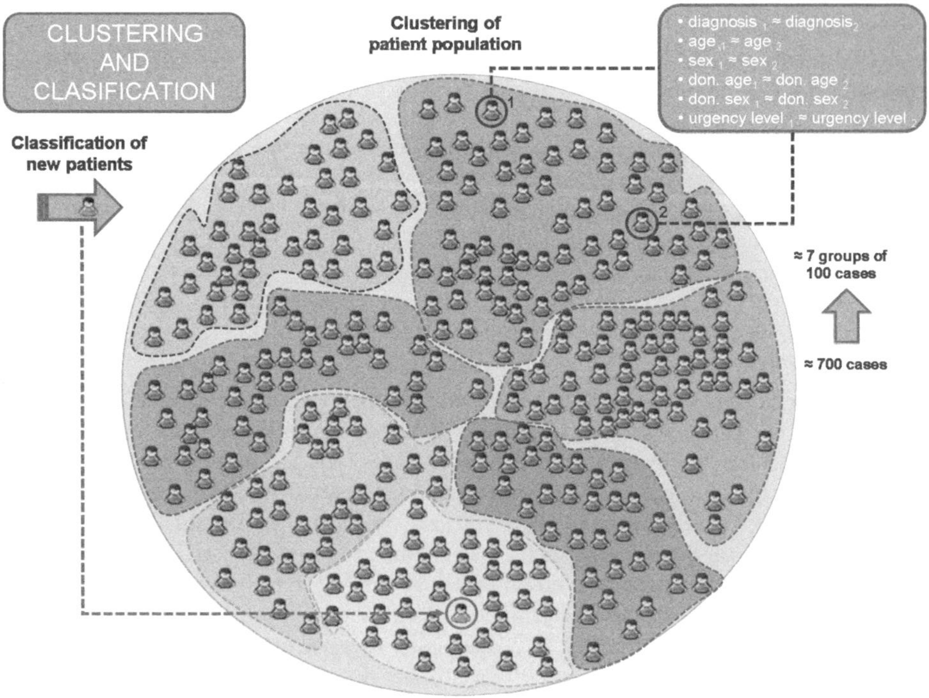

Figure 2: Clustering and classification

Once the groups are defined the SVM will be trained with them. Each patient will have a label so the SVM can identify to which group it belongs. After the training, the system will be capable of choosing the correct group for any patient presented. If the clustering process is done correctly, the selected group or cluster will contain patients with similar characteristics to the one selected. As it was explained above, each one of these patients has a record of events (usually comorbidities). Event data contains date, type and description. This information allows us to draw survival curves for each type of event managed. If we analyze the events for the group our SVM classifier has selected, we will obtain useful information about the probable evolution of the patient.

Each patient is a particular case and it is quite clear that no final conclusions can be extracted from this information. What we try to obtain here is the most accurate probabilistic information possible, with a model flexible enough to allow different insights. This will give the specialist up-to-date statistical information about the historical records based on a population with a set of similar characteristics.

Different sets of characteristics can be defined to obtain sets of clusters that will focus on phases or aspects of the transplant. To explain this we list some of the possible situations this system could be useful in and which sets of variables could be used to obtain the clusters.

- **Patient on waiting list:** the patient is not transplanted yet, so the data collected is scarce (diagnosis, age, sex, height, weight, alcoholism, number of cigarettes, etc.). Using just this set of basic variables we can group our records from already transplanted patients and extract the data to give the patient personalized information about the risks he is taking if he decides to be transplanted.
- **Patient on waiting list with possible donor:** in this case the patient is not transplanted yet but there is a possible donor. We can generate the clustering using the same variables as before plus the information obtained from the donor. If we make this kind of analysis for each of the patients on our waiting list we could list the patients that present lower comorbidity probabilities.
- **Patient with no immunosuppression:** the patient is about to be transplanted but the induction immunosupression he should receive has not been decided yet. If we make clustering based on the most significant data we know from the patient, our system can give us the group of patients that best matches the patient characteristics. This group can be subdivided depending on the immunosuppression taken. Study of the evolution for each subgroup can give us important information about which one renders best results. In this case, only patients with a constant immunosuppression can be studied, since, if the main treatment is changed, new events could be caused by the replacing treatment.
- **Patient transplanted:** the system estimates the group that best matches the patient characteristics, considering all the information contained in its record. This information could vary from the initial personalized risk report given since it considers a bigger set of variables. This information should be in the final report given to the patient, to let him know the possible problems that may occur and how to prevent them.

It's important to notice that these statistics are from the same hospital where the patient will be transplanted and that data collection and analysis takes place every day to count recent cases. We expect this information to be accurate since the system is assuming the same technical environmental conditions and it is always up-to-date.

4. Conclusions

Patient data is collected daily at hospitals giving us a source of knowledge in constant renewal. The challenge comes when we want to analyze this data and extract conclusions. Automating clustering of patients by a predefined group of variables will let us produce up-to-date statistical data from reference sets with similar characteristics. Using classification techniques we can estimate the closest group for any new patient and therefore predict possible comorbidities.

This information can be open for other health centre's queries. If the collected data is based on standardized protocols, this type of systems can allow the creation of networks where statistics would be based on a much larger database. These queries are quite fast since the classification process, in a previously trained system, is not time demanding.

Using real patient data to obtain new knowledge requires comparison. It is only after grouping our patient population by the relevant characteristics of the protocol studied when we will be able to extract conclusions. Learning machine techniques provide the necessary tools to carry out this process and standardize it. Once generalized, we will be able to apply it on any database we want.

References

[1] Uckun S. Intelligent systems in patient monitoring and therapy management. Int J Clin Monit Comput 1994;11:241-253.
[2] Mora FA, Passariello G, Carrault G, Le Pichon J-P. Intelligent patient monitoring and management systems: a review. Engineering in Medicine and Biology Magazine IEEE 1994;(12)4: 2
[3] Van Looy S. A novel approach for prediction of tacrolimus blood concentration in liver transplantation patients in the intensive care unit through support vector regresion. Crit Care 2007;11(4):R83.
[4] Sepúlveda-Sanchis J, Camps-Valls G, Soria-Olivas E. Support Vector Machines and Genetic Algorithms for Detecting Unstable Angina. 2002.
[5] Furey TS, Cristianini N, Duffy N. Support vector machine classification and validation of cancer tissue samples using microarray expression data. 2000
[6] Toth-Pal E. Computer decision support systems for opportunistic health screening and for chronic heart failure management in primary health care. 2007. ISBN: 978-91-7357-435-8
[7] JBoss Drools. [Online]. Available from: URL: http://www.jboss.org/drools/ (Last access: 08/01/2010).
[8] Hayes-Roth B, Washington R, Hewett R, Hewett M, et al, Intelligent monitoring and control. In: Proc. 11th International Joint Conf. on Artificial Intelligence. 1989. Detroit (MI); 243-9.
[9] López B, Zufia FJ, Ruiz R, et al. Seguimiento del paciente trasplantado: recomendaciones desde Atención Primaria. Medifam, ago.-set. ISSN 1131-5768. 2001; 11(8):46-50.
[10] Ansermino M. The future of intelligent monitoring. IHE. [Online]. Available from: URL: http://www.ihe-online.com. May 2009.

Medical and Care Compunetics 6
L. Bos et al. (Eds.)
IOS Press, 2010

doi:10.3233/978-1-60750-565-5-89

Effective e-Learning for Health Professional and Medical Students: The Experience with SIAS-Intelligent Tutoring System

Diana C. MUÑOZ[a], Alexandra ORTIZ[a], Carolina GONZÁLEZ[a,b, 1], Diego M. LÓPEZ[b,c], Bernd BLOBEL[b]
[a] *Software Engineering Research Group, University of Cauca, Colombia*
[b] *eHealth Competence Center, University Hospital Regensburg, Regensburg, Germany*
[c] *Telematics Engineering Research Group, University of Cauca, Colombia*

Abstract. Current e-learning systems are still inadequate to support the level of interaction, personalization and engagement demanded by clinicians, care givers, and the patient themselves. For effective e-learning to be delivered in the health context, collaboration between pedagogy and technology is required. Furthermore, e-learning systems should be flexible enough to be adapted to the students' needs, evaluated regularly, easy to use and maintain and provide students' feedback, guidelines and supporting material in different formats. This paper presents the implementation of an Intelligent Tutoring System (SIAS-ITS), and its evaluation compared to a traditional virtual learning platform (Moodle). The evaluation was carried out as a case study, in which the participants were separated in two groups, each group attending a virtual course on the WHO Integrated Management of Childhood Illness (IMCI) strategy supported by one of the two e-learning platforms. The evaluation demonstrated that the participants' knowledge level, pedagogical strategies used, learning efficiency and systems´ usability were improved using the Intelligent Tutoring System.

Keywords. E learning, evaluation, adaptability, intelligent tutoring systems, health education.

Introduction

In the last years, e-learning has been used to support training and education of students in different disciplines, including medical ones. Despite successful experiences, many open issues still exist. The Information Management Research Institute at the University of North-Umbria [1][2] addressed a study to identify problems in virtual education for health professionals and students. The results were classified in categories including the organizational, software and pedagogical levels. At the organization level, the main issues to be addressed are the long time for developing and adopting e-learning programs, and the lack of quality standards and trainers with skills

[1] Corresponding Author: Carolina González, PhD, Associate Professor; Systems Department, Universidad del Cauca; Calle 5 Número 4-70, Popayán, Colombia; Phone: +57-2-8209800 ext 2117. Fax: +49-2-8209810. Email: cgonzals@unicauca.edu.co; http://www.unicauca.edu.co

to develop e-learning materials. At the software level, the main problem is related to the usability of e-learning platforms including support for students' guidance and feedback as well as the reduced attention to the platform's evaluation process. From the pedagogical perspective, e-learning content is of poor quality and mostly incomplete. Furthermore, there is a resistance against changing teaching methods, for example, students need appropriate content and different alternatives for teaching strategies according to their learning styles.

Summarizing the aforementioned problems, for effective e-learning to be delivered in the health context, collaboration between pedagogy and technology is required. The content needs to be relevant and logically organized. Furthermore, it should be flexible enough to be adapted to the students' needs. The systems developed should be evaluated regularly, easy to use and maintain and provide students' feedback, guidelines and supporting material in different formats. In the context of health education, training sessions for patient and healthcare professionals have been recognized as one of the most important methods for patient empowerment improving health promotion and diseases prevention programs. However, current e-Learning systems are still inadequate to support the level of interaction, personalization and engagement demanded by clinicians, care givers, and the patient themselves (these 3 groups of participants are subsequently referred to as students) [3][4].

This paper describes the evaluation of an approach to improve the learning experience of medical students by providing personalized tutoring and tailored curriculum. The approach is supported by an Intelligent Tutoring System (ITS), which is a computer-based instructional system, created to dynamically adapt the content or learning style to each individual student. The ITS was used in one course on the WHO Integrated Management of Childhood Illness (IMCI) strategy [5], offered to medical students at the Faculty of Medicine, University of Cauca, Colombia. The aim of the IMCI strategy is to reduce death, illness, and disability of, and to promote improved growth and development among, children under five years of age. Moreover, this approach also can be used for providing patients with educational information according to the Health Empowerment Initiative [6].

The paper presents the implementation of the ITS, and its evaluation compared to a traditional virtual learning platform. The evaluation was carried out as a case study, in which the participants were separated in two groups, each group attending a virtual course on IMCI strategy supported by one of the two e-learning platforms. The evaluation criteria selected were the participants' knowledge level, pedagogical strategies used, learning efficiency and systems´ usability. The paper is organized as follows: In Section 1, each of the aspects related to virtual learning is revised. The methods are introduced in Section 2. In Section 3, the metrics for the evaluation are described. In Section 4, the case study design is presented including details of the participants involved and de software and tools used. Finally, the results of the evaluation are analyzed. Finally, in Section 6, the conclusions and future work are presented in Section 5.

1. Related Work

Intelligent Tutoring Systems (ITS) are computer-based instructional systems with models of instructional content that specify what to teach, and the teaching strategies that specify how to teach (Wenger 1987). They make inferences about a student's mastery of topics or tasks in order to dynamically adapt the content or style of instruction to the student's profile. ITS support a style of learning best categorized as ''learning by doing''. As students work on computer-based problems or simulations of real-world tasks, the ITS offers guidance, points out errors, and organizes the curriculum to address the needs of that individual learner [7].

In the last decade, ITS have left the research laboratories, now being incorporated into classrooms and workplaces to demonstrate their effectiveness [8]. The same is true in the medical domain. Crowley et al [9] describe SlideTutor, an ITS that teaches visual classification problem solving based on a cognitive model of expertise in the domain of inflammatory skin diseases. Nevertheless, medical terminology used in the system is highly specialized, therefore being used only by domain experts. COMET (Collaborative Medical Tutor) [10] was developed using the medical problem-based learning strategy. This system presents the same contents to all the students regardless their profile. Its performance has not yet been evaluated. IRIS-D is a diagnosis system that can be adapted to any environment, however not providing personalized instruction according to the student profile or learning styles. Curilem et al [11] describe a tutor for training patients with Diabetes Mellitus on all aspects related to this disease. The main objective is to support the learning process related to the disease and to achieve better quality of life for patients. The approach incorporates different mechanisms to improve usability aspects, adaptability and quality of the information managed. Other systems have been developed for different medical domains (anatomy, pathology, radiology), but a formal evaluation of their performance in real environments has not been provided so far.

2. Methods

2.1. Intelligent Tutoring Systems (ITS)

Intelligent tutoring systems (ITS) take into account the entire scope of a student's knowledge on the subject being taught, and even the personality features of the student in choosing each successive teaching action when they are faced to an-learning system. So, an ideal ITS must be able to provide impressive educational gains for students of many knowledge domains [12].

SIAS is an Intelligent Tutoring System developed for training students in the ICMI strategy. This system uses Bayesian Networks [13] to represent the student model. The tutor model in SIAS is represented as a Multi-agent System [14] which allows to monitor the student's progress and to assess the student's knowledge in every section of the course. Each course is created by health domain experts and stored in the domain model as an XML document.

The main feature of this approach is the adaptability provided through the student model. The SIAS-Tutor facilitates the implementation of an initial test in order to determine the initial student's knowledge level. According to the student's knowledge level identified, the system organizes the contents and the teaching strategies. SIAS-Tutor applies the questionnaire Honey-Alonso CHAEA Learning Styles [15] to identify the student's learning style (active, reflexive, theoretical, and pragmatic). Figure 1 describes each one of the components of SIAS.

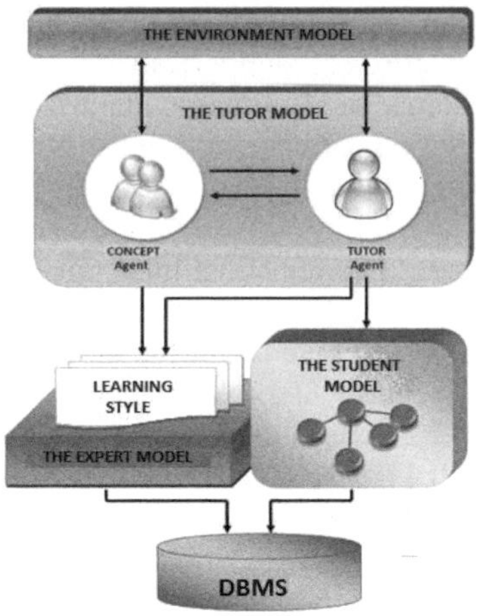

Figure 1. SIAS-ITS architecture

The Student Model. It uses Bayesian Networks to represent each one of the elements which define the course structure. Besides, it facilitates the diagnosis process about the student progress during the learning process.
The Expert Model. It contains information about the student's learning styles and the information about the domain to be taught.
The Tutor Model. It is structured as a multi-agent system consisting of two agents (concept agent and tutor agent) supporting the learning process.
The Environment Model. It presents information to the different users of the system (i.e. student, teacher, and administrator) facilitating the development of activities for each user.

2.2. Learning Management Systems (LMS)

A Learning Management System (LMS) is special software, generally used in most institutions for providing web-based learning [16]. An LMS facilitates management, delivery, tracking, testing, communication, registration and scheduling processes. There are many LMS systems on the market that can be freely used (i.e. Moodle, Claroline, ATutor, etc) or commercial systems (Blackboard, WebCT, and many others). Because of the large number of e-learning systems available everywhere, a mechanism to evaluate the quality, efficiency, and the performance of LMSs is needed (as the one presented in this paper). LMS Systems usually have big number of features and it becomes tedious to perform an evaluation of their real performance in learning processes.

2.3. Learning Styles: Honey-Alonso's Learning (CHAEA)

Learning styles are described as a set of cognitive, affective, and physiological features that serve as a set of stable indicators on how the students perceive, interact, and respond to the learning environment. These features are considered to be factors that influence the academic performance [17]. The Honey-Alonso learning questionnaire has been used during several years as diagnosis instrument about learning styles of medical students and health professionals. Therefore, its reliability and validity has been proven.

3. ITS Evaluation

In this section, we will discuss the criteria used for the evaluation of the ITS introduced in the previous section. To effectively evaluate the performance of SIAS-Intelligent Tutoring System in a health education learning process, we consider four criteria:

1. Knowledge Level: the student's initial knowledge on the course topics;
2. Pedagogical strategies: pedagogical quality of the course content, methodology, and student's profile;
3. Efficiency: the amount of time or effort required to perform the learning process;
4. Usability Level: the quality of user interfaces in terms of ease navigation and information readability.

In the evaluation process, we analyzed all the aforementioned criteria, measuring the performance of the proposed eLearning platform (SIAS-Tutor) against a traditional Learning Management System (Moodle). Moodle was chosen because it is the most used platform for virtual teaching and learning in different domains [18], and because no single evaluation of its performance against ITS has been demonstrated so far.

3.1. Knowledge Level

For reasons of simplicity, a great number of e-learning systems assume that the students know nothing or they have the same previous knowledge about the topics to be taught. In our approach we estimate each student's previous knowledge by using an exhaustive pre-test that contains questions related to each topic in the domain. With precision and objectivity, the pre-test measures the knowledge or current performance of a student. Then, a *post-learning test* is performed to compare the student's knowledge level at the end of the course.

The *preliminary test* consisted of 9 multiple choices questions with single answer which were structured by domain experts (medical faculty members). SIAS-ITS also assigned a score for each question. Moreover, the questions corresponding to the *post-learning test* were 10 and also designed by medical experts. Questions in the *post-learning test* are obviously more complexity, because the students are expected to increase their knowledge level.

3.2. Pedagogical strategies

The pedagogical model leads to the specification of teaching strategies that must be permanently evaluated. In order to evaluate the teaching strategies, we adapted the virtual questionnaire for course evaluation proposed by Arias [19]. In the questionnaire, the author classifies the learning material (i.e. platforms, virtual courses, and didactical units) and defines a metrics set for evaluating each type of system. The questionnaire has been selected by experts considering their reliability and relevance in the domain. According to the categories defined by Arias [20], we selected the pedagogical quality category to evaluate the teaching strategies used in the learning process. Table 1 presents the pedagogical quality category with their respective metrics.

Table 1. Pedagogical Quality Category.

Category	Metrics
Pedagogical Quality	Guidelines. Methodology. Content organization. Content quality. Didactic resources. Motivational skills. Multimedia. Language Style. Discrimination and values. User Singularity.

3.3. Efficiency

The efficiency is measured in terms of the effort required to perform a task within the course, the time spent by the student in a single task, and his progress during the learning process., In traditional systems (i.e. LMS), this criteria is usually measured by the human tutor which estimates the time necessary for a student to learn the topics included in the course. To flexibly evaluate this criteria, SIAS-ITS allows the course teacher to adjust the time estimated for each task according to the student's progress and performance.

3.4. Usability Level

The success of an ITS depends on the adequate consideration of different aspects during the design and implementation phases. In order to evaluate the usability level for this approach, we also used the metrics defined by Arias and that are described in Table 2.

Table 2. Usability Level

Category	Metrics
Usability	Ease navigation. Information readability. Esthetic quality of the general interface

4. Case Study Design

In this section, we discuss the case study performed, detailing the case study planning and implementation. To create an effective plan, we will refer again to the four criteria described in section 3: knowledge level, pedagogical strategies, efficiency, and usability level.

4.1. Target Population and Software Evaluated

A total of 40 volunteers participated in the case study. All the participants were medical students at the Faculty of Medicine, University of Cauca, Colombia. Some of the participants were familiar with virtual learning environments; however, no one had any particular expertise with intelligent tutoring systems. The case study was conducted using two groups. The first group covered 22 participants who used the LMS- Moodle. Among the participants using Moodle, 72.7% were female, and 27.3% were male gender. The average participant age was 23.45 years, with an age range between 20 and 29 years. Figure 2 (a) shows the participants using Moodle.

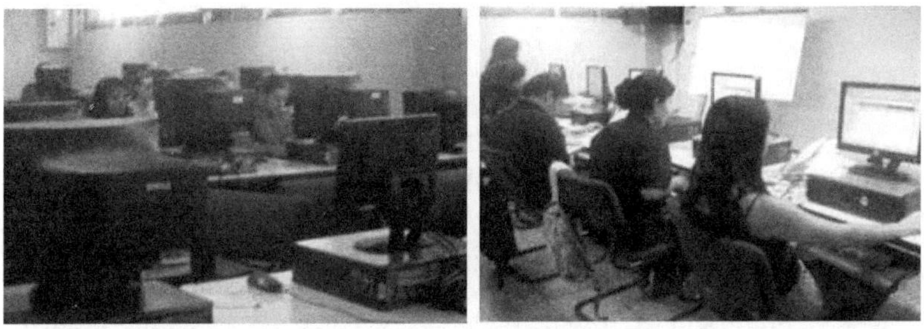

(a) Participants using Moodle (b) Paticipants using SIAS-ITS

Figure 2. Target Population

The second group covered 18 participants who used the SIAS-ITS. Among the students using SIAS-ITS, 44.4% were female, and 55.6% were male gender. The average participant age was 24,35 years with an age range between 23 and 30 years. The figure 2 illustrates the target population. Figure 2 (b) illustrates the participants using SIAS-ITS.

Each group was trained in the course "Integrated Management of Childhood Illness (IMCI)" introduced as part of the medical curriculum at the faculty of medicine. The course's content was structured by the professors responsible for the course.

4.2. Case Study Implementation

First Group. Participants in this group used the Moodle LMS. The course structure in Moodle was divided in six main topics: (i) IMCI introduction, (ii) Children growth and development, (iii) children's evaluation and classification, (iv) treatment, (v) resuscitation, and (vi) children's from 0 to 5 years. Figure 3 shows the course structure.

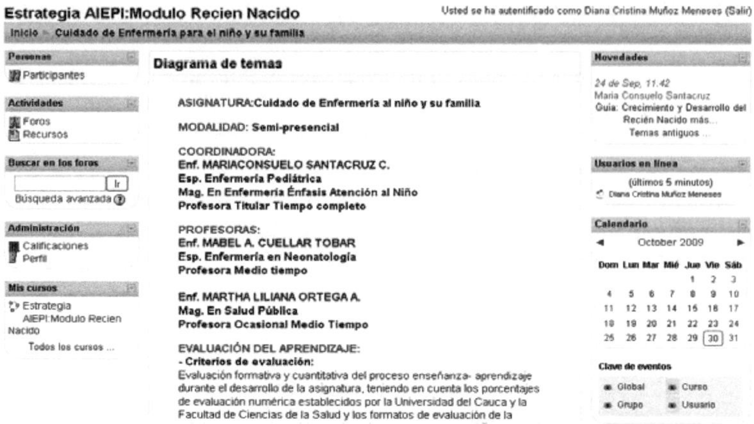
Estrategia AIEPI:Modulo Recien Nacido
Usted se ha autentificado como Diana Cristina Muñoz Meneses (Salir)
Inicio Cuidado de Enfermería para el niño y su familia
Personas
Participantes
Actividades
Foros
Recursos
Buscar en los foros
Ir
Búsqueda avanzada
Administración
Calificaciones
Perfil
Mis cursos
Estrategia AIEPI:Modulo Recien Nacido
Todos los cursos ...
Diagrama de temas
ASIGNATURA:Cuidado de Enfermería al niño y su familia
MODALIDAD: Semi-presencial
COORDINADORA:
Enf. MARIACONSUELO SANTACRUZ C.
Esp. Enfermería Pediátrica
Mag. En Enfermería Énfasis Atención al Niño
Profesora Titular Tiempo completo
PROFESORAS:
Enf. MABEL A. CUELLAR TOBAR
Esp. Enfermería en Neonatología
Profesora Medio tiempo
Enf. MARTHA LILIANA ORTEGA A.
Mag. En Salud Pública
Profesora Ocasional Medio Tiempo
EVALUACIÓN DEL APRENDIZAJE:
- Criterios de evaluación:
Evaluación formativa y cuantitativa del proceso enseñanza- aprendizaje durante el desarrollo de la asignatura, teniendo en cuenta los porcentajes de evaluación numérica establecidos por la Universidad del Cauca y la Facultad de Ciencias de la Salud y los formatos de evaluación de la
Novedades
24 de Sep, 11:42
Maria Consuelo Santacruz
Guia: Crecimiento y Desarrollo del Recién Nacido más...
Temas antiguos ...
Usuarios en línea
(últimos 5 minutos)
Diana Cristina Muñoz Meneses
Calendario
October 2009
Dom Lun Mar Mié Jue Vie Sáb
Clave de eventos
Global
Curso
Grupo
Usuario

Figure 3. Course Structure in Moodle Platform

Second Group. Participants in this group used SIAS-ITS. The course structure was organized as a tutorial containing a single theme consisting of nine (9) concepts. Each concept consisted of a variable number of explanations which are presented according to the teaching strategy used. Each theme has different associated learning resources (i.e. text, video, photos, etc) which are presented according to the student profile. Figure 4 shows the course structure in SIAS-Tutor. Table 3 describes the themes and concepts offered.

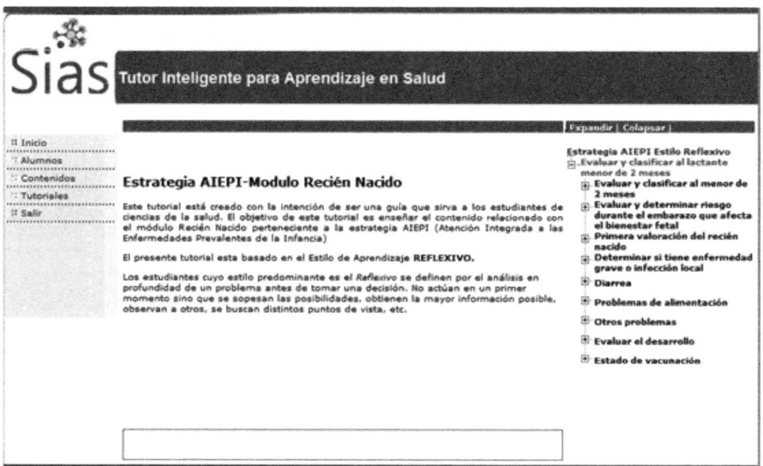

Figure 4. Course Structure in SIAS-ITS

Table 3. Course Structure in SIAS-ITS Platform

IMCI: Newborn Module		
Item 1: Assess and classify the infant under 2 months	**Concept 1:** Assess and classify children under 2 months.	Assess and classify children under 2 months.
	Concept 2: Assess and determine risk during pregnancy.	To assess risk during pregnancy. Determine risk during pregnancy. Classify the risk during pregnancy which affects fetal welfare. Case Studies.
	Concept 3: First assessment of the newborn.	How to make the first assessment of the newborn Determine gestational age. Sorting by weight and gestational age. How to classify the first evaluation of the newborn.
	Concept 4: Determine if the children have severe diseases or local infections.	How to evaluate a child with severe disease or local infection (part 1). How to evaluate a child with severe disease or local infection. (part 2). How to classify a child with very severe disease or local infection.
	Concept 5: Diarrhea	How to assess a child younger than 2 months with diarrhea. How to classify diarrhea.
	Concept 6: Feeding Problems	How to evaluate a child with low weight. Assess breastfeeding. How to classify food.
	Concept 7: Other problems	Assess other problems.
	Concept 8: To evaluate grow up.	How to evaluate a child. How to classify growing up problems
	Concept 9: Vaccination status.	Assess immunization status.

The case study was carried out by each participant on an individual basis, and according to their availability (time and internet facilities). Participants were permitted to take breaks between tasks. A fixed workplace was not required. After each course, the participants were requested to respond to questionnaires to collect the data established in the evaluation metrics. When the case study was completed, all data collected by the e-learning systems were analyzed.

5. Results

In this section, the results of the evaluation of Moodle and SIAS Tutor are presented, following the four criteria defined in section 3: knowledge level, pedagogical strategies, efficiency, and usability level.

The Knowledge Level. Figure 5 shows the resulting values obtained in the pre-test and post-learning test using Moodle and SIAS-Tutor, respectively.

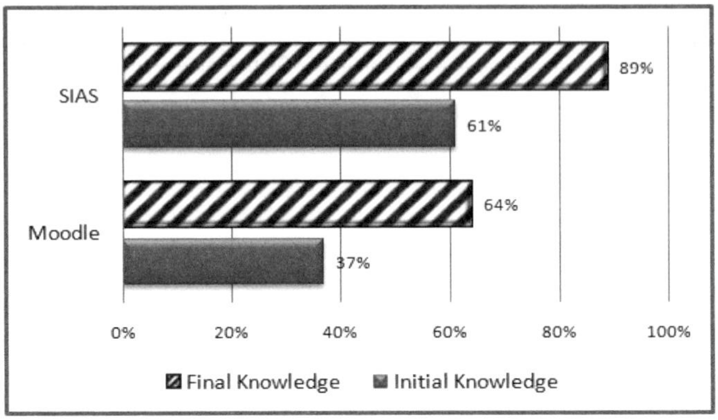

Figure 5. Knowledge Level Moodle vs. SIAS

Pedagogical Strategies. The strategies are evaluated according to the pedagogical quality metrics introduced in Section 3. The scale used ranges from 0 to 4 where 0 is the lower assessment and 4 the higher. Table 4 describes the results obtained for each metric. The first column presents the mean of responses to the survey for the SIAS system. The second column presents the mean of responses for the Moodle system. The difference is calculated as a percentage (SIAS-Moodle /4 =%).

Table 4. Results obtained for each measured indicating the percentage difference

Indicator	SIAS	Moodle	Difference (%)
Guidelines.	3.66	3.63	1
Methodology.	3.15	3.05	3
Content organization.	3.48	2.96	13
Content quality.	3.17	2.77	10
Didactic resources.	3.01	2.74	7
Motivational skills	2.83	2.81	1
Multimedia.	3.19	3.13	2
Language style.	3.27	2.93	9
Discrimination and values.	3.44	3.45	0
User Singularity.	3.25	2.9	9

Usability Level. Table 5 shows the results obtained after the evaluation of the usability criterion.

Table 5. Results obtained in Usability Category.

Indicator	SIAS (%)	Moodle (%)	Difference (%)
Ease navigation.	3,21	3,02	5
Information readability.	3,18	3,19	0
Esthetic Quality of the general interface	3,17	3,11	2

6. Discussion

In the following subsections, a discussion the results obtained for each one of the quality criteria is presented.

6.1. Knowledge Level Data Analysis

From the analysis of the results it is possible to conclude that the acquired knowledge level using SIAS-Tutor is 25% higher than that achieved with Moodle. This, especially because SIAS is taking into consideration the initial student knowledge to provide adapted contents, allowing the student to increase his knowledge level at the end of the tutorial.

6.2. Pedagogical Strategies Data Analysis

Taking into consideration the results obtained about pedagogical strategies, it is possible to identify the following advantages of using SIAS against Moodle:

Content Organization. The information presented in both approaches is updated. In the SIAS-Tutor however, the contents classification and organization is 13% higher, allowing the students to easily identify the relevance of the information presented.

Content Quality. Quality of the content is measured in terms of the degree in which the content is dynamically presented according to the student's learning preferences. This approach allows preparing different activities to stimulate the student's formative process. Quality of content is 10% higher in SIA-Tutor. Contrary, in Moodle, content is presented as hyperlinks, and the activities and tasks are presented without taking into consideration the student's learning preferences.

User Singularity. The results show that SIAS-Tutor specially addresses the specific student's learning characteristics, providing flexibility to the students to organize their time freely. Therefore, user singularity is 9% higher in SIAS-ITS. Moodle only considers the student's personal information.

Didactical Resources. This measure evaluates the adaptation level of the systems in terms of the number of learning guides provided, the mechanism used to present the content, and the feedback provided. The results prove that SIAS-Tutor provides different learning guidance according to the student's characteristics. The contents are presented with an adequate strategy and employ different learning resources. Furthermore, SIAS provides advices according to the student's evolution, allowing the students to explore all their skills. On the other hand, Moodle uses the same strategy to present the contents to the students. This strategy is defined by the teacher, and do not provide support or feedback to the student about the topics being taught. Summarizing, we can conclude that SIAS is 7% more adaptable than Moodle.

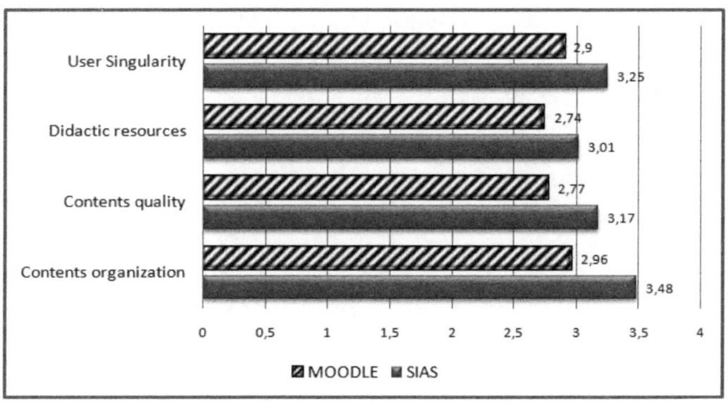

Figure 6. Results pedagogical quality with SIAS and Moodle.

Figure 6 presents a graphical comparison of the aforementioned results. The results show that the pedagogical strategies in SIAS are in general better addressed compared to Moodle .

6.3. Efficiency Data Analysis

This measure was not possible to be performed in Moodle because all tasks have to be mandatorily programmed by the teacher assigning a fixed time frame for its completion. Furthermore, in Moodle it was not possible to track the student's progress during the course. On the other hand, SIAS provides a complete report on the time employed by the students for each activity or task during the learning process. Besides, SIAS provides complete information about students' evaluation, their strengths and weaknesses, allowing tracking the students' progress in the tutorial. Figure 7 shows the time employed and estimated for one student to learn the concepts in SIAS-ITS.

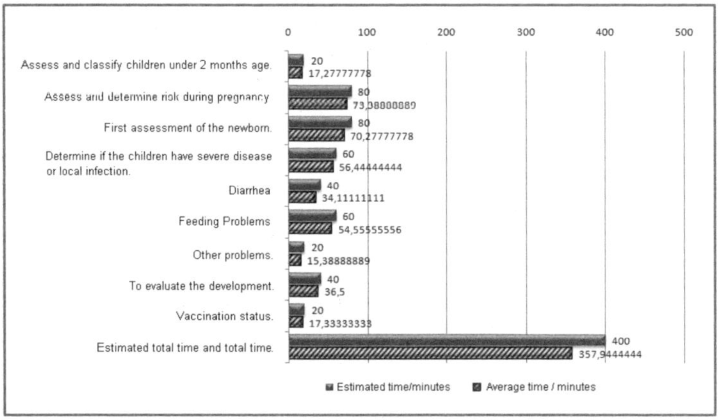

Figure 7. Time employed and estimated in SIAS-ITS

6.4. Usability Data Analysis

In terms of usability, Figure 8 shows that SIAS is in general better than Moodle in esthetic quality and ease to navigation. In relation to readability of the information, the two approaches are almost similar. The experience with the use of SIAS shows that it is more efficient to use and easier to learn. Unlike SIAS, Moodle offers many information and functionalities which often confuse the users, therefore decreasing the motivation for using the virtual platform.

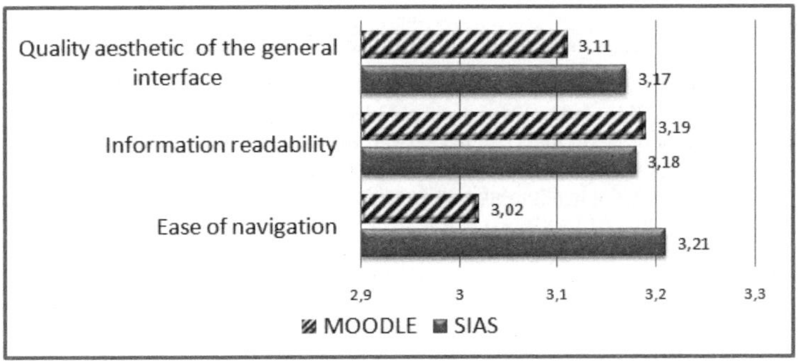

Figure 8. Results about usability in SIAS and Moodle.

7. Conclusions and Future Work

In this paper a comparative evaluation of two learning systems has been presented: Moodle and SIAS-Tutor. This evaluation was carried out within a course at the faculty of Medicine at the University of Cauca in Colombia with 40 medical students where 22 students used Moodle and 18 students used SIAS. Four evaluation criteria were used: the knowledge level, pedagogical strategies, efficiency and usability level. The results showed that the use of SIAS-Tutor had a positive impact on the participants and their learning process. The participants improved their knowledge level due to the SIAS adaptation level, which provided personalized instructions adapting the contents and presentation according to the participant's characteristics (i.e. learning styles, initial knowledge level of the student, etc). Moodle assumes that all the participants begin with the same knowledge level, therefore it presents the same contents without taking into account the individual participant`s characteristics. SIAS allowed tracking the time spent by the participant in each activity programmed in the course. This aspect is very important to measure the participant`s progress.

In relation to the system usability, the results showed that SIAS is easier to use, because the contents are distributed adequately and are presented to the participants using a simple user interface.

In the future, we plan to extend the work by developing a new approach that considers computerized adaptive tests and the student`s psychological characteristics. Additionally we would like to further explore the usability of the SIAS-Tutor for training of patients, clinicians and caregivers in issues related to the promotion and prevention of infectious diseases.

8. Acknowledgments

This work has been supported by the Health Education Network, funded by Conselho nacional de envolvimento cientifico e tecnologico brasileiro No. 490528/2007-4. The authors also wish to acknowledge the experts in Medicine and Pedagogy at the University of Cauca, along with all the medical students who voluntarily participated in the study.

References

[1] Learning for Health adn Social Care. NHSU. Elearning for Health: A discussion paper. Towards a strategy for NHSU, SHAs, partners and stakeholders. London: NHSU; 2004.

[2] Department of Health. Working Together – Learning Together. A Framework for Lifelong Learning in the NHS. London: Department of Health. [Online]. Available from: URL: http://www.dh.gov.uk/PublicationsandStatistics/Publications/PublicationsPolicyAndGuidance/PublicationsPolicyAndGuidanceArticle/fs/.

[3] Qiao Y, Lin X, Weatherburn G, Chen H, Guo L, Fletcher H. Adaptive tele-education for pressure ulcer prevention using rich Internet application. HC 2009;1-3.

[4] Erah P, Dairo E. Pharmacy Students Perception of the Application of Learning Management System in Patient-oriented Pharmacy Education: University of Benin Experience. International Journal of Health Research 2008;1(2);63-72.

[5] Patwari A, Raina N. Integrated Management of Childhood Illness (IMCI): A robust strategy. Indian Journal of Pediatrics 2002;69(1):41-8.

[6] Health Empowerment Initiative. [Online]. Available from: URL: http://www.healthempowermentinitiative.com/. (Last accessed Feb 2010).

[7] Sleeman D, Brown J. Introduction: Intelligent Tutoring Systems. In: Sleeman D, Brown JS, editors. Intelligent Tutoring Systems. Academic Press. 1998. p. 1-11.

[8] Lajoie S, Derry SJ. Computers as cognitive tools. Hillsdale (NJ): Lawrence Erlbaum; 1993.

[9] Crowley R, Legowski E, Medvedeva O, Tseytlin E, Roh E, Jukic D. Evaluation of an Intelligent Tutoring System in Pathology: Effects of External Representation on Performance Gains, Metacognition, and Acceptance. J Am Med Inform Assoc 2007;182-90.

[10] Haddawy P, Suebnukarn S. Comet: A collaborative Tutoring System for Medical Problem-Based Learning. IEEE – Intelligent Systems. 2007;22(4):70-7.

[11] Curilem S, Barbosa A, De Azevedo F. Intelligent Tutoring Systems: Formalization as Automata and Interface Design Using Neural Networks. Computers & Education. 2004.

[12] Li-zhen L, Min-hua W, Hua W, Liang G. Design an applied student model for Intelligent Tutoring System. International Symposium on Medicine and Education. 2009;1;485-9.

[13] González C, Burguillo JC, Llamas M. A qualitative comparison of Techniques for Student Modeling in Intelligent Tutoring Systems. Proceedings Frontiers in Education. IEEE. 2006. p. 13-8.

[14] Wooldridge M. Review of An Introduction to Multi-Agent Systems. Applied Spatial Analysis and Policy 2008;484.

[15] Alonso C, Gallego D, García J. Cuestionario Honey-Alonso de Estilos de Aprendizaje, CHAEA Estilos de Aprendizaje, 2006. [Online]. Available from URL: http://www.estilosdeaprendizaje.es. (Last Accessed: Feb 2010).

[16] Cavus N. The evaluation of Learning Management Systems using an artificial intelligence fuzzy logic algorithm. Advances in Engineering Software 2010;41:248-54.

[17] Galdames I. Learning Styles and its correlation from academic Performance on Human Normal Anatomy. International Journal of Morphology. 2007.

[18] Nagi K. Use of moodle reports for knowledge management, planning and eTraining in SMEs. IEEE International Conference on Management of Innovation and Technology. 2008. p. 946-50.

[19] Arias MJ, Evaluación de la calidad de Cursos Virtuales: Indicadores de calidad y construcción de un cuestionario de medida. Aplicación al ámbito de asignaturas de Ingeniería Telemática, Tesis Doctoral. Universidad de Extremadura. España. 2008.

[20] Arias MJ. Anexo II. Validación por Expertos. Departamento de ciencias de la educación, Universidad de Extremadura, Mérida, España. 2008.

Knowledge Representation and Ontologies

Medical and Care Compunetics 6
L. Bos et al. (Eds.)
IOS Press, 2010

doi:10.3233/978-1-60750-565-5-105

A Communication Standards Ontology Using Basic Formal Ontologies

Frank OEMIG[a 1], Bernd BLOBEL[b]
[a] *Agfa Healthcare, Bonn, Germany*
[b] *eHealth Competence Center, University Hospital Regensburg, Regensburg, Germany*

Abstract. Working interoperability not only requires harmonized system's architectures, but also the same interpretation of technical specifications in order to guide the development process. This paper analyses the commonly used structures of communication standards elaborated with HL7 Version 3 and proposes an ontological structure resulting in the so-called Communication Standards Ontology (CSO). As such a solution has to be developed within an architectural framework, the approach is aligned with the Generic Component Model (GCM).

Keywords. Interoperability, Communication Standard, HL7 Version 3, Ontology, Generic Component Model

Introduction

Enhanced communication and cooperation in healthcare as enforced by jurisdictional requirements in different countries normally require the utilization of communication standards. Not always a real "standard" is used, but a proprietary specification is established for solving the needs of either a user or a vendor. However, both – communication standards and proprietary specifications – require the fulfillment of the same kind of details.

In the following we will try to elaborate on those details exemplifying it using HL7 V3. But these generic details may be applicable for other standards as well.

1. Methods

To help with the development of a generic formal ontology for communication standards, a fine-grained analysis of communication standards is a necessary prerequisite. As mentioned before, this is done based on HL7 Version 3. This generic model is roughly verified with HL7 v2.x at the end of this paper. In the following, the Generic Component Model (GCM, [1]) as the reference framework for this analysis is presented.

Ontologies incorporate terminologies [2] with interrelated terms. Furthermore, a key feature of ontologies is to reuse ("import") other ones. One possible reuse is a mapping to other ontologies [3]. To support this fundamental approach, developing

[1] Corresponding Author: Frank Oemig, Agfa HealthCare GmbH, Konrad-Zuse-Platz 1-3, 53227 Bonn, Germany; Phone: +49-228-2668-4781. Email: frank.oemig@agfa.com; http://www.agfa.com/healthcare

new ontologies on the same basis is not only helpful but facilitates reuse and harmonization. For this purpose the Basic Formal Ontology (BFO, [4] is introduced.

1.1. The Generic Component Model (GCM)

The Generic Component Model (GCM) offers a generic architectural framework to any kind of system, not being restricted to ICT (Fig. 1). The scope goes far beyond and therefore incorporates other frameworks like the ISO 10746 Reference Model – Open Distributed Processing (RM-ODP) [5] as well.

The GCM provides three dimensions to present structure and behavior of any system in question. Depending on the perspective, the development process can be described reflecting the RM-ODP, another one is the architectural view considering composition and decomposition of components, and last but not least the separation of different domains.

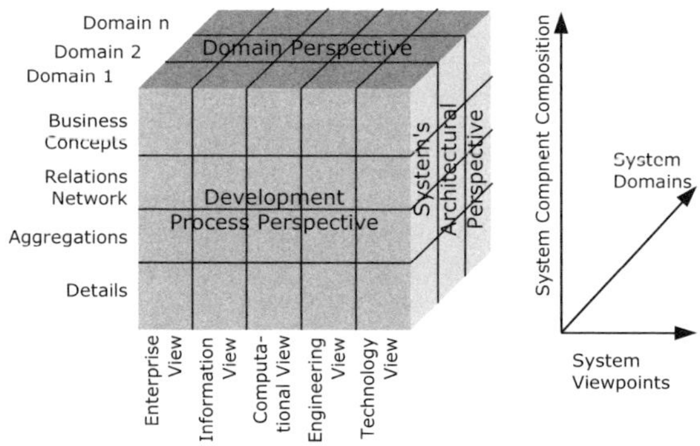

Figure 1. The Generic Component Model (GCM)

According to the GCM, communication standards represent different domains at different granularity levels, thereby being restricted to the enterprise and information view. Therefore, the appropriate model derived from the GCM can be reduced to the first two views in the development process. These views are shown in Fig. 3.

1.2. The Basic Formal Ontology (BFO)

From its origin, the Basic Formal Ontology (BFO) has some kind of philosophical orientation. Nevertheless, it provides an upper ontology which can therefore be used as a foundation for other ontologies [4]. Numerous research groups are utilizing BFO this way. Gene Ontology and Protein Ontology are examples resulting thereof.

One of BFO's primary advantages is its size. It is very small and comprehensive, so that ontology developers can easily align their concepts into it.

BFO groups everything below "entity" which acts as the root to the whole tree (Fig. 2). On the next level, everything is divided into entities that continue or persist through time (objects, qualities, functions) which is named "continuants" as the most generic concept. The other branch provides the entities for events or happenings (processes) in which continuants participate. It is named "occurrents".

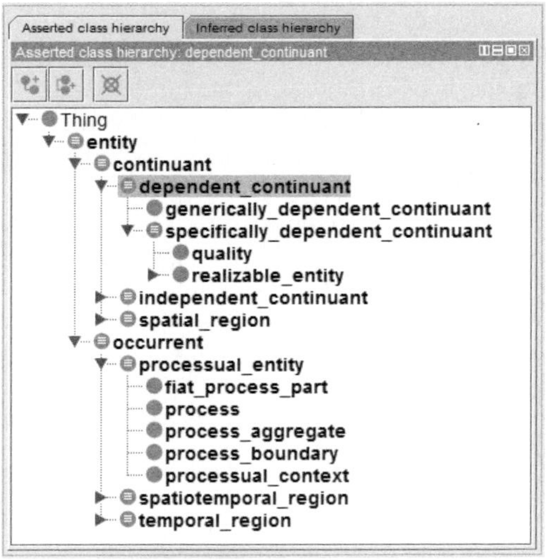

Figure 2. The Basic Formal Ontology (BFO)

2. Results

The introduced reference framework (GCM) is used to align the different HL7 V3 [6] elements (Reference Information Model (RIM), Data Types, Common Message Elements Types (CMETs), domain models (DMIMs), vocabulary, interactions, application roles, etc.) with.

In the first phase, the mentioned HL7 V3 elements are analyzed to obtain a deeper insight revealing their components and interrelations. These components are then aligned with the GCM. In the second phase, these components are also associated with the underlying basic formal ontology (BFO). The result of this process is herewith introduced as the Communication Standards Ontology (CSO).

However, the CSO only provides the generic concepts and the fundamental relationships. Therefore, the following sections guide through an introduction of the details, which have to be based on an architectural framework as well. As the GCM applies for any system despite the complexity level, it can also be used here.

Starting the described exercise, an investigation of available BFO based ontologies has revealed the Information Artefact Ontology (IAO) [7]. This paper does not further elaborate why IAO is not suitable for this task. Instead, a separate new ontology has been developed.

2.1. Analyzing HL7 Version 3

The HL7 V3 specification roughly talks about three different foundational parts: the reference information model (RIM), the data types, and the vocabulary. These parts are further enhanced with the domain models (DMIM) and their refinements (RMIM), application roles, and interactions.

An ontology maintains fine-granular concepts and their relationships [8], so that the aforementioned elements must be split into their conceptual parts which are explained as follows.

The RIM comprises of a set of classes with attributes and some basic interrelations. The "standard" ontological procedure would recommend modeling the RIM classes as different concepts with the RIM attributes as their properties. However, this approach does not seem reasonable, as the different attributes are comprised of datatypes as well. Therefore, an individual relationship between them should be established so that each element is represented as a class of its own.

This also counts for the attributes (elements) the Data Types are composed of.

The vocabulary is divided into vocabulary domains. These domains are in principle hierarchic constructs, enabling the identification of different entry points into this hierarchy to constrain the usage onto a subset only. On the other hand, these vocabulary domains are related to value sets identifying the individual values, possibly coming from different code systems.

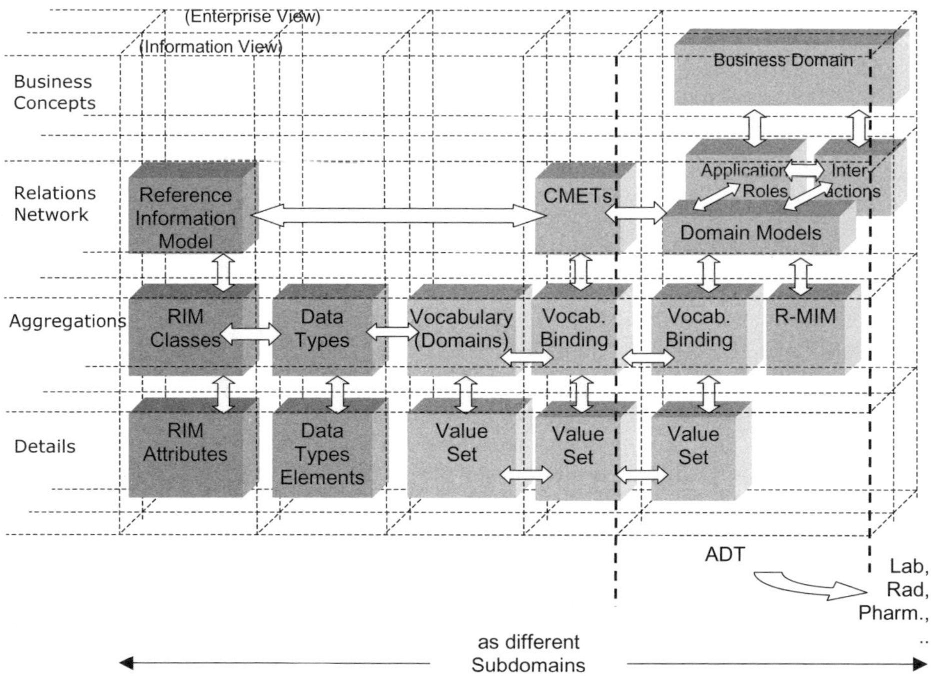

Figure 3. Analysis of HL7 V3 (based on GCM)

The Common Message Element Types (CMETs) are aggregations of some RIM classes which can be re-used in their entirety within other models. That way, one has to express, what a "patient" is, only once. CMETs can constrain the use of vocabulary by binding it to a certain subset.

Administration, billing, pharmacy, radiology, laboratory, order entry, medication etc., provide their own domain model. In terms of the GCM, they form a domain of their own. This is demonstrated in Fig. 3 for ADT (Admission, Discharge, Transfer) which represents a special domain and is related to the first domain with the "core concepts". All other domains can be placed adjacent to it, as is demonstrated by the white arrow.

The domain model reuses the other elements and is therefore set into relationship with those elements. Furthermore, it specializes and constraints not only the RIM classes with their attributes, but also the binding to special vocabularies and the domain model as a whole for specific use cases, e.g. "inpatient encounter management" within ADT. In HL7 V3, application roles are introduced together with the appropriate interactions and events resulting in message exchange. Those messages are constructed from the domain models.

The business domain explaining the rules and logic behind the different interactions is not made explicit within HL7, so that the business concept layer is not really populated. In Fig. 3, it is included for completeness.

Almost each element introduced so far has some kind of allowed usage and behavior in real message instances. The concepts to represent those details are introduced as information object quality and explained later. Finally, different paradigms like messaging and documents must be supported.

2.2. The Communications Standards Ontology

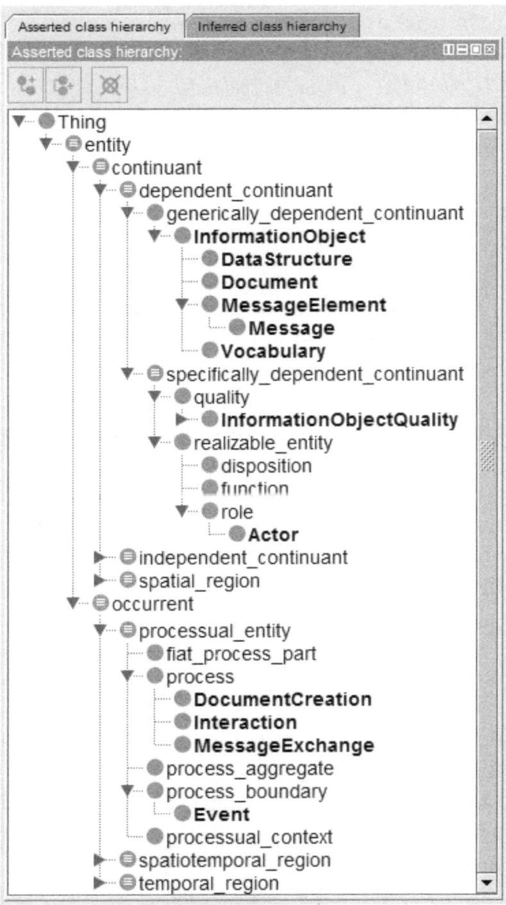

Figure 4. The Communication standards Ontology (CSO) in Protégé

In the second phase of this project, the identified elements are aligned with BFO as presented in Fig. 4.The primary elements are provided underneath a common concept called "Information Object":

- document
- message element (contents)
- message (entry point)
- vocabulary
- data structure

Two concepts does not fall directly into this hierarchy, nevertheless representing continuants:

- actor
- information object quality (optionality, null flavors, ..)

The process related information is assigned to processual entities below occurrents:

- message exchange
- document creation
- interaction
- event
-

2.3. Relationships

As mentioned, an ontology is distinguished from a terminology by the introduction of relationships among the concepts [2]. In order to support the use of intelligent agents, arranging them relationships in form of a hierarchy is essential. (Such a hierarchy is missing in BFO.)

Therefore, a root relationship (*hasRelationship*) with different specializations is the best way to achieve this goal (Fig 5). If different specializations share the same parent, it can be assumed that they have something in common, so that an agent can use the same logic to process the information, although different restrictions are applied to the siblings. A good example is the *hasParent* relationship, which introduces a link to the element which uses it as a component in a hierarchic structure, e.g. the message structure. Another example is the *isAttributeOf* relationship for the attributes of data types.

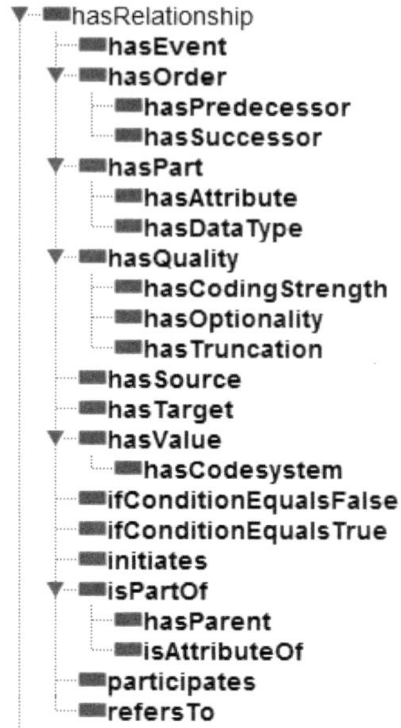

Figure 5. The Relationship of CSO (in Protégé)

This way, evaluating the hierarchic structure can be done by the same software component.

2.4. The HL7 V3 Ontology based on CSO

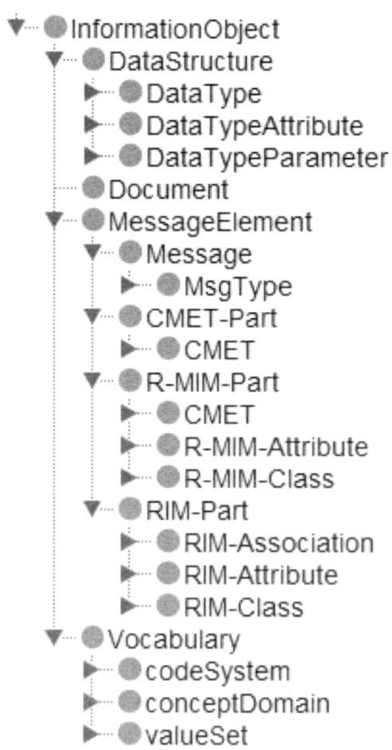

Figure 6. The V3 Ontology based on CSO

Taking the elements and components as identified by the aforementioned analysis and assigning them to the generic structure of CSO results in the hierarchy shown in Fig. 6. However, some elements occurring in this graphic require an additional explanation:

OWL allows for representing is-a relationships in form of class hierarchies. Hence, RIM classes, data types, messages and the vocabulary details are represented by such a hierarchy.

The associations between different RIM classes are represented by individual classes linking the RIM classes together, so it is possible to assign special qualities (attributes) to each relationship.

Data types not only consist of individual attributes, but they can also be used in a generic way to form sets, bags and lists. Furthermore, some data types like physical quantity (PQ) need parameters (nominator and denominator). Both are expressed separately.

The aforementioned V3 classes are primarily interrelated by the relationships provided by CSO. But some relationships like the attributes to data types are represented by their own specialized relationship. An example thereof is "hasDataTypeAttribute" as shown in Fig. 7.

The same is true for the special links between the vocabulary details *codeSystem*, *vocabDomain* and *valueSet*.

2.5. Information Object Qualities

As mentioned before, the use of ontology concepts requires an assignment of certain qualities like optionality, coding strength, etc., to information objects (Fig 8).

First, Tab. 1 introduces the usage of those classes within the different communication standards:

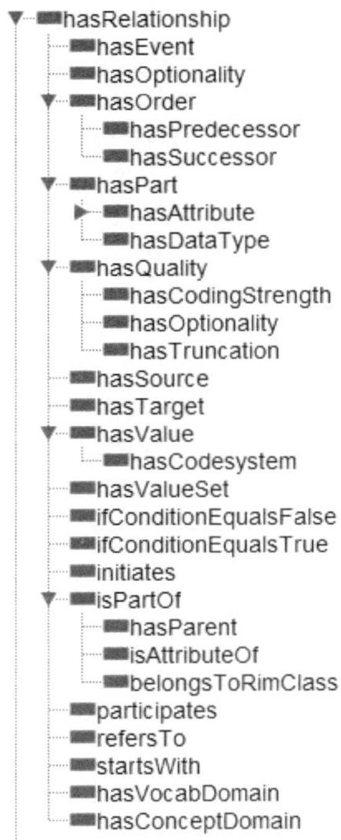

Figure 7. The Relationships of the V3 Ontology

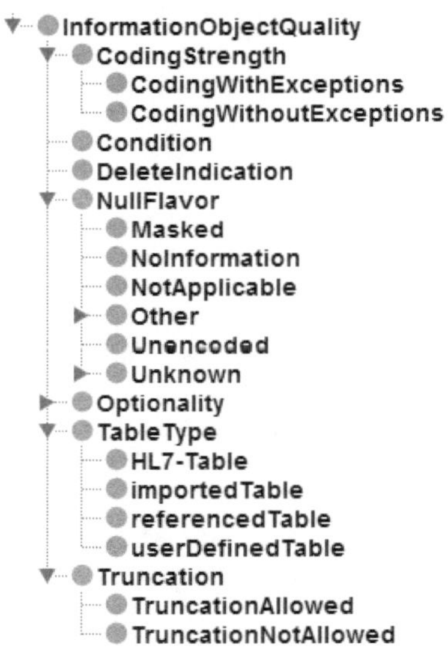

Figure 8. Information Object Qualities

Table 1. quality assignments

Concept	HL7 v2.x	HL7 V3
coding strength	X	X
condition	X	
delete indication	X	
null flavor		X
optionality	X	X
table type	X	
truncation	X	

The coding strength is applied to coded information and specifies whether site-specific codes are allowed to be used in message/document instances or not.

Especially in HL7 V3, the different specializations of null flavor are highly relevant. They form a hierarchy of its own, which is represented by individual classes.

The cardinality can be represented using the minCardinality and maxCardinality property of OWL.

The allowed length (min/max) of the classes can be established using constraints on data properties.

The optionality is the most important quality of information objects, as it applies to most of them, whereas other qualities are very limited in their use. Unfortunately however, the different specializations differ in their semantic meaning although the name/label is the same. Fig. 9 lists the names so that the same name may appear several times. The hidden namespace (represented in OWL) allows for an explicit assignment so that an exact equality between them can be established.

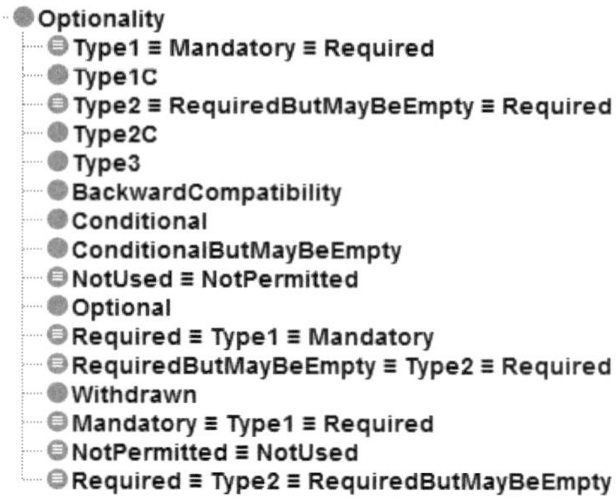

Figure 9. Optionality

A good example is HL7 v2.x "required" which equals V3 "mandatory" which in return is equal to the DICOM "Type 1" [9].

2.6. The HL7 v2.x Ontology based on CSO

The expanded ontology for HL7 v2.x reuses the same generic structure, but different specializations are necessary according to the details revealed by a separate analysis. As such, *MessageElement* and *Message* are directly used to establish a deeper hierarchy using *Message* as entry points. Furthermore, *Vocabulary* is refined by tables and table values, whereas data elements and components are a refinement of *DataStructure*.
A deeper elaboration would exceed the limited scope of this paper.

3. Discussion

During the development of CSO, the missing hierarchy of relationships turned out to limit the merits of BFO. This is caused by the lack of an architecture framework ontology systems have to be built on. Therefore, it should be discussed with the authors of BFO whether this can be changed. The presented hierarchy can be used as a starting point. Afterwards, the CSO relationships should be aligned with BFO.

Another issue is the mapping to other formal ontologies like DOLCE. It would be a nice exercise to provide this examination as well.

Last but not least, it would be an interesting task to test CSO against other communication standards like DICOM [9] and the German specific xDT [10].

4. Conclusions

It could be demonstrated that communication standards share the same principle structure. Therefore, CSO should be established as another top-level ontology within the OBO foundry [4].

5. Acknowledgment

The authors are indebted to their colleagues from HL7 for their kind collaboration.

References

[1] Blobel B. Application of the Component Paradigm for Analysis and Design of Advanced Health System Architectures. Int J Med Inform 2000;60(3):281-301.
[2] Oemig F, Blobel B. Harmonizing the semantics of technical terms by the Generic Component Model. 10th International Special Topic Conference of the European Federation for Medical Informatics; 2010 Jun 2-4; Reykjavík, Iceland. http://www.sky.is/efmi-stc-2010-.html, (accepted paper.)
[3] Oemig F, Blobel B. An Ontology Architecture for HL7 V3: Pitfalls and Outcomes. In: Proceedings of the World Congress 2009. Munich: Springer; 2009.
[4] The Open Biomedical Ontologies. [Online]: Available from: URL: http://www.obofoundry.org/.
[5] International Organization for Standardization: ISO/IEC 10746-2: 1996 Information technology – Reference Model for Open Distributed Processing - Part 2: Foundations. Geneva. ISO/IEC IS 10746 / ITU-T x.901. [Online]. Available from: URL: http://www.rm-odp.net/. (last accessed 17.03.09)
[6] HL7 Version 3. [Online]. Available from: URL: http://www.hl7.org/ctl.cfm?action=ballots.home.
[7] Information Artefact Ontology. [Online]. Available from: URL: http://www.obofoundry.org/cgi-bin/detail.cgi?id=information_artifact. (last accessed 14. 2.10)
[8] Gruber T. A Translation Approach to Portable Ontology Specifications. Knowledge Acquisition 1993;5(2):199-200.
[9] DICOM: Digital Images and Communication in Medicine. [Online]. Available from: URL: http://www.rsna.org/Technology/DICOM/index.cfm.
[10] KBV: .xDT: 2001, http://www.kbv.de/ , http://www.zi-koeln.de/ and http://www.zi-berlin.de/, http://www.kbv.de/ita/4274.html.

Medical and Care Compunetics 6
L. Bos et al. (Eds.)
IOS Press, 2010

doi:10.3233/978-1-60750-565-5-114

User-Specific Perspectives on Ontologies

Mathias BROCHHAUSEN[a1], Laura SLAUGHTER[b,c] Holger STENZHORN[d], and Norbert GRAF[d]

[a]*Institute for Formal Ontology and Medical Information Science (IFOMIS), Saarland University, Saarbrücken, Germany*

[b]*Department of Computer and Information Science, NTNU, Trondheim, Norway*

[c]*The Interventional Centre, Rikshospitalet University Hospital, Oslo, Norway*

[d]*Department of Paediatric Oncology and Haematology, Saarland University Hospital, Homburg, Germany*

Abstract. Ontologies are more and more used in clinical informatics in different settings and supporting different functionalities. Most experts see the role of ontologies as operating in a black box and being invisible for the end-user. With respect to some of the systems that have recently been developed this is only partly possible. Therefore, we provide a methodology to create an end-user perspective on a clinical ontology. This will foster participation of the clinical expert in both ontology exploitation and ontology maintenance. This methodology does not only provide the basis for a better integration of the experts into the ontology-based system, but it can be used to support patient empowerment by helping the patient to understand the content that is stored and partake in its management.

Keywords. Clinical Ontologies, Ontology-based Clinical Information Systems, Patient Information

Introduction

Ontologies are among the key strategies for semantic integration of distributed data. However, their success hinges on the technical quality of the reality representation they provide. This leads to problems for both medical professionals and patients to understand the ontologies which is a pre-requisite to use and evolve the ontology in question.

Ontologies cannot only be used to integrate data, but they are more and more used to capture data [1]. These tasks are putting the strategy of keeping the ontology in a black box from the end-user on a test. We argue that there are easy to use techniques to represent the types in an ontology in a user-oriented way, without compromising the theoretical soundness of the ontology as such. Our approach cannot only be used to foster usage of ontologies in clinical information systems, but it provides the basis for patient-oriented, ontology-based IT for the eHealth arena.

Keeping patients informed about their health situation and conveying this kind of information quickly, in a flexible way and tailored to specific life situations is one of the necessities regarding empowerment of patients in the future. Hitherto there is a certain amount of neglect regarding the automatic transfer of patient data into patient understandable form.

[1] Corresponding Author. mathias.brochhausen@ifomis.uni-saarland.de.

We will demonstrate how the structure already existent in a domain or application ontology can be used not only to create a user-specific view of the data structure, but also to enable inference from the knowledge captured in the ontology. Our strategy is to use Web Ontology Language (OWL) to create formal artefacts supporting this kind of functionality.

1. Best practice in ontology development and the clinical domain

With respect to ontology-based strategies to collect and store data a basic distinction must necessarily be made: The ontology provides the representation of types or classes in the domain. The data are instances or members of the aforementioned. Best practice ontology development demands that the structure of the ontology is derived from ontological criteria and not from epistemological states [2]. Thus, the structure that provides the basis of the data collection and storage process is a highly specialised one, namely an ontological one.

Basically, ontologies are representations of the entities in reality and the relations between them. Most commonly ontologies are built around a taxonomy which is the representation of entities ordered according to their subsumptions (formal is_a relation) (e.g. a bacterium is_a organism is_a physical object).

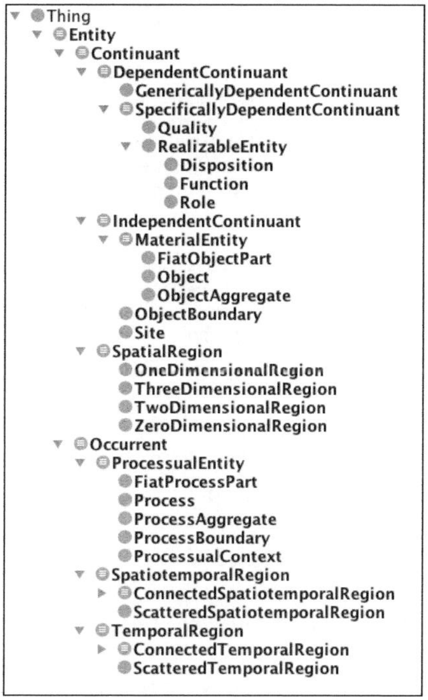

Figure 1: The entities of Basic Formal Ontology (BFO).

The gap between the world of medical practice and its ontological representation partly arises from using Upper Ontologies. The IEEE defines an Upper Ontology as a representation of universals and classes that are not domain specific, but general [3].

The use of Upper Ontologies is a major strategy to foster harmonization of existing ontologies and it supports purely ontological classification [4]. Taking a look at one instance of an Upper Ontology, namely *Basic Formal Ontology* (BFO) [5] it is easy to see that the entities represented by it are far from the practical world of both clinician and patient (Figure 1). Many existing and widely used medical terminologies are not built on sound ontological principles, but are representations of specific perspectives of the medical world [6, 7]. The latter may accommodate the wishes and expectations of end-users nevertheless they fail to provide a non-arbitrary representation of the domain.

For the reasons described above ontologies built in accordance with sound ontological principles look alien to domain experts and end-users, for instance clinicians. Figure 2 shows the branch of occurrents in the ACGT Master Ontology [8, 9], a clinical ontology built as extension of BFO.

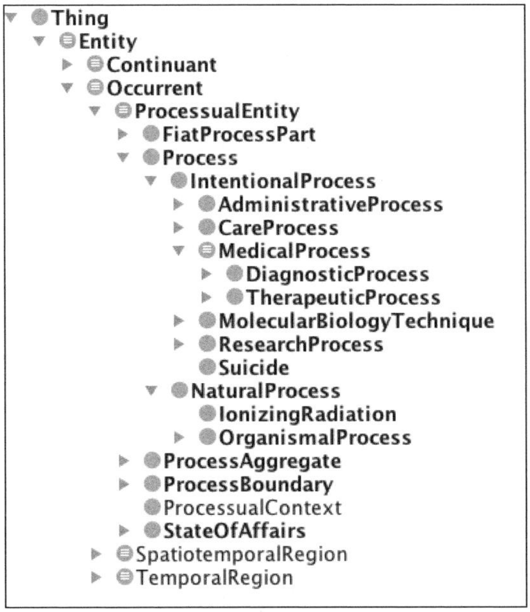

Figure 2: Occurrent Branch of ACGT Master Ontology

However, for most ontology-based systems this does not create a problem since the general strategy is to keep the ontology in a black box and keep it invisible from the end-users.

2. The ACGT approach towards a clinical view of the ACGT Master Ontology

One aim of the ACGT consortium is to provide an ontology-based clinical trial management system (ObTiMA). This entails strategies to annotate data immediately in accordance with the ACGT Master Ontology. However, the result of this process is that clinical users of ObTiMA, at least the chair person of a clinical trial or the technical staff administrating the data, needs to get into contact with the ontology. This is, of course, contrary to the black box strategy mentioned above.

One of the key issues in developing ObTiMA was the question whether we could do something with the ontology itself to facilitate the work of the software engineers providing the graphic user interface (GUI) for the system. The first step was to collect end-user requirements of GUIs for clinical systems, emphasizing the management and control of clinical studies. Figure 3 shows a detail from the proposals made by the clinical partners in ACGT. We call this view on the data collection and management process the ACGT clinical view. It provided the basis for our approach to render a specific perspective on the ontology for the end-user.

The key restriction we accepted was that the ontology could not be altered in its structure to accommodate the user requirements. Changing the ontology design from being based on non-arbitrary ontological decisions to representing task specific perspectives in only one set of end-users, would have resulted in compromising the quality criteria which were embraced in the beginning of the ACGT MO development.

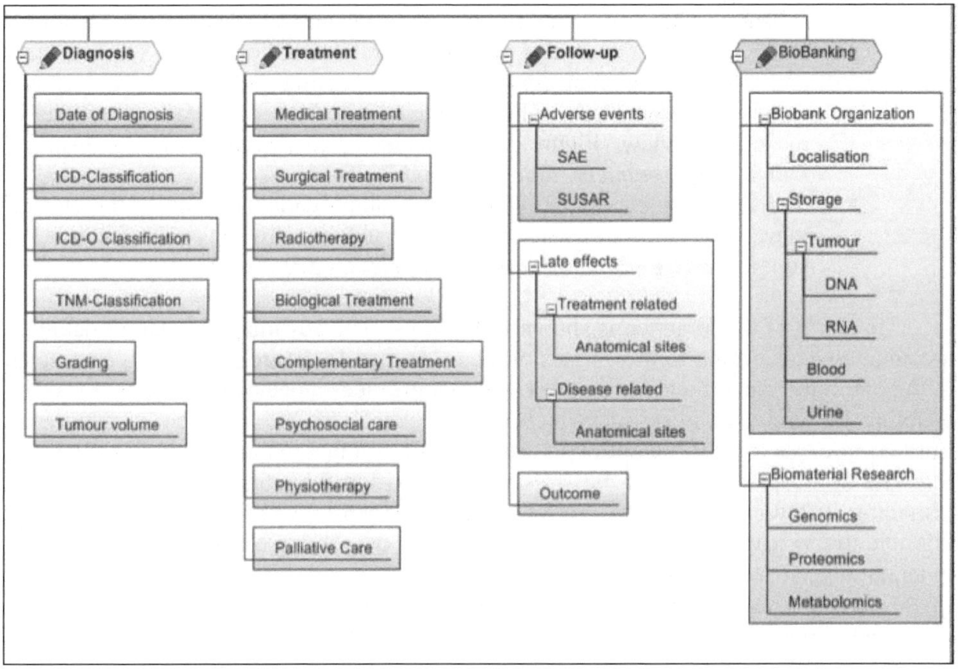

Figure 3: Detail from a clinical view on trial administration.

3. Flexible ontological perspectives on ontologies: a user- and situation-oriented solution

One prerequisite of the solution we propose is that the ontology on which we want to allow different perspectives is deployed via the Internet (this ontology will be called *target ontology* in the following). This is the case for the ACGT Master Ontology. For our solution we use the Protégé ontology editor, a free software to create OWL files and that can be downloaded from the Internet [10]. So once our target ontology can be downloaded we start with creating a new OWL file.

Note that we do not speak of an ontology when addressing the second OWL artefact. We will stick to this practice since we will need to create multiple inheritances within that OWL file to achieve our aim. However, we hold that multiple inheritance is not good ontological practice. Thus we will refer to the second OWL file which renders the perspective on the target ontology as an *OWL artefact*. In the following we will give a step by step description of the creation of an OWL implementation of the clinical view and its connection with the target ontology, more specifically the ACGT Master Ontology.

- *Step 1:* To create the OWL artefact we start with importing the entire target ontology from the Internet. Protégé provides easy means to accomplish this [11]. For the case study at hand we import the ACGT Master Ontology from http://www.ifomis.org/acgt/1.0. Since this ontology is using BFO as Upper Ontology, the import results in subsuming bfo:Entity and its subclasses as only subclass to owl:Thing.
- *Step 2:* In order to create an OWL implementation of the clinical view and link it to the classes of the pre-existing ontologies we create a subclass of owl:Thing called *ClinicalView*. Now we add the sections in the clinical view (Figure 3) as subclasses to *ClinicalView*, for instance *Diagnosis*, *Treatment*, *Follow-up* and *Biobanking*.
- *Step 3:* Those classes of the target ontology which are part of the clinical view are defined as having the matching clinical view section as superclass (e.g. *Radiotherapy* has superclass *Treatment*).

The result of this practice is shown in Figure 4. The advantage is that all data that are annotated according to the classes of the target ontology, are in fact only annotated to the ontology. Nevertheless, the OWL artefact provides an easy to use basis for GUIs enabling the end-user to decide which kind of data is to be collected or integrated. Furthermore, we foresee the option to use the OWL artefact in ontology-maintenance.

The key aspect that must be stressed here, is that this strategy is not limited to providing different professional views on a given ontology, but that it is absolutely possible to use it to support patient information on data that are collected or integrated in an ontology-based manner.

Again, we want to stress that we do not claim that the result of the practice described above is an ontology. Figure 4 clearly shows why this is not the case: The selected class *acgt:Radiotherapy* has two superclasses, namely *acgt:TherapeuticProcess* and *Treatment*. The criterion of avoiding multiple inheritance is therefore not realized in the OWL artefact.

Some might think that rooting this solution on the Internet provides a critical issues with respect to the universality of applying it. Yet, we hold that the solution is based on the way ontologies are expressed and that the target ontology can be imported from were ever it is stored. The Internet is only presenting the most open and easiest to connect to option.

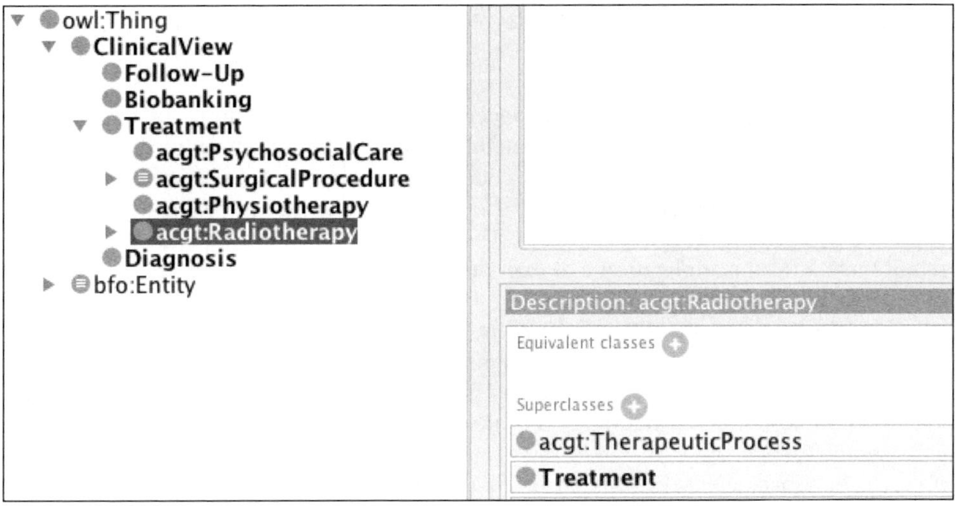

Figure 4: Detail from screenshot of ACGT Clinical View in the OWL artefact

4. From expert views to patient language

The aim of the method described above is to enable the end-user, e.g. a clinician, to partake in the process of ontology exploitation and ontology maintenance in a more active role than this has hitherto been the case. The latter is of key importance since the clinicians form the group of users with the best in-depth knowledge regarding the domain of clinical medicine. If we only rely on novel insights published in journals our ontology maintenance is restricted to a relatively slow pace. The goal is to harvest experiences from clinical research as quick as possible. Therefore, to enable the clinician to actively guide the development of the ontology by the curator is an absolute necessity.

While the use-case for the development of our methodology to create user-oriented perspective on an ontology focused on the clinician, we hold that the same technique can be used to enable the patient. Towards this aim we see three aspects of how the patient needs to be enabled:

- Understanding the content that is stored in a clinical information system;
- Keeping up to date his/her own records as far as possible;
- Managing data deployment, if necessary.

Regarding our use-case here, the management of clinical trials, we hold that the clinical view will provide a huge step towards patient empowerment with respect to these three issues. The only thing that surely needs to be accomplished is to foster automatic translation from expert language to patient language

Brochhausen and Slaughter [12] stressed that the latter is a problem that calls for solutions of the problem of how patient language can be mapped unto an expert ontology. The key question is whether patient language is referring to an ontology at all, or whether it represents a web of belief that is incommensurable with reality-based ontological representation.

5. Remarks on architecture and the development of ontologies in the eHealth domain

When addressing architectural issues concerning ontologies, it is important to state that an ontology does not provide a functionality. We can talk about ontologies as "lazy" artifacts. What an ontology provides is coded information on the world and semantics. The functionality to produce meaningful information for the user needs to be carried out by an application (e.g. a query tool). The business process of the system defines the requirements for the application that exploits the ontology and thus determines the kind of information or service provided.

The main reason to use ontologies is the conviction that these can be universal artifacts to be re-used in multiple systems, thus creating something like a standard universal representation of reality as a basis for semantic reference domain by domain.

Nevertheless, we see that many mistakes regarding semantics in eHealth stem from a mismatch of semantic resources (e.g. ontologies, terminologies) and the business process. For instance, MESH is an artifact created to only annotate texts and give a library science-inspired order of them [4] and ICD was created to report causes of death. Despite these facts both are used to support other functionalities alien to their origin.

One of the key challenges for the future of ontologies in eHealth is to bring together the need for universal reality representations and functionality-focused artifact aimed at specific business processes. One strategy that might help us to overcome this gap is to view the information systems we aim to create in a more systemic way and set up ontology developments embedded into the strategy of the Generic Component Model (GCM) [13]. Nevertheless, we need strategies to ensure that not every business process makes use of a specific ontology and therewith of a specific semantic, and we need to maintain the aim for unification of semantic reference, since this is a key strategy with respect to the *Semantic Web*.

Conclusion

The ever growing acceptance and use of ontologies for clinical information systems and other medical applications makes it necessary to provide ontologies to a multiplicity of users of the data. Thus, we need to provide techniques to allow different action or role dependent views on the ontology. One of the possible use-cases is providing a view specifically geared to patients in order to help them to understand the schemata in accordance to which their data are being collected and stored.

The strategy of the OWL artefact that creates specific views on a pre-existent ontology deployed over the Internet provides one way to facilitate the development of interest group specific views. The methodology can be used on any kind of ontology that is deployed via the Internet. Using the ontology in the OWL artefact to provide user-oriented views will not compromise the quality of reality representation in the ontology itself. Different perspectives can be provided for different user groups. For instance, it is absolutely possible to provide perspectives on an ontology exploited by a clinical information system for clinical users, trial chairpersons, IT staff and patients. The extent to which the OWL artefacts can be used to support maintenance of its target ontology has to be investigated.

Regardless of the advancement of patient empowerment that can be provided by this methodology, one key issue that remains to be resolved is the problem of mapping patient language onto expert-aimed ontologies.

References

[1] Weiler G, Brochhausen M, Graf N, Hoppe A, Schera F, Kiefer S. Ontology Based Data Management Systems for post-genomic clinical Trials within an European Grid Infrastructure for Cancer Research. In: Proceedings of the 29th Annual International Conference of the IEEE EMBS; 2007 Aug 23-26; Lyon, France. IEEE; 2007. p. 6434-7.

[2] Bodenreider O, Smith B, Burgun A. The Ontology-Epistemology Divide: A Case Study in Medical Terminology. In: Varzi A, Vieu L, editors; Formal Ontology and Information Systems. Proceedings of the Third International Conference (FOIS 2004). Amsterdam: IOS Press; 2004. p. 185-95.

[3] [Online]. Available from: ULR: http://suo.ieee.org/ (last accessed: 07.03.2010).

[4] Smith B, Brochhausen M. Establishing and Harmonizing Ontologies in an Interdisciplinary Health Care and Clinical Research Environment. In: Blobel B, Pharow P, Nerlich M, editors; eHealth: Combining Health Telematics, Telemedicine, Biomedical Engineering and Bioinformatics on the Edge. Global Expert Summit Textbook. (Health, Technology and Informatics, 134). Amsterdam: IOS Press; p. 219-34.

[5] Grenon P, Smith B. SNAP and SPAN: Towards Dynamic Spatial Ontology. Spatial Cognition and Computing 2004;4:69-103.

[6] Smith B, Ceusters W, Temmerman R. Wüsteria. Proceedings Medical Informatics Europe 2005, Geneva. Stud Health Technol Inform. 2005;116:647-52.

[7] Ceusters W, Spackman K, Smith B. Would SNOMED-CT Benefit from Realism-Based Ontology Evolution? Proceedings of the Annual Symposium of the American Medical Informatics Association; Chicago, IL. 2007. p. 105-9.

[8] [Online]. Available from: URL: http://www.ifomis.org/wiki/ACGT_Master_Ontology (MO) (last accessed: 07.03.2010).

[9] Brochhausen M, Weiler G, Martín L, Cocos C, Stenzhorn H, Graf N, Dörr M, Tsiknakis M, Smith B. Applications of the ACGT Master Ontology on Cancer. In: Meersman R, Tari Z, and Herrero P, editors. Proceedings of 4th International IFIP Workshop On Semantic Web & Web Semantics (OTM 2008: Workshops); LNCS 5333; 2008. p. 1046-55.

[10] [Online] Available from: URL: http://protege.stanford.edu/ (last accessed: 07.03.2010).

[11] Horridge M, Jupp S, Moulton G, Rector A, Stevens R, Wroe C. A Practical Guide To Building OWL Ontologies Using Protégé 4 and CO-ODE Tools Edition 1.1. [Online]. Available from: URL: http://www.co-ode.org/resources/tutorials/ProtegeOWLTutorial-p4.0.pdf (last accessed: 07.03.2010).

[12] Brochhausen M, Slaughter L, Patient Empowerment by Ontology-Based Multi-lingual Systems. IFMBE Proceedings 2009;25/XII:439-42.

[13] Blobel B. Architectural approach to eHealth for enabling paradigm changes in health. Methods Inf Med 2010; 49,2:123-34.

Medical and Care Compunetics 6
L. Bos et al. (Eds.)
IOS Press, 2010

doi:10.3233/978-1-60750-565-5-122

Management of Knowledge Gaps: Concept Representation of Things We Don't Know

Juerg P. BLEUER[a,1], Daniele TALERICO[b], Kurt BÖSCH[b], Vincent LAMPÉRIÈRE[b], Christian A. LUDWIG[b]
[a]*Healthevidence GmbH, Berne, Switzerland*
[b]*Suva, Lucerne, Switzerland*

Abstract: Suva (Swiss National Accident Insurance Fund) is the most important carrier of obligatory accident insurance in Switzerland. Its medical division supports doctors working in inpatient and outpatient care with comprehensive case management and with conciliar advice. The Suva hospitals provide inpatient rehabilitation. In 2002, Suva started the InWiM project. InWiM is an acronym and stands for "Integrierte Wissensbasen der Medizin", which can be translated as "Integrated Knowledge Bases in Medicine". Information retrieval within InWiM is achieved by means of the MeSH Index (Medical Subject Headings), the thesaurus of the United States National Library of Medicine (NLM). InWiM has now been extended towards the management not only of publications but also of areas where sound knowledge is missing, so called "knowledge gaps": Knowledge gaps are indexed with MeSH terms in a similar way to publications. This improves knowledge management: In particular it is possible to search and find knowledge gaps and solutions covering the same or a similar topic, thus allowing adequate collating and it prevents duplication of work. Furthermore, literature search strategies for the NML are predefined and do not need every time to be reinvented from scratch.

Keywords: Knowledge management, information retrieval, MeSH index, concept representation, knowledge gap.

Introduction

Suva (Swiss National Accident Insurance Fund) is the most important carrier of obligatory accident insurance in Switzerland. It is an independent, non-profit-making company under public law. Among the 2'904 employees there are about 150 medical doctors and 130 case managers working in 19 agencies, 2 hospitals and one back office in the headquarter in Lucerne, Switzerland. Suva's medical division supports doctors working in inpatient and outpatient care with comprehensive case management and with conciliar advice. The Suva hospitals provide inpatient rehabilitation.

In 2002, Suva started the InWiM project. InWiM is an acronym and stands for "Integrierte Wissensbasen der Medizin", which can be translated as "Integrated Knowledge Bases in Medicine". It comprises the definition and documentation of all

[1] Corresponding author: Juerg P. Bleuer, MD, MPH, Healthevidence GmbH, P.O. Box 6551, CH-3001 Berne, Switzerland; Email: bleuer@healthevidence.ch

processes in the field of medical knowledge management as well as the implementation of the InWiM knowledge management application. The latter is based on the concept Schreyögg and Geiger called "an approach to knowledge inspired by information theory"[1]: Knowledge is represented as a multidimensional link-up of information entities. Annotations allow one to add a narrative description to each link. Details of the implementation and the underlying knowledge representation model are described elsewhere[2]. Information retrieval is achieved by means of the MeSH Index (Medical Subject Headings), the thesaurus of the United States National Library of Medicine (NLM). The InWiM implementation of MeSH supports all features including subheadings and limits. It allows users to search the in-house document repository as well as to access the online literature service of the NLM (www.pubmed.org) through the same graphical user interface (GUI). As far as the authors are aware, InWiM is currently the only implementation worldwide – except for the NLM and its national representatives - which supports all MeSH features for in-house retrieval. Currently, InWiM addresses only Suva health professionals but it is envisaged to target a larger audience. Via internet it will support professionals in in- and outpatient care as well as inform patients about their conditions.

1. Knowledge Gaps and Knowledge Solutions

The term "Knowledge Gap" has different meanings: Tichenor, Donohue and Olien used it already in the 70's to denominate differences in knowledge between groups with different socio-economic status[3]. In this publication, the term means "area of lack of knowledge" and not the difference in knowledge between groups of individuals.

David Sackett defined evidence-based medicine (EBM) as "the conscientious, explicit, and judicious use of current best evidence in making decisions about the care of individual patients" and he pointed out the importance of identifying personal knowledge gaps when practicing and teaching EBM: He stated that "... to guide the learner in transforming knowledge gaps into well-built clinical questions" is one of four key steps in teaching how to ask questions for EBM[4].

Localizing "knowledge gaps" is also important for institutions: We define "Corporate Knowledge Gaps" as areas of knowledge, where there are no defined and valid answers to specific questions within an institution. Various reasons can be found for this: The scope ranges from "Nobody ever explicitly asked this question" to "Science can not give an answer". Thus, the term "Corporate Knowledge Gap" stands for different things such as areas of activity governed solely by tacit knowledge as well as domains with scarce or entirely missing scientific evidence.

The term "tacit knowledge" refers to the part of knowledge which cannot be codified, but can only be transmitted via training or gained through personal experience. A good example of tacit knowledge is the ability to ride a bicycle, which is more "know-how", than "know-why".

Because it is difficult to verbalize and to transfer to another person, tacit knowledge is a challenge for every knowledge management initiative within an organization. Areas of tacit knowledge are domains of selfhood and they favour kludges over evidence-based approaches. Medicine is still full of tacit knowledge resulting not seldom in a vast diversity of opinions about the facts of a case. Insecurity about the appropriateness of any actions and concerns among doctors and patients are the consequences. In insurance medicine, there is an additional risk of different decisions about financial aspects, e.g. whether a health problem is covered by the accident insurance or not. Lawsuits may be the consequence. Tacit knowledge should therefore be transferred to explicit knowledge whenever possible.

Encouraging employees to ask a question makes only sense if somebody will answer them. This answer is what we call a "knowledge solution". Knowledge solutions may vary in extent and comprehensiveness: Depending on the subject, they may answer simply a particular question or contain profound scientific treatises (e . g. evidence-based guidelines). Furthermore, a knowledge solution may cover only a certain aspect of a reported knowledge gap or answer more than one reported clinical question resulting in a somehow fuzzy n:m relation between knowledge gaps and knowledge solutions.

2. Managing Corporate Knowledge Gaps

Since its beginnings in the late 1970s at McMaster University (Hamilton, Ontario) evidence-based medicine has emerged worldwide and was adopted by various institutions, among them health regulatory authorities such as the National Health Service (NHS) in the UK. The philosophy of EBM is also part of Suva's knowledge management efforts and namely the InWiM project, and the skill in "transforming knowledge gaps into well-built (clinical) questions" is trained in the framework of continuous medical education.

Management of corporate knowledge gaps within a large institution is not trivial: Employees apprehend knowledge gaps in the course of daily work and often under time pressure. Writing out clinical questions in full is therefore not always their utmost concern. Identified knowledge gaps should be reported to one single place in order to allow their efficient management: Some reports may cover the same or a similar topic and the answer to the clinical questions may be the same. Limited resources may impose the assignment of priorities and to put some questions on hold.

Over time, knowledge gap reports can become numerous in an enterprise with more than 200 users which makes it difficult to keep track of open, fully or partially answered questions, knowledge solutions under way etc. and their mutual dependencies. Facing the need of an appropriate management tool, we started to modela future reporting and management process of knowledge gaps and to define the requirements for a software module called "knowledge gap manager": Knowledge gaps are defined as entities identified and reported by employees with the help of a web based reporting tool. In order to facilitate further processing each reported knowledge gap shall allow for indexing with keywords according to its content. The same applies for knowledge solutions, where indexing with keywords shall be implemented as well.

Given the full implementation of MeSH in the InWiM application, it was self-evident to use MeSH terms for indexing. However, with regard to knowledge gaps not all MeSH terms and features make sense. That's why MeSH terms where restricted to the "Disease Category" tree. This part of the MeSH index covers all diseases and allows mapping of issues to specific health problems.

3. The Knowledge Gap Manager

Writing knowledge solutions follows various workflows. Depending on complexity some questions may be answered by one single person. Others require a collaborative approach, sometimes even an international collaboration. There are however some landmarks in processing of knowledge gaps and solutions: Once a collaborator has localised a knowledge gap by asking a specific question, an editorial board will review it and assign it to an expert. This expert will subsequently take over responsibility. In particular he will be in charge of the appropriate use of MeSH terms and he will perform an initial literature search in order to prepare a recommendation for further processing. Based on the expert recommendation, the editorial board will decide about the next steps. Decisions on how to proceed may depend not only on a specific problem but also on general conditions such as available resources, urgency of other problems etc. Eventually, one or several knowledge solutions will be available and the expert will then link them up with the related knowledge gaps.

The majority of Suva employees speaks German. We therefore implemented the GUI of the release candidate presented here in German only. Translations in French and Italian will follow. Within the InWiM user interface, the hyperlink with the caption "Wissensbedarf" opens the graphical user interface of the Knowledge Gap Manager (see Figure 1).

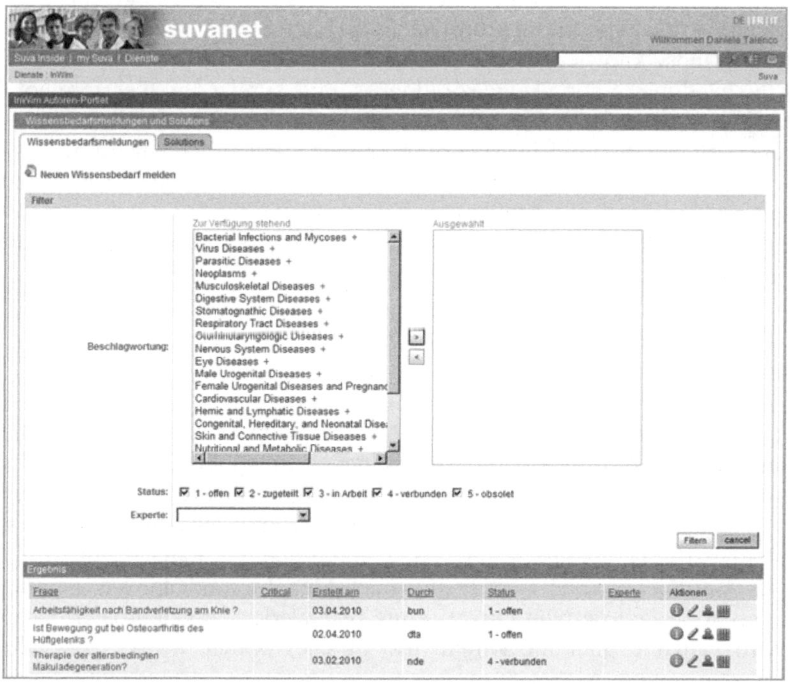

Figure 1. Graphical user interface of the Knowledge Gap Manger with MeSH filter, status filter and expert selector for reported knowledge gaps.

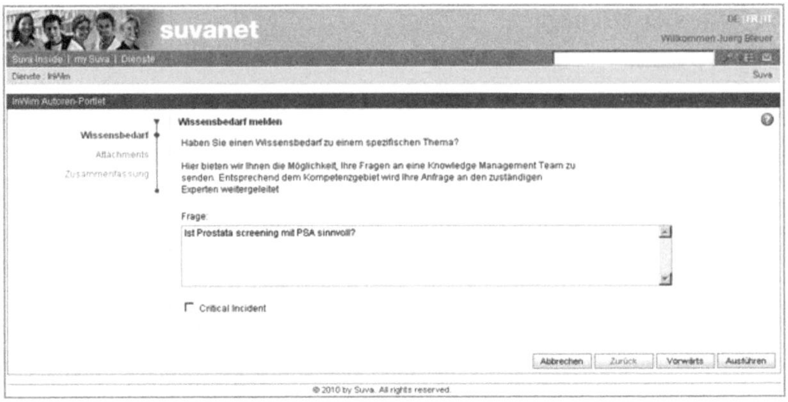

Figure 2. Reporting wizard for knowledge gaps

The left window in the filter section displays the subset of MeSH terms available for indexing. Selecting MeSH terms brings them to display in the right windows. The status selector below the two MeSH windows allows for selection of knowledge gaps which are "open", "assigned to expert", "work in progress", "linked to a knowledge solution" or "obsolete". The lower part of the screen displays knowledge gaps already reported. By clicking on the "Filter" button, the listing of knowledge gaps is restricted to knowledge gaps with the appropriate MeSH terms and statuses. If an expert is selected, only those knowledge gaps will be displayed which are assigned to him. The GUI for the handling of knowledge solutions is quite similar and therefore not depicted here. It can be accessed by means of the tab "Solutions" on top of the screen.

Figure 2 shows the GUI for reporting knowledge gaps. A wizard guides the user through several steps which include formulating the question, attaching additional documents and indexing with MeSH terms: The GUI for the latter is similar to Figure 1 and shows the available MeSH terms in the left and the selected MeSH terms in the right Window.

4. Discussion

Extending knowledge management to knowledge gaps is innovative. As far as the authors are aware, the InWiM knowledge management application is the first one with such functionality and a paragon is therefore missing. Compared to asking questions by email or phone, the solution presented here has several advantages, especially with regard to the MeSH feature. MeSH is a controlled vocabulary with over 25'000 descriptors and it is based on concepts[6]: Each MeSH term denotes a specific concept which refers to a well defined object in the real world. This approach makes MeSH much more valuable than the simple use of cues which always goes along with ambiguity in meaning. MeSH terms are hierarchically structured with superordinate concepts and subordinate concepts thus allowing appropriate representation of real world objects within the scope of healthcare and research. MeSH's primary purpose is information retrieval for medical literature. The extension towards indexing of knowledge gaps allows a "semantic capture" of an issue just at the beginning of its life cycle, just when the corresponding question arises. Indexing a knowledge gap with MesH terms facilitates handling at every further stage of processing: In particular it is possible to search and find knowledge gaps and solutions covering the same or a similar topic, thus allowing adequate collating and it prevents duplication of work. Furthermore, literature searches for the NML (www.pubmed.org) are predefined and do not need every time to be reinvented from scratch.

The question remains open if the restriction to MeSH terms of the “Disease Category” makes sense. Although it simplifies indexing, additional dimensions for indexing might be essential. In case the usability tests will confirm this, further MeSH categories will be added, in particular MeSH terms which refer to medical actions and judgments such as “aetiology”, “diagnosis”, “therapy” and “prognosis”.

Acknowledgments

The authors would like to thank all the members of the project group for their work and valuable input: Klaus Bathke, Erich Bär, Viktor Bydzovsky, Fiorenzo Caranzano, Massimo Ermanni, Bruno Ettlin, Pius Feierabend, Roland Frey, Franziska Gebel, Carlo Gianella, Raphael Good, Ulrike Hoffmann-Richter, Roland Jäger, Sönke Johannes, Bertrand Kiener, Hans Kunz, Jürg Ludwig, Wolfgang Meier, Bettina Rosenthal, Jan Saner, Rita Schaumann-von Stosch, Felix Schlauri, Holger Schmidt, Fred Speck, Klaus Stutz, Benno Tobler, Felix Tschui, Walter Vogt. A special vote of thanks is due to Renato Reinau, Suva Linguistic Services, for his valuable assistance.

References

[1] Schreyögg G, Geiger D. Wenn alles Wissen ist, ist Wissen am Ende Nichts?! Vorschläge zur Neuorientierung des Wissensmanagements. In: Zeuch A, editor. Management von Nichtwissen im Unternehmen. Carl Auer 2007. p. 69–89.

[2] Bleuer JP, Bösch K, Ludwig CA. InWiM: Knowledge Management for Insurance Medicine. Stud Health Technol Inform. 2008;137:141-6.

[3] Tichenor, PJ, Donohue GA, Olien CN. Mass Media Flow and Differential Growth in Knowledge. Public Opinion Quarterly 1970;34:159-70.

[4] Straus SE, Richardson WS, Rosenberg W, Haynes RB, Sackett DL. Evidence-Based Medicine: How to Practice and Teach EBM. 2nd ed. Edinburgh: Churchill Livingstone; 2000.

[5] National Library of Medicine. [Online]. Bethesda, Maryland: Fact Sheet. Medical Subject Headings (MeSH) [updated 2008 Dec 15; cited 2010 Mar 26]. National Library of Medicine; [1 screen]. Available from: URL: http://www.nlm.nih.gov/pubs/factsheets/mesh.html

Medical and Care Compunetics 6
L. Bos et al. (Eds.)
IOS Press, 2010

doi:10.3233/978-1-60750-565-5-128

An Ontology-Based Tool for the Correspondences between Specialist and Consumer Medical Lexicons for the Geriatrics Domain

Stefano BONACINA[a,1] and Francesco PINCIROLI[a]
[a]*Dipartimento di Bioingegneria, Politecnico di Milano, Milan, Italy*

Abstract. New services devoted to improve personalized healthcare are emerging from information technology developments. Personal health record systems allow the patients to participate actively in their healthcare process. However, the dissemination and use of personal health record systems face with some barriers, for example low health literacy that leads to discrepancy in understanding medical concepts. While it is important to present health information using consumer-familiar terms in consumer applications, consistently converting medical terms to consumer-familiar ones is a challenging task. We designed and developed both an ontology-like taxonomic structure devoted to the Geriatrics domain for the outpatient and a software tool, for carrying out the matching between the medical vocabulary of the consumer and that of the doctor from the outpatient's and their family point of view.

Keywords. Terminology and ontology challenges, communication between caregivers and patients, Protégé, databases

Introduction

Recently developed patient- and consumer-centered health record systems allow the patients to participate actively in their healthcare process by collecting and managing their digital health documents and information [1-3].

However, terms used by the medical professionals and consumers are quite different. Therefore, the dissemination and use of personal health record systems face with some barriers [4]. One of them is the consumer's low health literacy [5]. Health literacy has been defined as "the degree to which individuals have the capacity to obtain, process and understand basic health information and services needed to make appropriate health decisions" by the US Institute of Medicine (IOM) [6]. Low health literacy leads to discrepancy in understanding medical concepts and affects therapy adherence [7], even more when patients are elders. Therefore, while it is important to present health information using consumer-familiar terms in consumer applications, consistently converting medical terms to consumer-familiar ones is a challenging task [8]. We designed and developed both an ontology-like taxonomic structure devoted to

[1] Corresponding Author: Stefano Bonacina, Ph.D., Dipartimento di Bioingegneria, Politecnico di Milano, Piazza Leonardo da Vinci 32, 20133 Milan, Italy; E-mail: stefano.bonacina@biomed.polimi.it.

the Geriatrics domain for the outpatient and a software tool, for carrying out the matching between the medical vocabulary of the consumer and that of the doctor from the outpatient's and their family point of view.

1. Methods

1.1. Modeling an Outpatient Perspective

In this paragraph, we explain the perspective of the outpatient. When a citizen shows some symptoms, reasonably he goes to the general practitioner (GP) or to the Specialist doctor, too. To diagnosis, the doctor examines the patient or prescribes examinations, too. When the diagnosis is performed, the doctor assigns therapy. Depending on the diagnosis, the therapy can be surgical, drug-based, and rehabilitative. The pathologies involve some body part, system, or organs.

The Figure 1 represents the Unified Modeling Language (UML) class diagram for describing the static aspects of the health status of a patient at the household. UML is a language for specifying, visualizing, constructing, and documenting the artifacts of software systems, as well as for business modeling and other non-software systems [9]. Class diagrams show static structure of concepts, types, classes and class-class relationships. While in software development, UML classes becomes software components of the system, here we used that representation as a support to develop an ontology-like taxonomic structure, as explained in the paragraph 1.3.

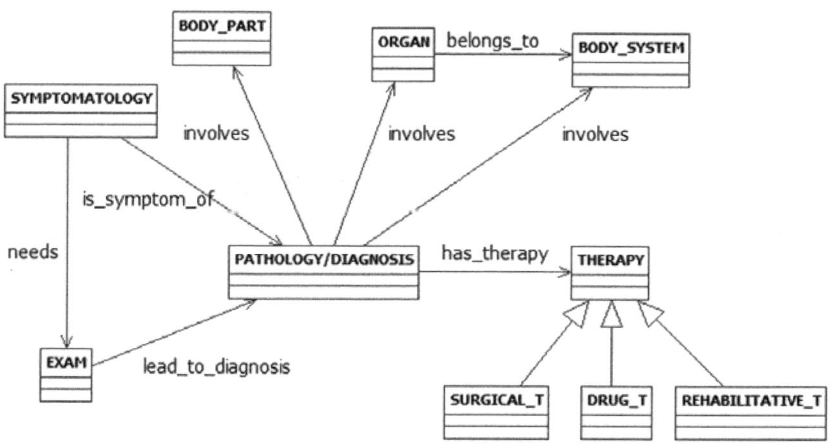

Figure 1. The classes and their relationships. The unlabeled relationships are IS_A.

1.2. Modeling the Approach

In this paragraph, we explained the approach we followed (Figure 2), starting from some considerations about medical dictionaries devoted to consumer. There are many biomedical dictionaries developed by professionals and devoted to professionals (all of which are gathered by the US NLM Unified Medical Language System (UMLS) [10]), whereas the number of the electronic medical dictionaries devoted to consumers is small [11]. One of them is the open access Consumer Health Vocabulary (CHV) [12]. It is an electronic medical dictionary devoted to consumers and whose terms and concepts are mapped to the UMLS Metathesaurus concept terms. However, the CHV is in English language only; therefore, we design a framework to obtain the matching between the medical vocabulary of the consumer and that of the doctor in Italian language, too.

The Figure 2 represents the conceptual approach of our project, considering CHV as an available resource. "Balloon a" is the "Specialist Medical Source/ Textbook in Italian", i.e. a specialist medical source. The Italian specialist medical lexicon in Geriatrics (balloon b), which represent the healthcare professional's lexicon, is connected to the Italian consumer medical lexicon for Geriatrics (balloon c). The Italian consumer medical lexicon has been built first, asking relatives of people acknowledged and authors, terms and concept related to Geriatrics; then, adapting gathered information and definitions from Dorland Medical Dictionary to a lower level and merging the two sets of terms.

The bolded arrow indicates the adaptation of information to a lower level for helping the consumer to comprehend (Figure 2). We named this process "Case Conceptual Correspondence". In addition, the open access CHV (balloon e) helped us to enrich the Italian consumer medical lexicon in Geriatrics, by translating the original terms.

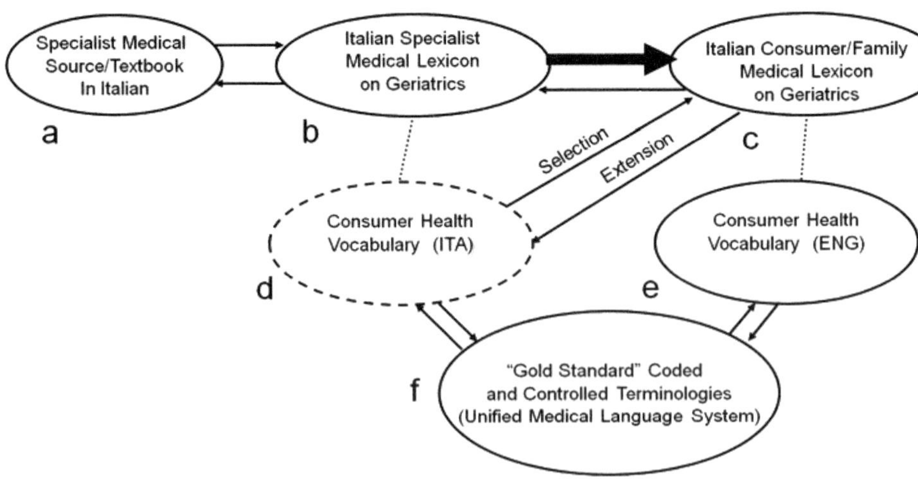

Figure 2. The conceptual approach for building a tool for the correspondences between Specialist and Consumer Medical Lexicons.

At present, an Italian version of the CHV is not available (lined balloon d), however we considered it within the conceptual schema. In fact, while the balloon c represents the consumer/family lexicon for the geriatrics domain - coming from unstructured knowledge too -, the balloon d has to be considered as relating to all the medical specialties, like the CHV in English language [12]. In addition, as the CHV contains information about preferred terms – which are the most used terms to express a concept - the balloon d should contains analogous information. Then, balloon c and balloon d are connected each other (Figure 2). The connection starting from balloon c and ending in balloon d describes an "Extension" action: terms originated from and used within the families are coded, organized, and added to the Italian CHV. The connection starting from balloon d and ending in balloon c describes a "Selection" action: originated from Specialist Lexicon of Geriatrics too, terms become common within the family/consumer environment.

The black arrow in Figure 2 connects balloon b (Italian Specialist Medical Lexicon for Geriatrics) to balloon c (Italian Consumer/ Family Medical Lexicon). From the perspective of involved actors in the Healthcare domain, we identified some language contexts [13-14]. The language contexts (layers) form something like a hierarchy starting with the Specialist Medical Lexicon to the Consumer Medical Lexicon (Figure 3). Each language context (layer) receives "messages" from the layer above, adapt them depending on the layer and pass them down to the next language context [13-14]. In our approach, we considered the adaptation between the most distant layers: the "Case Conceptual Correspondence" (black arrow in Figure 3). The dotted lines indicate that there is not a sharp bound between a layer and the following one.

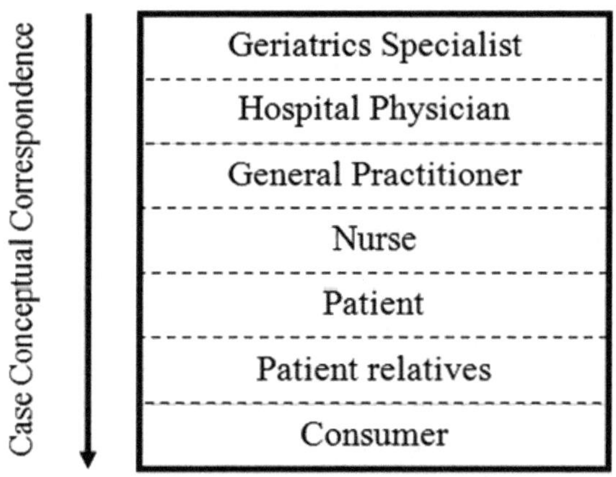

Figure 3. Language contexts for Healthcare domain actors.

1.3. Designing an Ontology-like Taxonomic Structure

Using an Italian edition of the Dorland's Medical dictionary as specialist medical source (balloon a), we developed an ontology-like taxonomic structure for the Geriatrics domain. In the field of computer science: "An ontology defines (specifies) the concepts, relationships, and other distinctions, that are relevant for modeling a certain domain" [15].

The process we adopted to create an ontology for the "Geriatrics" domain of the outpatient can be summarized as it follows:

1. Considering the Italian edition of the Dorland's Medical dictionary and the pair CHV- UMLS, in English language, as specialist medical sources.
2. Apply human term recognition techniques to those sources.
3. Extract geriatrics concepts, terms and their relationships (considering the first level classes and relationships as showed in Figure 1).
4. Assemble those terms into an ontology-like taxonomic structure considering both Italian and English languages. We used the Protégé software tool [16] that is a free, open source ontology editor and knowledge-base framework.

The extracted concepts were grouped in three object categories within Protégé. First category is "Endurant" i.e. continuants, are "entities that endure through time while maintaining their identity and that are fully present at one single point in time" [17]. The second is "Perdurant" i.e. occurrences, which are like processes, are "entities that never fully present at anyone given moment in time, but unfold themselves in successive phases, or temporal parts" [17]. The third category is "Quality", which defines entity's characteristics.

Examples of "Endurant" are "Body Part", "Exam", "Therapy" and "Pathology". Examples of "Perdurant" are diagnostic procedures such as "Encounter" and "Exam execution". The "Medical History", "Risk Factors", and "Gender" are examples of "Quality". Then, the existing relationships between concepts were defined and inserted as concept's properties into two Protégé project files: one in Italian and another in English.

1.4. Designing a Relational Database and a Graphical User Interface

We designed a relational database by Entity – Relationship (E-R) diagrams (conceptual model). The significant entities we defined are:

1. The "Familiar Medical Term" which is described by the attributes "Term Description", "Term Definition" and "Source".
2. The "Specialist Medical Term" which is described by the attributes "Term Description", "Term Definition", "Source" and "Characteristic" – i.e. one of the classes shown in Figure 1.
3. The "CHV Term" which is described by the attributes "Term Description", "UMLS CUI Code" and the Boolean "Preferred" – that is "true" when a term is the preferred one to indicate a concept [8] (CUI stands for Concept Unique Identifier).
4. The "UMLS Term" which is described by the attributes "Term Description", "UMLS CUI Code", "Term Definition" and "Source".

To allow the storage of relationships, one or more, between concept terms, we defined E-R recursive binary relationships for the "Specialist Medical Term" and "Familiar Medical Term" entities. In addition, there are relationships among the entities to allow the construction of correspondences. Then, we transformed the E-R model to Structured Query Language (SQL) and implemented a database using the MS Access®; finally, we populated the database.

In addition, we designed a graphical user interface (GUI) able to make the database inquiry by using buttons instead of SQL scripts.

2. Results

The results are presented in two sub-sections following the order of the Methods section: the first is related to the ontology and the second to the software tool, its interface and examples of correspondences between medical terms.

2.1. The Ontology-like Taxonomic Structure

Figure 4 contains two snapshots from the Protégé editor: the left represents the first level of the developed ontology in English language, the right some details about the "Amnesia" concept. The upper part contains the definition and the CUI code, while the lower part states that Amnesia belongs to Symptomatology class and has some relationships (for example, it is a symptom of Alzheimer's disease). Table 1 shows the elements composing the ontology: concepts, relations, and annotations (i.e. descriptions, see Figure 4).

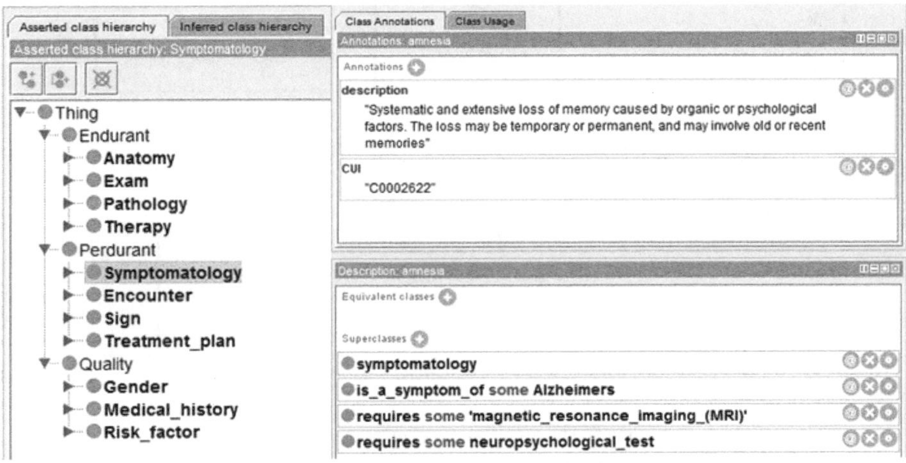

Figure 4. Snapshots from Protégé: left, first level concepts; right, annotations and description about "Amnesia".

Table 1. Elements composing the present version of the ontology.

Headings	Ontology in Italian Language	Ontology in English Language
Number of Concepts	108	106
Number of Relationships	211	209
Number of Annotations	165	168

2.2. The Tool and the Graphical User Interface

We developed a tool - based on a relational database - able to show the defined correspondences between the family medical lexicon (balloon c, Figure 2) and that of the doctor (balloon b). In addition, the UMLS concepts and their definitions (balloon f, Figure 2) are available for browsing. We populated the database with 150 terms, their definitions for each lexicon, and defined the relating correspondences. The graphical user interface of the system was designed and implemented to ease filling research's objects and better comprehension of displayed information (Figure 5).

The text area 'Object to search' is where to insert the query string, e.g. a term, a concept, or a UMLS Concept Unique Identifier (CUI). Clicking on one button launches the query within a specific lexicon, while clicking on one of the arrows shows the correspondences between two lexicons, e.g. from "Specialist Medical Lexicon" to "Consumer Medical Lexicon". This is what we named "Case Conceptual Correspondence".

When a term is inserted as 'Object to search' clicking on the 'Wide search' button returns the complete cycle of correspondences, not only the term matching between two lexicons. In this case, the result-set attributes are those listed in "Headings" column of Table 2. There, the "Record #1" column shows the results for the symptom "Male alle ossa" (bones pain) query string, while the "Record #2" column shows the results for the examination "Oftalmoscopia" (Ophthalmic examination) query string.

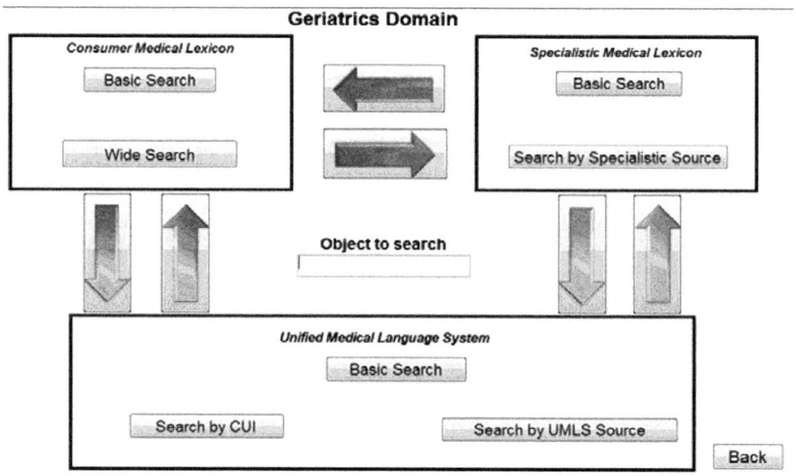

Figure 5. The graphical user interface of the tool.

Table 2. Some results of "Wide Search" inquiry.

Headings	**Record #1**	**Record #2**
Familiar Medical Term (in Italian)	Male alle ossa	Esame del fondo dell'occhio
Familiar Definition and Source (in Italian)	Dolore alle ossa	Esplorazione dell'interno dell'occhio tramite uno strumento chiamato oftalmoscopio
Specialist Medical Term (in Italian)	Dolore osseo	Oftalmoscopia
Specialist Medical Definition (in Italian)	Dolorosa sensazione nelle ossa (Dorland's Medical Dictionary - Italian Edition)	Esame della regione interna dell'occhio mediante un oftalmoscopio (Dorland's Medical Dictionary - Italian Edition)
UMLS Concept Unique Identifier (CUI)	C0151825	C0200149
UMLS Concept Term	Bones pain	Ophthalmic examination and evaluation
UMLS Term Definition	Painful sensation in the bones. (NCI Thesaurus/A7637436)	A test performed by an ophthalmologist or optometrist assessing vision and ability to focus on and discern objects, as well as other tests and examinations pertaining to the eyes. (MeSH/A0094898)

The first query string belongs to the Familiar Medical Lexicon, while the second belongs to the Specialist Medical Lexicon. In addition, the “Search by Specialist source” allows returning all the terms coming from a particular source, while the “Search by UMLS source” allows returning all the terms coming from a particular dictionary within UMLS (Table 2, “UMLS Term definition” row). Further, a “Search by UMLS CUI” is available. This was devoted to the caregiver instead of to the patient.

3. Discussion

Because health literacy is a barrier for the active participation of the patients in their healthcare [18,19], overall, the designed and implemented tool can be considered significant for an essential step towards effective personal health record systems and home care services [20].

Healthcare is a complex environment where the communication occurs between different actors, such as clinicians, doctors, nurses, and patients. The communication deals with complex and interconnected concepts, and is often affected by uncertainty, in the sense that the education degree, domain knowledge, environment, and skills held by the involved actors - senders and receivers- affect the message tailoring [13-14]. In Figure 3, we charted a layer-like schema to represent the different contexts of medical language. As health information needs to be clear and easy to understand [21], we performed the adaptation between the most distant contexts of medical language: the first relates to the hospital environment, while the last relates to the household.

The presented tool can help for bridging the literacy gap between patients and doctors. Depending on the health literacy and computer skills, the developed tool can be used by patients and consumers on their own or during patient-doctor encounters. In the latter cases, the doctor can guide the patients and explain specialized medical terms to them.

The built ontology does not exhaust the specialist Geriatrics domain, and needs to be updated and maintained; however, it was built considering both the medical vocabulary at the family level (i.e. the consumer as main beneficiary) and the first of well-formed ontology principles, that is “endurant”, “perdurant” and “quality” are the subclasses of “thing” class [17]. While adopting automatic knowledge acquisition methods can decrease the costs and time of ontology development [22], a human review of results must be taken into account [23].

The use of CHV allowed us both to include the standard medical language system UMLS, and to facilitate the correspondences between Italian Specialist Medical lexicon and the UMLS concept term identifiers. A next step of our researches will be to work on the development of an Italian Consumer Health Vocabulary (Balloon d, Figure 2). At present, we obtained some results regarding the medical lexicon within the family environment [24].

The implementation carried out by MS Access could lead to a wide diffusion within the household; however, the designed database can be implemented in other database management systems and web user interfaces can be designed and implemented, too.

In our previous work, we considered different approaches for building medical ontologies devoted to family or household environments [25]. As far as the ontology for the geriatrics domain is concerned, some advances have been achieved and are presented as it follows. First, we formalized the static aspects related to the health status of a patient at the household (Figure 1). Second, in the followed approach we involved the contexts of medical language (Figure 3) to take into account factors such as environment, skills and education [13-14, 21]. Third, the ontology built by Protégé software tool contains the number of elements shown in Table 1 now. Fourth, the design, modeling, implementation, and population of a relational database allow enquiring of terms, their relationship, and their definitions. Fifth, we defined a prototype of graphical user interface (GUI) considering the profile - skill and education - of candidate users: there is only a form field where to insert the query string, while there are some buttons to perform specific searches. The buttons were placed and labeled adequately (Figure 5). Finally, the tool based on the relational database and the GUI has been implemented.

A next step of our work will be the development of training materials or user manuals. They will be designed and developed hypothesizing both health literacy levels and computer skills held by different kinds of user. While training and education initiatives on information technologies devoted to healthcare professionals are growing [26-29], consumer's digital knowledge comes from educational paths or from common digital services such as home banking, internet browsing and social network applications, and management of digital pictures.

4. Conclusions

In this project, we considered the family environment that is characterized by verbal communication and not well-bounded knowledge domain in medical area. The medical language used by laypeople is very changeable and is affected by some factors: environment, skills, education. Attempting to represent such a language and matching professional medical language with it is a challenging task.

We designed and developed both an ontology devoted to Geriatrics for the Outpatient (in Italian and in English languages) and a tool, based on a relational database, for carrying out the matching between the medical vocabulary of the consumer and that of the doctor. This patient education tool can help in bridging the literacy gap during patient-doctor interactions or communications.

As new systems and services devoted to health information technologies are emerging, tools similar to the one here presented can be deployed on personal handle devices with little effort.

Acknowledgments

The authors would like to acknowledge the Biomedical Engineering students and Mathematical Engineering students of the 'E-Health Methods and Applications' course who contributed to develop the project.

References

[1] Mandl KD, Simons WW, Crawford WC, Abbett JM. Indivo: a personally controlled health record for health information exchange and communication. BMC Med Inform Decis Mak 2007;7:25.

[2] Kupchunas WR. Personal health record: new opportunity for patient education. Orthopedic nursing / National Association of Orthopedic Nurses 2007;26(3):185-91.
[3] Halamka JD, Mandl KD, Tang PC. Early experiences with personal health records. J Am Med Inform Assoc 2008;15(1):1-7.
[4] Lober WB, Zierler B, Herbaugh A, Shinstrom SE, Stolyar A, Kim EH, Kim Y. Barriers to the use of a personal health record by an elderly population. In: Proc AMIA Symp; 2006. Washington (DC); 2006. p. 514-8.
[5] Kim EH, Stolyar A, Lober WB, Herbaugh AL, Shinstrom SE, Zierler BK, Soh CB, Kim Y. Challenges to using an electronic personal health record by a low-income elderly population. J Med Internet Res 2009;11(4):e44.
[6] Institute of medicine. Health Literacy: a prescription to end confusion. Washington (DC): National Academies Press; 2004.
[7] Kripalani S, Robertson R, Love-Ghaffari MH, Henderson LE, Praska J, Strawder A, Katz MG, Jacobson TA. Development of an illustrated medication schedule as a low-literacy patient education tool. Patient Educ Couns 2007;66(3):368-77.
[8] Zeng QT, Tse T, Divita G, Keselman A, Crowell J, Browne AC, Goryachev S, Ngo L. Term identification methods for consumer health vocabulary development. J Med Internet Res 2007;9(1):e4.
[9] Object Management Group. The Unified Modeling Language™ Specifications. UML web site. [Online]. Available from: URL: http://www.uml.org/. 1997.
[10] Bodenreider O. The Unified Medical Language System (UMLS): integrating biomedical terminology. Nucleic Acids Res 2004;32(Database issue):D267-70.
[11] Zielstorff RD. Controlled vocabularies for consumer health. J Biomed Inform 2003;36(4-5):326-33.
[12] The Consumer Health vocabulary initiative. [Online]. Available from: URL: http://www.consumerhealthvocab.org/
[13] Gould M. Anyone here a doctor who speaks nurse? Health Serv J 2008;Jun:22-4.
[14] Carthey J. Involving and communicating with patients and the public. Nurs Stand 2006;20(17):50-3.
[15] Gruber TR. A translation approach to portable ontology specifications. Knowledge Acquisition (Special issue: Current issues in knowledge modelling) 1993;5(2):199-220.
[16] Protégé Ontology Editor. [Online]. Available from: URL: http://protege.stanford.edu/.
[17] Schulz S, Hahn U. Towards the ontological foundations of symbolic biological theories. Artif Intell Med 2007;39(3):237-50.
[18] Kim SP, Knight SJ, Tomori C, Colella KM, Schoor RA, Shih L, Kuzel TM, Nadler RB, Bennett CL. Health literacy and shared decision making for prostate cancer patients with low socioeconomic status. Cancer Invest 2001;19(7):684-91.
[19] Cutilli CC. Health literacy in geriatric patients: An integrative review of the literature. Orthop Nurs 2007;26(1):43-8.
[20] Eysenbach G. Medicine 2.0: social networking, collaboration, participation, apomediation, and openness. J Med Internet Res 2008;10(3):e22.
[21] Shaw A, Ibrahim S, Reid F, Ussher M, Rowlands G. Patients' perspectives of the doctor-patient relationship and information giving across a range of literacy levels. Patient Educ Couns 2009;75(1):114-20.
[22] Shamsfard M, Barforoush AA. Learning ontologies from natural language texts. Int J Hum Comput Stud 2004;60:17-63.
[23] Brewster C, Jupp S, Luciano J, Shotton D, Stevens RD, Zhang Z. Issues in learning an ontology from text. BMC Bioinformatics 2009;10(Suppl 5):S1.
[24] Bonacina S, Pinciroli F. Experiments of characterizations of the family medical lexicon for tele-homecare applications, In: M.H. Hamza, editor. Proceedings of the Second IASTED International Symposium on TELEHEALTH and ASSISTIVE TECHNOLOGY (TAT 2009); 2009 Nov 2-4; Cambridge (MA): ISBN 978-0-88986-815-1. Calgary (Canada): ACTA Press; 2009. p. 103-10.
[25] Bonacina S, Pinciroli F. Architectural Pros and Cons for Building Family Medical Ontology, In: M.H. Hamza, editor. Proceedings of the Second IASTED International Symposium on TELEHEALTH and ASSISTIVE TECHNOLOGY (TAT 2009); 2009 Nov 2-4; Cambridge (MA): ISBN 978-0-88986-815-1. Calgary (Canada): ACTA Press; 2009. p. 21-30.
[26] Alpay L, Russell A. Information technology training in primary care: the nurses' voice. Comput Inform Nurs 2002;20(4):136-42.
[27] Stepánková O, Engová D. Professional competence and computer literacy in e-age, focus on healthcare, Methods Inf Med 2006;45(3):300-4.
[28] Ward R, Stevens C, Brentnall P, Briddon J. The attitudes of health care staff to information technology: a comprehensive review of the research literature. Health Info Libr J 2008;25(2):81-97.
[29] Smedley A, The importance of informatics competencies in nursing: an Australian perspective. Comput Inform Nurs 2005;23(2):106-110.

Medical and Care Compunetics 6
L. Bos et al. (Eds.)
IOS Press, 2010

doi:10.3233/978-1-60750-565-5-138

Exploring the Link between Populomics and Knowledge Management: Patient-Oriented Case Exemplars

Rajeev K. BALI[a1] , M Chris GIBBONS[b]
[a] *Knowledge Management for Healthcare (KARMAH) research subgroup, Biomedical Computing and Engineering Technologies Applied Research Group (BIOCORE), Coventry University, UK*
[b] *Johns Hopkins Urban Health Institute, Baltimore, USA*

Abstract. The challenge of population-level health problems, such as healthcare disparities, encompasses socio-behavioural, community and biologic factors and advances in information and communication technologies (ICTs). These elements are reflected in the key ethos of contemporary knowledge management (KM), as knowledge emerges from the confluence of people, process and technology. This paper illustrates how knowledge-based health case studies can be used as effective exemplars to illuminate understanding and explore possible connections between populomics and KM.

Keywords. Populomics, knowledge, KM, ICT

Introduction

Knowledge Management (KM) embodies organizational processes that seek a synergistic combination of data and information processing capacity of information technologies, and the creative and innovative capacity of human beings. Populomics is a confluence of three seemingly disparate concepts (population science, medicine and informatics). This fusion has a direct parallel with the growing field of KM which, like Populomics, combines the essential components of people, process and technology. KM principles and methodologies provide researchers and practitioners with valuable analytic tools and a systematic approach to the integration of different types of data to enable novel knowledge-based insights and spur scientific advances in healthcare. This paper presents three patient-focussed healthcare case studies and discusses how KM and Populomics can be used in combination to produce better health outcomes.

1. Populomics

The term Populomics has emerged from the synthesis of the Population sciences, Medicine and Informatics [1,2]. Populomics is defined as an emerging discipline

[1] Corresponding Author. r.bali@coventry.ac.uk

focused on population level, transdisciplinary, integrative disease/risk characterization, interdiction and mitigation that rely heavily on innovations in computer and information technologies. Populomics seeks to characterize the interplay of socio behavioral pathways and biophysiologic and molecular mechanisms which work across levels of existence, to impact health particularly, at the population level.

2. The Efficacy of Knowledge Management for healthcare

KM solutions for healthcare and clinical environments actively incorporate primary and/or secondary care deliverers as facilitators who are in direct contact with target patients and populations. Changes in ICT products have developed with the evolution of the KM concept in organisational decision-making over the last forty years.

Contemporary organisations (including those operating in a healthcare environment) are facing a deluge of data and information whilst simultaneously lacking knowledge [3,4]. New ways of working and collaboration, and the prevalence of ICTs, have resulted in organisations being inundated with information to an unprecedented degree resulting in "information overload" [5-8]. This has major implications for clinical decision makers as they have to deal with increasingly large amounts of data. One of the major challenges that face managers is how to make effective decisions based on the data at hand. It is acknowledged that the selection of a particular direction is both constrained and influenced by the availability of data, the ability to transform data into information and then to make recognition of it by deriving knowledge from information.

Knowledge Management is a steadily maturing, yet often misunderstood management approach that is aimed at solving contemporary organisational challenges to increase efficiency and efficacy of core organisational processes while simultaneously incorporating continuous innovations. KM, via the use of various tools, processes and techniques, combines relevant organisational data, information and knowledge to create business value and enable an organisation to capitalise on its intangible and human assets so that it can effectively achieve its primary business goals, as well as maximise its core business competencies [9,10]. Adoption of KM has been spoken of as a solution to the massive problem of information overload. It is our contention that transferring knowledge to the primary care deliverers requires seamless integration within routine clinical process. The seamless transfer should address the issue of communicating knowledge to these healthcare professionals while avoiding the problem of information "inundation". This would pave the way in refining and making well informed evidence-based clinical decisions.

3. Case exemplar #1: Breast Screening

Breast cancer is the most common cancer in women with over forty thousand women being diagnosed with the disease each year in the UK [11]. Any information related to the breast can largely affect a women's consciousness and a threat of breast cancer will have varying impacts on women psychology. Typically breast cancerous cells originate in the mammary glands (lobules) or in the ducts connected to these glands or in other tissues around these glands [12]. When in close proximity to the lymphatic system, these cells can result in being carried to other organs of the body. This subsequently results in cancerous growth in that organ and is described as metastatic breast cancer [12]. Although many causes had been identified for breast cancer, the knowledge of finding a cure is still not within the reach of modern medicine.

Breast cancer should ideally be diagnosed at the earlier stages of its development. Possible treatments include removing or destroying the cancer cells to avoid the spread of the affected cells. Breast Self-Examination (BSE) is an effective and non-intrusive type of self diagnosis exercise for checking any abnormalities/lumps in the breast tissue. Unfortunately this greatly depends on the size of the lump, technique and experience in carrying out a self-examination by the woman. An ultrasound test using sound waves can be used to detect lumps but this is usually suited for women aged below thirty-five owing to the higher density of breast tissue [12]. Having a tissue biopsy via a fine needle aspiration or an excision is often used to test the cells for cancer. These tests are mostly employed in treatments or post-treatment examination and as second rung diagnostic confirmation methods. Performing a Computed Tomography (CT) or a Magnetic Resonance Imaging (MRI) scan would result in a thorough examination of the breast tissue but this technique is not favoured due to reasons including that it may not be economical, needs preparation, noisy, time consuming and images may not be clear.

Breast Screening Programme

Mammography is a technique for detecting breast tissue lumps using a low dosage of X-ray. This technique can even detect a three millimeter sized lump. The X-ray image of the breast tissue is captured and the image is thoroughly read by experienced radiologists and specialist mammogram readers. Preliminary research suggests that women aged fifty five and above are more susceptible to breast cancer; mammography is more suited to the women aged fifty five and above (due to the lower density of breast tissue) [13]. Even though mammography has its critics - mainly due to its high rate of false positives and false negatives [14] - it has still become the standard procedure for screening women by the National Health Service (NHS) National Breast Screening Programme UK [15]. Mammography is the best and most viable tool for mass screening to detect cancer in the breast at an early stage [16]; however, the effectiveness of diagnosis through screening is directly dependent on the percentage of women attending the screening programme. The NHS Breast Screening Programme, catering to the entire eligible women population is funded by the Department of Health in the UK and is the first of its kind in the world. It covers nearly four million women and detected more than thirteen thousand cancers in the screened population for the year 2005 [17]. Currently the screening programme routinely screens women between the ages of fifty and seventy, and employs two views of the breast, medio-lateral and cranio-caudal. The lack of breakthroughs in finding a definitive cure means that preventive medicine is the only viable alternative to reduce deaths due to breast cancer.

The UK National Health Service (NHS) National Breast Screening Programme (NBSP) is unique as it provides free breast screening for the female population aged between 50 and 70 at a national level [15,18]. The recent increase of the upper age limit from 63 to 70 for screening and making a two-view mammogram mandatory has greatly increased the efficiency of benign or malignant tumor detection. The NBSP currently runs a massive screening programme catering to almost two million eligible women across the UK [18]. This programme runs on a call/recall cycle which screens all eligible women in a three year interval. The information published by the UK Government Statistical Service (NHS Health and Social Care Information Centre) in its Community Health Statistics report for the year 2006 agrees that, for the past ten years since 1995, the uptake has remained constant at around 75%. The number of non-attendees has been significantly increasing and has reached half a million. Simple projection of this data submits that nearly 4,000 cancer incidences would not have been diagnosed. Even if a small percentage of these non-attendees could be made to attend, it would result in the saving of significant lives. Indirectly we can also infer that, despite focussed efforts on these non-attendees for the past ten years, there was no real effect on their attendance. Moreover, early stage cancer detection would have a huge impact in reducing cancer related deaths. From these facts and data, we see that the primary concern is to reduce non-attendance [19].

These challenges can be addressed by a resource saving strategy which has better healthcare at its core. The first component in the proposed strategy is related to knowledge via Artificial Intelligence (AI), employing Neural Network (NN) algorithms. This strategy also includes a Service Oriented Architecture (SOA) to deliver the envisaged knowledge as the second component. This research proposes to unify the existing National Breast Screening Computer System (NBSS) software onto a single platform and create prototype software component based on Open Source technologies. The proposed prototype software would be automated to produce the pre-processed data and eventually normalise the data for AI (neural network) assimilation. These activities would be performed sequentially without human involvement for repeatability, reliability and accuracy. The Java Based Attendance prediction by Artificial Intelligence for Breast Screening (JAABS) model itself would be simulated on the Open Source technology platform. This model incorporates all additional transformations occurring within the screening process (including the change in the screening upper age limit). The prototype framework proposed will incorporate the AI model for creating a list of predicted non-attending women. The prototype combines the demographic data pertaining to the non-attending women and information related to her General Physician (GP) as a messaging package. This package triggers the generation of an electronic message based on the Health Level 7 (HL7) version 3 standards and utilises Service Oriented Architecture (SOA) as the message delivering technology.

The objective of this work was to identify the challenges which are being faced by the UK NHS' national breast screening programme and find approaches to alleviate these impediments and eventually reduce mortality due to breast cancer. Based on JAABS algorithm's negative prediction value (for the first to sixth episode) the number of non-attendees correctly predicted *a priori* to screening date would be at least 42 women for every 100 screening non-attendees. When such knowledge is shared with the GPs (with whom the women are registered) can initiate interventions. Such interventions can educate the non-attending women and clarify their attitudes and beliefs. The expected outcome is that the women commits to a positive informed decision, which would culminate in attending the screening appointment. This work not only confirms that breast screening attendance can be predicted through an automated software solution, but also can be leveraged to increase screening attendance by employing emerging KM tools and techniques. This research work draws its strength from such KM tools and techniques. This work is also one such initiative addressing the NHS' breast screening attendance through efficient KM methodologies. A 25% success in GP interventions will result in saving more than 350 women's lives per year. Even if one women's life can be saved by our approach, this approach can be deemed as a success. The new bespoke software prototype, incorporating JAABS algorithm can be easily converted and integrated in to the NBSS software.

4. Case exemplar #2: Maternity Services

At its conception in 1948, the UK's National Health Service (NHS) held three core principles: (a) to meet the health care needs of everyone, (b) free at the point of delivery and (c) based on clinical need, and not the ability to pay. The aim was to create an uniform service combining all hospitals under one central system with the ideal that healthcare should be available to all regardless of wealth status. Sixty years on, the NHS is relatively uniform but with significant inequalities in service and quality of care with access to treatment. This case will examine some of the various KM issues induced by the introduction of ICTs into the NHS with a particular focus on Maternity Services.

Maternity Services were not particularly affected by various changes in policy and NHS maternity care is given without charge at the point of delivery. However, in comparison to other European countries, the UK Government has contributed approximately 1-1.5 per cent less to healthcare on an annual basis. This has been a contributory factor in the inadequacies of healthcare provided by the NHS today [20]. The NHS organization consists of multiple layers of health service providers each responsible for the procurement of their own IT systems. This has led to a vast amount of systems that have not been introduced in a coherent approach, therefore integration and sharing of information between providers and across the services has not been efficient or effective. In order to increase efficiency, effectiveness, equity and reduce risk, particularly at the point of care, The National Programme for Information and Technology (NPfIT) was introduced in 2002. Connecting for Health (CfH) is the Government agency responsible for the implementation of NPfIT. It is the largest civil technology program undertaken and is intended to unite separate NHS organizations. This is a centrally driven mandate.

The aim is to electronically connect all 50 million plus patient records, allowing access by patients and health professionals in over 30,000 General Practitioners (GP) Practices and 300 hospitals. It was envisaged that during an incremental period of ten years, NPfIT will bring modern computer systems into the NHS changing the way the NHS works to improve patient care and services. However, the formation of a single demographic database gives rise to many concerns. In particular, how this information will be used, by whom and how patient confidentiality and security will be maintained are common themes amongst those resistant to a national database. Many patients and clinicians are concerned that the system is not secure [21]. A number of clinicians are skeptical of the need for integrated records via a national database, as systems already exist for locality data sharing between relevant GP's and hospitals 'without the need to leave a copy of the information on the nationally accessible database' [22]. In order to satisfy patient concerns and control access, the consequence of illegal misuse of data from the databases may require greater legal penalties than the current financial ones.

4.1. Proposed changes within Maternity Services

Current NHS reforms aim ‘to develop a patient led NHS that uses available resources as effectively and fairly as possible to promote health, reduce health inequalities and deliver the best and safest healthcare’ [23]. Maternity organizations must therefore supply accessible, efficient, quality care. Services should provide care that is women focused considering individual needs of health status, culture, religion, social needs and disabilities. High quality, efficient Maternity Services are essential in contributing the attainment of the Department of Health’s Public Service Agreement (PSA) targets [24]. In relation to Maternity Services, the PSA targets include: (a) reduction by 10% of health inequalities, measurable by infant mortality and life expectancy at birth, (b) a substantial reduction of mortality rates, (c) reduce by 1% per annum women who smoke in pregnancy, (d) reducing the under 18 year old conception rate and (e) increase breastfeeding rates by 2% per annum.

In addition, the Department of Health produced the *Maternity Standard, National Service Framework (NSF) for Children Young People and Maternity Services* (2004) identified as best practice guidance. The NSF is based on a care pathway approach which place value on women-focused care rather than meeting the needs of the service. In doing so, an emphasis is placed on evidenced-based procedures and guidelines representing a method for continuous quality improvement. Maternity care pathways will provide a system through which services will be integrated between primary, secondary and social services to provide comparable high quality effective clinical care.

The large scale and constituents of the work force will have a major impact of change within the NHS. In comparison to other countries the UK has a lower number of health care professional per population [20]. Recruitment and retention of staff in some services, particularly midwifery, create significant difficulties and can seriously effect patient care. The NHS Plan proposes new ways of working to reduce professional barriers resulting in a more flexible workforce between staff groups. In addition, it aims to increase the amount of skilled workforce. Nurse Practitioners/Midwives could assume 20 per cent of doctor’s work, whilst Health Care Assistants (HCAs) could perform duties of the Nurse/Midwife workload. This skill mix change would increase the workforce capacity. However significant investment in IT would reduce administration time allowing increased time providing patient care.

4.2. Patient Expectations

Patients today are better informed with access to better information regarding treatment, management and prevention of illness and diseases. Patients have rights to informed consent but also demand informed choice of type and place of their care. Healthcare does not meet patient expectations particularly regarding access of care and waiting times for treatment. In addition, the health service is not yet sufficiently patient-centered; the Wanless Report included survey evidence showing that patients commonly feel that they have insufficient involvement in decisions, there is not one to talk to about anxieties and concerns, tests ant treatment are not clearly explained with insufficient written information provided. A survey by the Department of Health (2005) observed that women using NHS Maternity Services would have preferred more choice in type of care and place of delivery.

In addition, there is a commitment from the Department of Health to improve paticnt information, in particular, the areas of consent. Moreover, the NHS Litigation Authority risk management standard, Healthcare Commission Standards, and the Department of Health Toolkit for producing patient information, provide national standards that Trusts must adhere to. Certain geographical locations have experienced an increase in European migrants which has had an impact on Maternity Services, particularly with language difficulties. For local Trusts there are cost implications involving translators and written forms of communications that are not met centrally. With widening access to current maternity health care information, for example via the Internet, the general public are more assertive and better informed to demand change within Maternity Services.

5. Case exemplar #3: Lifetime Health Record

In trying to propel Malaysia into a "developed nation" status, the Government of Malaysia has formulated vision and mission statements such as the Malaysian Vision 2020 as well as the Malaysian Healthcare Vision. In trying to actualize both these visions into reality, the government and the Ministry of Health of Malaysia (MOHM) have started preparing itself through the *Integrated Telehealth Initiative* where the Lifetime Health Record (LHR) is used as the basis for continuous care. The LHR correlates each episode of care for an individual into a continuous health record. It is the summarized health record of every individual compiled from their electronic medical records. These records refer to a patient's electronic medical records that are cumulatively derived from the clinical support system (such as clinical information system, laboratory information system, pharmacy information system and patient management system) and it can be collected and gathered from the various spectrums of health information systems and healthcare levels.

5.1. Current healthcare delivery system

The Malaysian public healthcare system is structured in a hierarchical pyramid-based concept. At the base of the pyramid is a broad array of primary healthcare services (such as health centers, polyclinics, mobile clinics and maternal and child clinics) spread throughout the country. The next level consists of district hospitals in every one of 120 districts, feeding into state general hospitals in each state capital. At the top of the pyramid lies the Hospital Kuala Lumpur which is the national tertiary reference centre which provides specialist and super specialist services for the nation [26,27]. In term of the physical healthcare facility setup, the healthcare premises are normally developed within the area where the most population is living [28]. Since 1998, 95% of the population were living within a 5-kilometre radius of the nearest healthcare facility. This setup enables patients from anywhere in the country to be referred to the appropriate hospital, to access and visit several healthcare facilities through a nationwide network of clinics, hospitals and other health programs in a convenient manner.

5.2. Background of Outpatient Clinics

The outpatient clinics department administratively reports to the Family Health Division of Public Health Services of MOHM. Healthcare services are provided through various health centers and community polyclinics strategically located in the most populated areas in the district. The health centers and community polyclinics comprise the first level of service made available to the community. The services provided are comprehensive at this level, essentially comprising maternal health, child health, acute care of diseases, chronic care of diseases, mental health, geriatric care, community-based rehabilitation, well person services and health promotion. These services are provided as outpatient treatments. In order to support such services, there are laboratory services and also radiological services. The pharmaceutical services are also provided in-house. With these comprehensive services and workflows, it was a significant reason that the outpatient clinic department was selected as a case study organization for advancing knowledge on the case under study. The selected organization will cover most of the processes of consultation and medical diagnosis workflow in outpatient clinic. The healthcare setting provides relevant evidences and extensive information about patient demographic and clinical data that would contribute in developing the LHR components and structure.

5.3. The proposed LHR data sets

Based on inputs and evidences obtained from the case study, the LHR was divided into three components: (1) Patient Master Information, (2) Health Condition Summary and (3) Episode Summary.

5.3.1. Patient Master Information (PMI)

Patient Master Information comprises of administrative records and the required information to identify and distinguish the patient across healthcare facilities and levels. It often used to locate patient identifier, including patient demographic and the related health administration information. The patient master information comprises the following set of information including demographic record, next of kin record, birth record, family health record, medical insurance record, employment record and organ donor record. It was noted from the findings of the primary data collection, the analysis of patient demographic information to be viewed by doctors during consultation) that the patient demographic information is highly required during consultation and medical diagnosis workflow. The demographic information is indicated as compulsory due to the fact that the demographic information is a key identifier for the patient. The administrative records (examples are next of kin record, birth record, family health record, medical insurance record, employment record and organ donor record) could be included in the patient information as optional records.

5.3.2. Health Condition Summary

The Health Condition Summary comprises of records, which summarize the illness and wellness condition of the patient. Each condition has a status indicator to indicate whether the condition is active or inactive. This summary of a patient's condition will enhance the continuity of care by providing a method for communicating the most relevant information about a patient and providing support for the generation of LHRs

[29,30]. It was noted from the primary data collection that the first step of patient care or treatment was that the doctor will gather information about the patient's current health status. Here, many types of information were collected about the patient and placed in the patient's health record. By giving the latest health condition summary of the patient at the beginning of a first doctor-patient encounter, the accuracy, quality, safety and continuity of care would be given. The health condition summary component could be added and enhanced in future and the set of information given below are the initial information revealed from the primary data collection and system analysis. The health condition summary comprises such information as chronic disease record, allergy record, immunization/vaccination record, social history record, surgical medical procedure record, disability record and obstetric record.

5.3.3. Episode Summary

The Episode Summary is comprised of data for a particular episode or visit. If required, it provides the necessary data for reference to the source of the information where details of the episodes are stored. It comprises the following information; episode record, encounter record, symptoms record, diagnosis record, lab test record, radiology record, medication record, vital sign record and health plan record. The LHR components defined above provide the conceptual structure of LHR information and it is envisaged that the many LHRs could be collected and generated continuously from telehealth applications and various health information systems. The integrated telehealth system, via its role as the premier database repository for patient's LHR in the country, will function as the health knowledge platform from which a variety of research and development activities within the healthcare domain can be launched. These research and development initiatives will spearhead the development and establishment of initiatives which will produce innovative healthcare products and services of national and international significance.

5.3.4. Knowledge Management

The KM implications and practice in this case are varied. The integrated telehealth system, by way of its role as the premier database repository for patient's LHR in the country, will function as the health knowledge platform from which a variety of research and development activities within the healthcare domain can be launched [31]. These initiatives will spearhead the development and establishment of initiatives which will produce innovative healthcare products and services of national and international significance. In terms of health group data services, the LHR's standardized data sets would ensure effective mining (data, information and knowledge). The LHR repository would be a premier health database repository in the country and would become an important source for health knowledge data mining purposes [32]. rough judicious use of standardized KM applications, personalized health plans could be formulated [33].

6. Moving towards a link between KM and Populomics

The healthcare domain not only provides challenging opportunities for managing knowledge but also is one of the areas where it is often most poorly understood and deployed. This predicament is slowly being addressed as more and more KM-focussed projects are initiated and healthcare professionals (and other stakeholders) with better understanding of KM are being involved. The three provided case studies have a strong orientation towards established KM tools and technologies and the emerging discipline of Populomics.

More family and community residents are becoming "caregivers" and "care providers". This shift is enhancing the impact of social, behavioral, community and economic realities on their therapeutic regimens and provider relationships. In short, the social and behavioral sciences, which traditionally had not been considered within the domain of healthcare, are increasingly recognized as fundamentally linked to illness, health and healthcare outcomes [25] while the need for an integrated approach to health research and healthcare is gaining appreciation, thinking across disciplinary lines can be challenging.

The growing realization of healthcare disparities is forcing clinical researchers to think about disease causation not only among individual patients, but also across entire groups or populations of people. Among patients who have vastly differing cultural beliefs and practices, diets, educational or literacy levels and socioeconomic resources, clinical practitioners and researchers developing interventions that ignore these sociocultural realities may struggle to demonstrate or maintain therapeutic efficacy across increasingly multicultural populations of patients. Focussing on electronic health care records, a growing number of patients want both access and control of their own information, large employers are exploring new methods to improve employee (and beneficiary) health while reducing healthcare costs and leading technology companies are anxious to offer an effective technology solution.

Increasingly, scientific evidence suggests that disease causation results from complex interactions of social, environmental, behavioral and biologic factors which simultaneously and often cooperatively act across more than one level of existence over time [34]. Thus a comprehensive understanding of health and disease requires the integration of knowledge derived from the bench, sociobehavioral and population sciences. Most historic and contemporary conceptual models of health though, have often been derived either from the socio-behavioral sciences *or* the biomolecular sciences. With the exception of those pathways based on stress (neuro-immunological) mechanisms, the published frameworks in the behavioral sciences and epidemiological literature largely lack clearly stated, causal biologic connections to observed health outcomes [35-39]. On the other hand, most biologically oriented formulations poorly account for socio-environmental and behavioral effect modifiers that may profoundly influence the pathogenesis of disease and the development of health disparities [40-43].

Populomics represents a new comprehensive way of studying health problems and crafting health solutions. It is being advocated by some officials at the National Institutes of Health as a new science that should be supported as the population level equivalent of genomics, which may lead to quantum leaps forward in understanding health challenges and developing new effective therapies and treatments [44]. The three case studies illustrate how KM and knowledge-based initiatives such as Populomics can be used to create powerful health outcomes.

7. Conclusion

Our current work includes additional research continuing to investigate linkages between Populomics and the field of KM (for all three case studies). For all of the given case studies, the knowledge created is useful for contemporary clinical and healthcare management. The outcomes leverage the knowledge created in order to share it with the healthcare deliverers to alleviate the particular predicaments faced, be they increasing uptake of breast screening, fostering better access to maternity services or compliance with national telemedicine initiatives. Such research has direct synergies with the central component of Populomics, one of the key aims of which is to reduce disparities and inequalities. Although the role and importance of KM for the three provided case scenarios is central to their success, their focus on large patient communities empowers Populomics to add its inherent value to the case studies. Socio-behavioural factors and community-wide risk profiles can be integrated into the existing knowledge-based initiatives as, in combination, Populomics and KM can come together to produce a powerful focus for current and future, patient-focused, practice. We encourage researchers in similar fields to include Populomics into relevant KM-based studies.

Acknowledgements

The authors would like to thank the following for the use of their case studies: Dr Vikram Baskaran (*Breast Screening*), Kim Davis (*Maternity Services*) and MAK Ghani (*Malaysian Telemedicine*). These cases appear courtesy of the Knowledge Management for Healthcare (KARMAH) research subgroup, BIOCORE, Coventry University, UK (www.coventry.ac.uk/karmah).

References

[1] Abrams DB. Applying transdisciplinary research strategies to understanding and eliminating health disparities. Health Educ Behav 2006;33(4):515-31.
[2] Gibbons MC. eHealth Solutions for Health Care Disparities. New York: Springer; 2008.
[3] Liebowitz J, Beckman T. Knowledge Organizations: What every manager should know. USA: St. Lucie Press; 1998.
[4] Sieloff C. If only HP knew what HP knows: The roots of knowledge management at Hewlett-Packard. Journal of Knowledge Management 1999;3(1):47-53.
[5] Yabroff KR and Mandelblatt JS. Interventions Targeted toward Patients to Increase Mammography Use. Cancer Epidemiol Biomarkers Prev 1999;8: 749-57.
[6] Bell TS, Branston LK, Newcombe RG, Barton GR. Interventions to Improve Uptake of Breast Screening in Inner City Cardiff General Practices with Ethnic Minority Lists. Ethn Health 1999;4(4):277-84.
[7] Cothrel J, Williams R. On-line communities: helping them form and grow, Journal of Knowledge Management 1999;3(1):54-60.
[8] Drucker P. The coming of the new organization. Harvard Business Review on Knowledge Managemen. USA: Harvard Business School Press; 1998.
[9] Swan J, Scarbrough H, Preston J. Knowledge Management – The Next Fad To Forget People? Proceedings of the 7th European Conference in Information Systems. 1999.
[10] Davenport T, Prusak L. Working Knowledge, Boston: Harvard Business School Press; 1998.
[11] Cancer Research UK. CancerStats Incidence-UK. [Online]. 2005; Available from: URL: http://www.cancerresearchuk.org/aboutcancer/statistics/statsmisc/pdfs/cancerstats_incidence_apr05.pdf (last accessed 10 August 2005).
[12] American Cancer Society Inc. Cancer Reference Information. [Online]. 2005. Available from: URL: www.cancer.org/docroot/CRI/content/CRI_2_4_1X_What_is_ breast _cancer_5.asp> (last accessed 10 August 2005).
[13] Blanks RG, Moss SM, McGahan CE, Quinn MJ, et al, Effect of NHS breast screening programme on mortality from breast cancer in England and Wales, 1990-8: comparison of observed with predicted mortality. BMJ 2000;321(7262):665–9.

[14] Burton G. Alternative Medicine. Washington: Future Medicine Publishing; 1997.
[15] Forrest P. Breast Cancer Screening - A report to the Health Ministers of England, Scotland, Wales and Northern Ireland. London: HMSO; 1986.
[16] Medicine net. Breast Cancer. [Online]. 2002. Available from: URL: http://www.medicinenet.com/breast_cancer/page3.htm (last accessed 10 August 2005)
[17] NHS Review. The Breast Screening Programme Annual Review 2005. [Online]. 2005. Available from: URL: http://www.cancerscreening.nhs.uk/breastscreen//publications/2005review.html (last accessed 14 July 2007)
[18] Cancer Research UK. Breast Cancer Factsheet. [Online]. 2004. Available from: URL: http://publications.cancerresearchuk.org/epages/crukstore.sf/en_GB/?ObjectPath=/Shops/crukstore/Categories/BrowseBySubject/BreastCancer (last accessed 18 September 2004)
[19] Bankhead C, Austoker J, Sharp D, Peters T, et al, A practice based randomized controlled trial of two simple interventions aimed to increase uptake of breast cancer screening. J Med Screen 2001;8(2):91-8.
[20] Wanless D. Securing our Future Health: Taking a Long-Term View. London : HMSO; 2002.
[21] Carvel J. NHS plan for central patient database alarms doctors. The Guardian 2006 Nov.
[22] Leigh D. What health professionals say about the new NHS database. The Guardian 2006 Nov 1.
[23] Department of Health, Health Reform in England: update and commissioning framework, London: HMSO; 2006.
[24] HM Treasury. Spending Review: Public Service Agreements 2005-2008. London: HMSO; 2004.
[25] Singer BH and Ryff CD. New Horizons in Health: An Integrative Approach. Washington (DC): National Academy Press; 2001.
[26] Abu Bakar MA. Malaysia Healthcare Delivery System. Personal Interview with MAK Ghani, Coventry University PhD candidate. March 2007
[27] Ariff KM, Teng CL. Rural health care in Malaysia. Aust J Rural Health 2002;10(2):99-103.
[28] Suleiman AB. The Untapped Potential of Telehealth, Int J Med Inform 2001;61(2-3):103-12.
[29] Medical Record Institute. Continuity of Care Record (CCR) - The Concept Paper of the CCR - Version 3. [Online]. 2006. Available from: URL: http://medrecinst.com/pages/about.asp?id=54 ((last accessed 2 April 2008).
[30] Ministry of Health Malaysia. Telemedicine Blueprint: Telemedicine Flagship Application. Government of Malaysia; 1997.
[31] Harun MH. Integrated Telehealth: What Does It All Mean? DTP Enterprise Sdn Bhd, 2002.
[32] Ministry of Health Malaysia. Concept Request for Proposal for Lifetime Health Plan: Telemedicine Flagship Application. Government of Malaysia; 1997
[33] Mohan J, Raja Yaacob RR. The Malaysian Telehealth Flagship Application: a national approach to health data protection and utilisation and consumer rights. Int J Med Inform 2004;73(3);217-27.
[34] Gibbons MC, Brock M, Alberg AJ, Glass T, LaVeist TA, Baylin SB, et al, The Socio-biologic integrative model: Enhancing the integration of socio-behavioral, environmental and bio-molecular knowledge in urban health and disparities research, J Urban Health 2007;84(2):198-211.
[35] Macintyre S. The Black Report and beyond: what are the issues? Soc Sci Med 1997;44(6):23-745.
[36] Acheson D. Independant Inquiry into Inequalities in Health. London: UK Department of Health; 1998.
[37] Williams DR. Race, socioeconomic status, and health: The added effects of racism and discrimination. Ann NY Acad Sci 1999;896:173-88.
[38] LaLonde M, A new perspective on the health of Canadians. 1981; Government of Canada.
[39] Evans RG, Stoddart GL. Producing health, consuming health care. Soc Sci Med 1990;31(12):1347-63.
[40] Burger R, Gimelfarb A. Genetic variation maintained in multilocus models of additive quantitative traits under stabilizing selection. Genetics 1999;152(2):807-20.
[41] PhillipsTJ, Belknap JK. Complex-trait genetics: emergence of multivariate strategies. Nat Rev Neurosci 2002;3(6):478-85.
[42] Sharma AM. The thrifty-genotype hypothesis and its implications for the study of complex genetic disorders in man. J Mol Med 1998;76(8):568-71.
[43] Meyer JM, Breitner JC. Multiple threshold model for the onset of Alzheimer's disease in the NAS-NRC twin panel. Am J Med Genet 1998;81(1):92-7.
[44] Gibbons MC. Healthcare Disparities Solutions Blog. [Online]. 2010. Available from: URL: http://hcdisparities.blogspot.com/2010/01/top-10-health-technology-trends-for.html (last accessed viewed 13 March 2010).

Electronic Health Records

Medical and Care Compunetics 6
L. Bos et al. (Eds.)
IOS Press, 2010

doi:10.3233/978-1-60750-565-5-153

Standardized Vectorial Representation of Medical Data in Patient Records

Wolfgang ORTHUBER [a,1] and Efthymios PAPAVRAMIDIS [a]
[a]*Department of Orthodontics at Universitaetsklinikum Schleswig-Holstein Campus Kiel, Germany*

Abstract. In this paper standardized vectorial (quantitative) representation of medical data is suggested for use in patient records. Vectorial representations are (as sequences of numbers) language independent, precise, directly comparable, and they allow advanced evaluation, e.g. similarity calculation using well defined distance functions. It is possible to search for a patient with a certain combination of diagnostic parameters on the Web records of patients with similar parameters. The information about chosen treatments and treatment outcome at these patients can be used anonymously or pseudonymously for decision support. Because patient records from all countries can be compared, in the long run this could open systematic access to a very large wealth of clinically relevant information. Here the technical principle is described and illustrated by examples (e.g. similarity search of heart sounds). Previously published material is integrated in parts for explanation of the motivation and background.

Keywords. similarity comparison, patient record databases, Vectorial Resource Descriptor, Vector Space Identifier, Vector Space Descriptor, Quantifiable Resource, QRI, Feature vectors, task sharing, metric databases, decision support

1. Introduction

Step by step it is becoming common to store information about anamnesis, diagnostics, treatment and treatment result in electronic patient records. Together these records summarize a huge and permanently increasing wealth of valuable information which by far exceeds the knowledge of any human doctor. It is clear that this should be used for decision support, according to the wishes of the patients (anonymously or pseudonymously). Until now, however, patient records are usually stored in separated databases in incompatible formats. To alleviate exchange of health data, much effort is invested in building standards for electronic interchange of clinical, financial, and administrative information among health care oriented computer systems [1], and huge vocabularies have been created. For example, SNOMED CT [2] is a medical ontology with increasing size that contains already today within its English version more than 300000 concepts, 900000 descriptions and 1300000 relationships. There are also large collections of identifiers available for exchange of quantitative data, e.g. LOINC® [19]. Quantitative data can help to improve the resolution of symbolic descriptions. This is desirable and welcome for decision support. Because optimal therapeutic decisions are the aim, the representation of medical data should be even designed for decision

[1] Corresponding Author: Arnold Heller Str. 16, 24105 Kiel, Germany; E-mail: orthuber@kfo-zmk.uni-kiel.de.

support. Here we propose a concept for this. It is designed to support the clinician in his *cycle of decision*:

a) The clinician makes measurements (in the broadest sense, also speaking with the patient and looking at a picture is a measurement).
b) The clinician focuses on those measurement results which are interesting for his therapeutic decisions (feature extraction).
c) The clinician compares these measurement results with experience. At this he may use rules or models which are derived from common experience.
d) The clinician decides for therapy, and measures the effect of his decision, i.e. the cycle starts again with (a).

Usually several measurements are done before therapeutic decisions, and so (a) can be a complex process which also requires decisions. The decision for the initial measurements has to be done by the clinician, together with the patient who tells the clinician his concerns. After this initial data acquisition the clinician has a rough impression and can select a keyword (a "rough diagnosis") or already provide certain measurement results to get support when he decides for further fine measurements. In 2.5 is described how this can be used to get help for steps (a) and (b). For support of steps (c) and (d) we propose standardized vectorial representation of medical data. *Vectors* or *feature vectors* (sequences of numbers) within a vector space (metric space) provide besides high resolution also multidimensional comparability. This is especially in step (c) important and allows high resolution search within a large collection of data.

The usage of vector spaces is (of course) not new in informatics, there are already well known applications e.g. in bioinformatics, biophysics, signal processing, imaging, and vector spaces are used for data integration within the framework of the Conceptual Space approach [3][4][5]. Conceptual Spaces follow a theory of describing entities at the conceptual level in terms of their natural characteristics similar to human cognition in order to avoid the symbol grounding issue [6]. They enable representation of resources as vectors within a geometrical space which is defined through a set of quality dimensions. For instance, a particular color may be defined as vector with the dimensions hue, saturation, and brightness. This is finer and more precise than a symbolic representation. Describing instances as vectors furthermore enables the automatic calculation of their similarity, in terms of their distance, in contrast to the costly representation of such knowledge through symbolic representations. Even complex data which describe e.g. faces, sounds, fingerprints and biometric data can be processed by feature extraction to vectorial form for similarity comparison and recognition. Generally, feature extraction is an essential pre-processing step to pattern recognition and machine learning problems. The resulting feature vectors open a large spectrum of applications for vector spaces [7].

It is possible to make precise diagnostic measurements on a patient, and to make feature extraction on decision relevant findings. The resulting vectorial representation could be standardized. This would allow to search worldwide (within all accessible data collections) the records of patients with similar diagnostic findings, to study possible therapies and their long term consequences with probabilities of failure and success, in order to support the clinician in making better decisions.

This motivated us to write this paper which proposes standardized vectorial representation of medical data. First we introduce the basics and describe the application of vector spaces for representation of quantitative properties and data integration in general. Then a framework for vectorial representation of medical data and efficient implementation of vectorial similarity search is presented.

2. Material and Methods

2.1. Appropriate resources for vectorial representation

The numbers which represent quantitative data can be regarded as components of a vector. Quantification is precondition for vectorial representation. To be suitable for vectorial representation, a resource must have one or several quantitative properties, i.e. one or several attributes which each have an inherent order (from "little" to "great"). We will call such a resource "*Quantifiable Resource*" (QR). If two QRs are represented by instances of the same quantitative property (or properties in case of many dimensions), these QRs are *comparable*. Their vectorial description belongs to the same vector space.

For example measurement results and numeric results of feature extraction are QRs. Important for similarity comparison is that small changes of the original are mapped to small changes of the representing numbers.

2.2. Vector space

The mathematics of *vector spaces* or *linear spaces* is focused in linear algebra and used in many areas. There are well known applications in nature sciences, e.g. in physics. Also in computer science vectors are used for representation of concepts or real world objects, e.g. in metric databases. All vectors which represent the same sort of data are comparable and belong to the same vector space. They can be added, multiplied and subtracted (which is important for comparison). Let n denote the dimensionality of a vector space V^n, then the coordinate vectors $\mathbf{e}_1 = (1, 0, ..., 0)$, $\mathbf{e}_2 = (0, 1, 0, ..., 0)$, to $\mathbf{e}_n = (0, 0, ..., 0, 1)$, form a *basis* of V^n, called the *standard basis*, so that any vector $(x_1, x_2, ..., x_n) \in V^n$ can be uniquely expressed as linear combination of these vectors:

$$
\begin{aligned}
&(x_1, x_2, ..., x_n) \\
&= x_1(1, 0, ..., 0) + x_2(0, 1, 0, ..., 0) + ... + x_n(0, ..., 0, 1) \\
&= x_1\mathbf{e}_1 + x_2\mathbf{e}_2 + ... + x_n\mathbf{e}_n.
\end{aligned}
$$

It is possible to define a norm [8] or "length" function on a vector space. Then the vector space can be called *metric space* [9]. Let $\| \ \|$ denote the norm and A, B two vectors, then the distance d between A and B is the length of the difference vector:

$$d(A,B) = \|A - B\|$$

With A and B also the difference $A - B$ is a vector. There are many norms and associated metrics (distance functions). Well known are the Manhattan metric and the Euclidean metric. For clarification we write the Euclidean metric here explicitly - without loss of generality. Let A, B denote two vectors with $A = (a_1, a_2, ... a_n)$,

$B = (b_1, b_2, \ldots b_n)$, $a_i, b_i \in \Re$, then the unweighted Euclidean distance between A and B is

$$d_u(A,B) = \sqrt{\sum_{i=1}^{n} (a_i - b_i)^2} \tag{1}$$

Different dimensions can have different variance and importance. Therefore it is adequate to define a weighting vector $W = (w_1, w_2, \ldots w_n)$, $w_i \in \Re \setminus \{0\}$ and the *weighted* Euclidean distance:

$$d(A,B) = \sqrt{\sum_{i=1}^{n} (w_i a_i - w_i b_i)^2} \tag{2}$$

If $w_i = 1$ for every dimension $i \in (1, 2, \ldots n)$, the unweighted distance (1) is identical to the weighted distance (2). Here by "distance" we always mean the weighted distance. The greater w_i, the more contributes dimension i to the distance. Formula (2) shows that $d(A,B) \geq 0$; the distance $d(A,B)$ is the greater, the more A and B differ, and $d(A,B) = 0$ if and only if $A = B$, i.e. $a_i = b_i$ for every dimension. So we see that (2) can be used to quantify similarity between two vectors.

2.3. Vectorial Resource Descriptors (VRDs)

The proposed data structure for representation of a QR is called *Vectorial Resource Descriptor* (VRD). We suggest a design with full integration into the Web of Linked Data, to achieve maximal efficiency within the current Web Infrastructure. The Resource Description Framework (RDF) can be used, with HTTP URIs (and not other URI schemes as URNs and DOIs) as identifiers, in agreement with the recommendations for Linked Data [10]. HTTP URIs provide as Web Addresses a simple way to create globally unique names[2] and task sharing without centralized management, and they work not just as a name but also as a means of accessing information about a resource over the Web. This is in many applications even necessary, in connection with the vectorial approach it is necessary to get immediate access to the definition of the valid distance function of the vector space for calculation of similarity.

The VRD structure is shown in Figure 1. It contains:

a) The identifier of the QR (QRI). It is a HTTP URI which points to the resource.
e) The Vector Space Identifier (VSI). It is a HTTP URI which points to the Vector Space Descriptor (VSD).
f) The feature vector (usually a sequence of numbers). It represents the quantitative properties of the resource.

Additionally it can contain:

g) Auxiliary data, e.g. date, keywords.

---

[2] These can integrate also names of existing definitions, e.g. codes of LOINC® [19] or DOIs, so systematic adoption of existing work is possible.

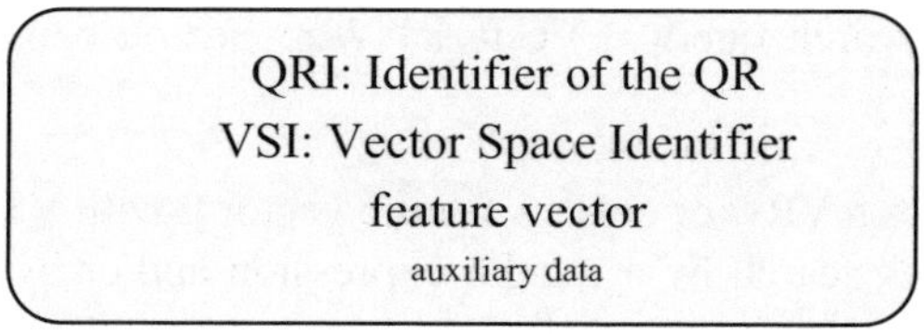

Figure 1. The Vectorial Resource Descriptor (VRD). It is the data structure for representation of a QR. The components QRI and VSI are both HTTP URIs.

The feature vectors of all VRDs with the same VSI are elements of the same vector space and comparable as described in 2.2. Similarity search is done within this space. As HTTP URI the VSI not only identifies the content of the feature vector, it simultaneously points to the *Vector Space Descriptor* (VSD, Figure 2) which provides all necessary information about the vector space, particularly about the metric for comparison, definitions of dimensions, templates for human readable representation of instances and links to further related Web content.

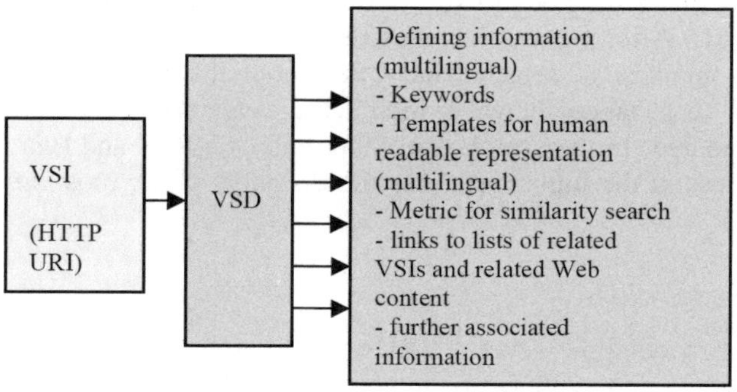

Figure 2. The *Vector Space Identifier* (VSI) points to the *Vector Space Descriptor* (VSD) which provides important information about all VRDs with this VSI.

VRDs are machine readable and can be embedded into the semantic Web as Linked Data [11]. They are uniformly comparable and searchable, and the usage of HTTP URIs makes it possible to share the work for definition of vector spaces and generation of VRDs among all domain name owners.

2.4. Vectorial Web Search

Subsequently we assume that the patient records are distributed over the Web and accessible according to the wishes of the patient. So the total Web is the database of patient records, therefore we use the term "search engine" for the tool which allows similarity search of patient records according to the wishes of the user. The VRDs are the fundament of Vectorial Similarity Search over the total Web (Vectorial Web

Search). Due to the standardized structure of the VRDs one and the same search engine can be used for all search queries. Vectorial Web Search consists of the following steps:

- User provides a VRD or only its feature vector F with VSI.
- User confines search by a regular expression and/or by a conventional word based search string S (optional)
- Search engine collects all VRDs
  - with the chosen VSI
  - optionally with string S at the associated resource (identified by QRI)

  via conventional word based search
- If a regular expression is given in step two, the collection is confined so that it fulfills this expression.
- Using the metric provided in the VSD (figure 2) the search engine calculates distances between the feature vector F and the feature vectors of the collected VRDs and sorts them according to distance.
- In the search result the rank of collected VRDs and associated resources is the higher, the smaller the distance is.

As it is apparent in the above list, Vectorial Web Search starts with word based search (for the VSI): After the user has provided a VSI and feature vector F, among all VRDs those with this VSI are selected and (after optional further confinement) used for comparison, i.e. the distances between their feature vectors and the searched feature vector F are calculated. In the search result the rank of VRDs and (via QRI, figure 1) associated resources is the higher, the less the distance is, i.e. most similar resources are listed first.

2.4.1. Combination of VRDs

It is possible to combine several VRDs in a search to find resources which are simultaneously associated with (resp. in the QRI field of) all VRDs. At this it is necessary to use a combined distance d_{comb} . It can be set to the weighted sum of the single distances:

$$d_{comb} = \sum_{i}^{n} m_i d_i$$

in which n is the number of combined VRDs, m_i the weighting factor and d_i the distance of VRD *i*. One cannot expect that the user provides appropriate weighting factors m_i, so there must be the option for automatic weighting. A possible solution is to set

$$m_i = \frac{1}{s_i}$$

in which s_i is the standard deviation of the distances of VRD *i*. This is a reasonable choice because it takes into account that the statistical significance of a fluctuation is the greater, the less the standard deviation of the concerned variable is.

2.5. Application in medicine

The here proposed application in the medical domain is the representation of decision relevant anamnestic and diagnostic (and past therapeutic, e.g. medication) data in vectorial form (as VRDs). As mentioned in the introduction (see 1), in the *cycle of decision* the clinician makes (unconsciously) feature extraction from all available measurements (also from complex measurements like MRI scans) and compares the result with experience. Important parts (of course not all) of this procedure can be mapped to database algorithms.

First the scientific community has to start a *diagnosis-VSI-database*: A list of important keywords or "rough diagnoses" must be defined or derived from existing ontologies like SNOMED CT [2]. Then to every[3] rough diagnosis standardized measurement combinations must be associated, which provide the most important data for therapeutic decisions, with standardized numeric representation of the results - as combination of elementary VRDs with appropriate VSIs[4], with combined distance function (default see 2.4.1). The combination of elementary VRDs with minimal dimensionality can be appropriate to facilitate flexible queries. After creation of the diagnosis-VSI-database the following workflow is possible:

- Select a rough diagnosis in the diagnosis-VSI-database.
- Get from the diagnosis-VSI-database the information about the combination of VSIs which is appropriate for this rough diagnosis, and make all necessary measurements to get the VRDs with these VSIs which are connected with this rough diagnosis.
- Optionally make further measurements which are interesting (relevant for therapeutic decisions.) and convert them to VRDs.
- Select all decision relevant VRDs and send them to the search engine to search patient records which have these VRDs with minimal distance (2.4.1).
- Look in the found patient records whether additional diagnostic measurements have been useful. If appropriate, make these measurements, convert these to VRDs and continue with the previous step.
- Look in the found patient records for the most successful therapeutic decisions. Statistical evaluation and mathematical modeling is possible.

3. Examples

3.1. VRD combination for vertebral (osteoporotic) compression fractures

Let us take as example "vertebral compression fracture" as rough diagnosis. We will reflect on a VRD combination, which could be associated to this rough diagnosis in the diagnosis-VSI-database. Aim is to pack most important decision relevant information in a sequence of numbers as short as possible. In case of orthopedic findings the geometry is usually important, for an osteoporotic compression fracture we can define the numbers v, c and d which show the relative remainders of the vertebral body

---

[3] It makes sense to start with most important and most expensive rough diagnoses.

[4] If the medical community defines a 3D reference coordinate system on an anatomical reference model, it is possible to use a VSI for localization of most diagnostic findings and the "rough diagnosis" need not contain localization information.

ventrally (*v*), centrally (*c*) and dorsally (*d*). Furthermore the number *a,* which shows the relative narrowing of the vertebral channel can be important, and the number *n* of the vertebra (numbered consecutively from head to sacrum). Let *d1, d2, d3, c2, v1, v2, v3, a1, a2, a3* denote the scalar lengths of the lines as drawn in figure 3. Then we can calculate the numbers *v, c, d, a* as follows:

$v=2*v2/(v1+v3)$,
$c=4*c2/(v1+v3+d1+d3)$,
$d=2*d2/(d1+d3)$,
$a=2*a2/(a1+a3)$.

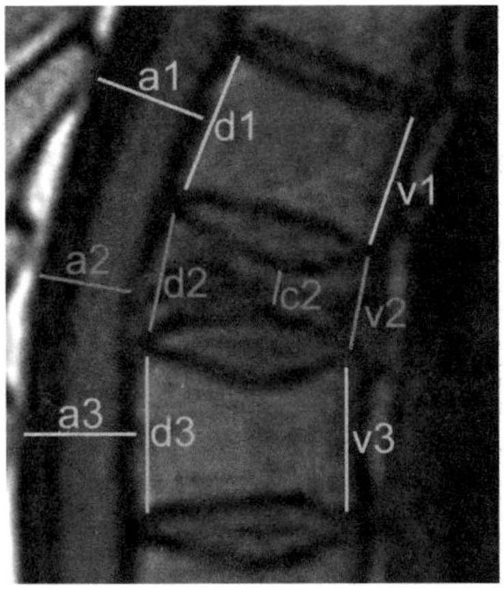

Figure 3. MRI scan of a vertebral compression fracture in the area of maximal compression. The lengths *a1,a2, a3, d1, d2, d3, c2, v1, v2, v3* are used for construction of the feature vector of this fracture as described in the text.

The VRD for the geometry of the compression has the 5 dimensional feature vector *(v,c,d,a,n)*. Additionally a representative measurement of the bone density *t* like the DXA T-score (at representative vertebra, e.g. L1) may be important, so that we could combine (2.4.1) the two VRDs with feature vectors *(v,c,d,a,n)* and *(t)* to search for patient records which contain similar parameters *v, c, d, a, n, t,* and for the most successful therapeutic decisions at these patients. It is clear that purely symbolic approaches cannot provide the resolution and precision of this method. For decision support, however, such precision is desirable.

3.2. Similarity search of heart sounds

We have built a software prototype to demonstrate the functionality of the approach also in case of nontrivial vectorial representations. Complex original data like sounds and pictures usually require an appropriate transformation as first step for calculation of feature vectors. In case of heart sounds a wavelet transformation proved to be useful, because it allows analysis of the signal at different scales and times [12][13]. This is implemented in our software. It consists of two program modules:

The first module (used for generation of searchable data) reads a sequence of heart sounds from a .wav file and displays it on the screen (figure 4). One period is reproducibly selected (figure 5) and a Daubechies wavelet transformation is performed. The smoothened absolute values of the transformation coefficients (figure 6) are used for building a searchable feature vector of the sound. This is stored as a VRD in a local database in an internal format.

The second program module (used for similarity search) calculates a VRD from the upload[5] and compares it with the VRDs of the database by calculating the distances to them. It generates the search result which is an ordered list of references to these VRDs (figure 7). The less the distance, the higher is the rank of a VRD in the search result list. This means that VRDs which represent the most similar sounds in the database have upper position in the search result. The main parts of the second program module could be used also for similarity search of other data which allow a vectorial description. This means that one and the same search engine can be used for similarity search in very different applications, if the searchable data are stored in an appropriate way.

Technical remarks: The finest scale for the wavelet transformation has been 2^{11} (figure 8). This resulted in $\sum_{i=1}^{11} 2^i = 4094$ coefficients. This is also the dimensionality of the feature vector, because all coefficients have been used in this application. As distance function we used

$$d(X,Y) = 1 - \frac{\sum_{i=1}^{n}(x_i - \bar{x})(y_i - \bar{y})}{\sqrt{\sum_{i=1}^{n}(x_i - \bar{x})^2 \sum_{i=1}^{n}(y_i - \bar{y})^2}}$$

in which n=4094 is the dimensionality, X, Y are the compared vectors, x_i, y_i their coordinates, i.e. the smoothened absolute values of the wavelet coefficients, and $\bar{x}$ the mean of the x_i resp. $\bar{y}$ the mean of the y_i. It is apparent that the distance function contains the correlation coefficient and ensures that the greater the correlation is, the smaller the distance becomes. So the rank of a heart sound is the greater in the search result, the more its wavelet decomposition correlates with the wavelet decomposition of the searched sound.

We want to underline that this implementation is designed for illustration purposes. All 4094 coefficients have been used, so that the time frequency distribution becomes well visible (figure 6). For more efficiency there would be much potential for compression and dimension reduction, because heart sounds have by far not the variability which 4094 coefficients provide. Moreover the process could be fully automated [14]. In contrast to this the workflow of figures 4, 5 and 6 shows the principle and demonstrates a typical half automatic feature selection. Especially in the initial state after introduction of VRDs the half automatic selection of features (or even manual selection like done in figure 3) can have advantages because it can help to keep overview, and introduction of software for feature vector and VRD generation can be accelerated. Later step by step more and more automation is possible, if wished.

---

[5] The module allows upload of original heart sounds as .wav files in compressed form. Because it is specialized to one kind of original data, it can convert these to VRDs before comparison without needing a VSI.

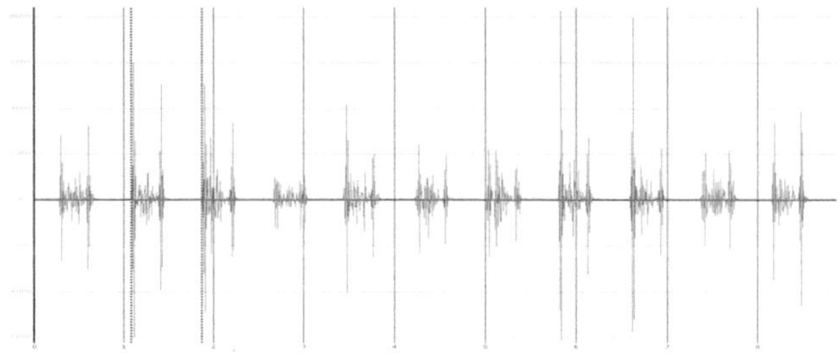

Figure 4. Sounds of a heart with aortic valve stenosis; vertical axis: relative amplitude, horizontal axis: time in seconds. The brown dashed lines have been set reproducibly by a catching algorithm after rough manual prepositioning (semi-automatic process). They show the bordering of a representative period.

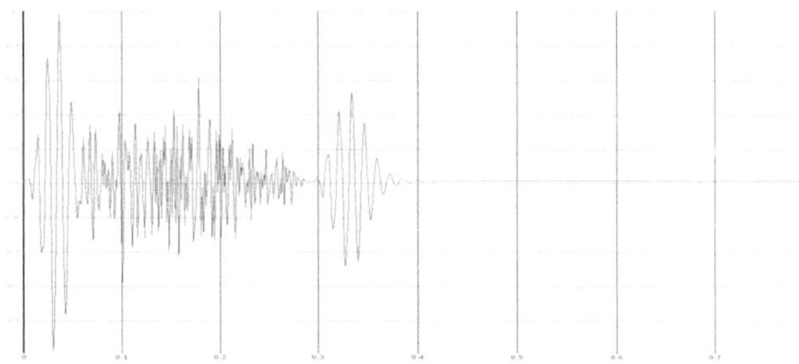

Figure 5. The bordered part of figure 4 is stretched so that one period remains, i.e. the length of the period is standardized. So heart sounds with different period length can be compared.

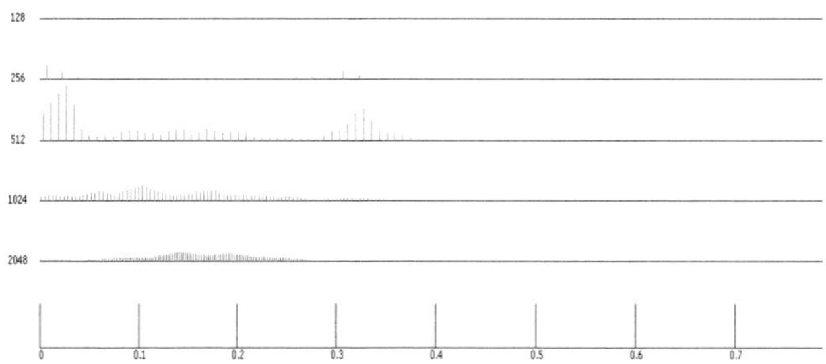

Figure 6. The sound of figure 5 after Daubechies wavelet transform; smoothened absolute values of the wavelet transform coefficients for five different scales. They can be directly used for building a searchable feature vector of this heart sound. Note the delayed appearance of the high frequency part which results from blood flow through the narrowed aortic valve during systole.

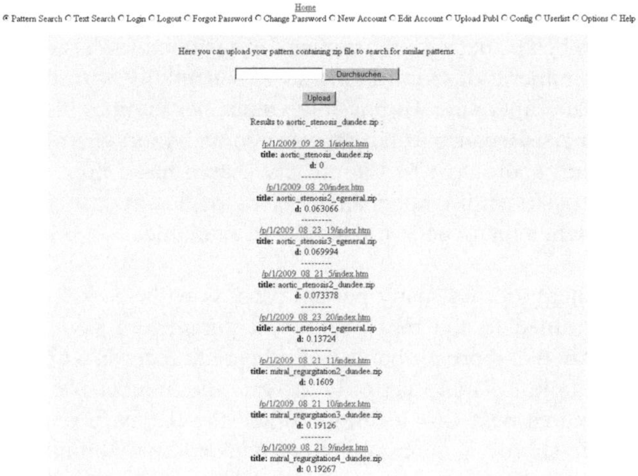

Figure 7. Exemplary output of our prototype. The VRD of the uploaded file represents the heart sound in case of aortic valve stenosis after wavelet transformation as shown in figure 6. Links to resources with most similar VRDs are listed first. The distance d quantifies the deviation, the first link points to a VRD which represents the same sound like the uploaded file, therefore the distance is zero.

4. Discussion

According to 2.4 similarity search of VRDs (Vectorial Web Search) is the sequence of two well known workflows:

1. Conventional word based search (for VRDs with the same VSI; this can be simplified using an index: To every VSI an index with all VRDs and their URLs can be collected beforehand).
2. Similarity comparison (of the VRDs' feature vectors, as done in metric databases or by our prototype)

Both workflows are established, so it has to be expected that also the sequence "one after the other" works. Of course the hardware requirement of the global Web application must be considered. For larger amounts of data we made a small experiment to get a hint about the necessary time for comparison of vectors using a C++ compiler on a single PC (Pentium® 4 CPU). The time for calculating 1 million weighted Euclidean distances of vectors with dimensionality 10 in double accuracy was between 0.20 and 0.21 seconds. Such calculation would be necessary if similarity search is done within VRDs with altogether 1 million 10 dimensional feature vectors with serial comparison. Depending on implementation, disk access would require additional time. To minimize the time for comparison, the total dimensionality (the sum of dimensions of all feature vectors) of the searched VRD combination should be minimized. This should be also done because the sparsity increases exponentially with the total dimensionality in case of a constant amount of data, with points tending to become equidistant from one another ("Curse of Dimensionality" [15] [16]). Parallel processing can substantially reduce the time for comparison because it is not necessary to calculate the distances sequentially.

We expect the most important problems in the beginning. Initially investment is necessary for creating the infrastructure, and initially there won't be enough patient records available for decision support. When the number of patient records grows, the situation becomes better, because the concept is designed for large data collections. The resolution of the numeric description grows exponentially with the dimensionality - it is well known that if there are 10 possible values per number, there are 10^k possible values for k numbers. Because usually there are much more than 10 possible values per number, it becomes soon clear that similarity search has a high resolution and can be highly selective even within huge amounts of data - at last a great advantage for decision support when many patient records are available.

As long as there are not many patient records with the selected rough diagnosis, one may be restrained to the most important parameters (low dimensional search), because in this way it is more probable to find patient records with "similar" parameters. In the above example 3.1 one may only provide the number *n* of the vertebra, to find compression fractures near this location. When the database returns more cases near this *n* than one can survey, it is possible to provide additional numbers (dimensions) for a more selective search.

Additionally to direct decision support the precise vectorial descriptions can be useful for skill enhancement (e.g. study of selected diagnostic constellations) and scientific research. Because the feature vectors of VRDs with the same VSI represent points within the same metric space, there is the possibility for "local statistics", i.e. statistics among VRDs whose vectors lay "near" (within a given distance from) a given point. For example it is possible to calculate within a given radius the average of a further dependent variable or the frequency of some incident. Such local statistics is not difficult to interpret, moreover it has the advantage that it can be quickly computed. But especially if there are only a few points (vectors) within the investigated radius, the result could be imprecise due to coincidental fluctuations and it can be more accurate to consider all available points (defined by feature vectors of all VRDs with appropriate VSI) for immediate regression analysis or for calculation of a mathematical model [17] (blue curve in Figure 8).

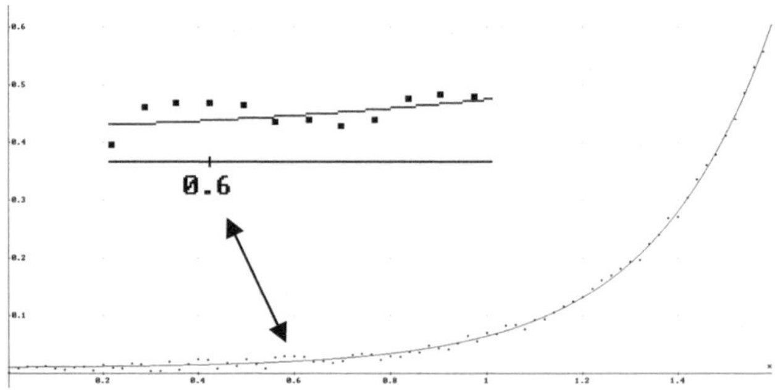

Figure 8. Local statistics can be used if there are many points „near" to the area of interest. If not, coincidental fluctuations, as shown in the enlarged detail, can become relevant and a mathematical model (blue curve), which takes into account all points, is more accurate.

We show a practical example of how such modeling can be used to "interpolate" at places where data are missing. Suppose patient records are available which contain VRDs whose feature vector describe the medication of a patient in the form (*t*, *x*) resp (*t*, *y*), in which *t* is the duration of the medication in days, and the numbers *x* resp *y* represent the daily dosage (e.g. in mg) of medicament X resp. medicament Y. Furthermore VRDs with another VSI provide the blood concentration z of a liver enzyme (which indicates damage of the liver). For modeling it is possible to select all patients with $t > t_{min}$ (e.g. $t > 30$ days, to ensure enough medication time), and to calculate from the found data points a function [18] which approximates the concentration z of the liver enzyme in dependence of the medication dosages x and y. A possible resulting function is shown in Figure 9. Because polymedication and drug interaction is an increasing problem (especially in geriatrics), the practical relevance of the approach is obvious.

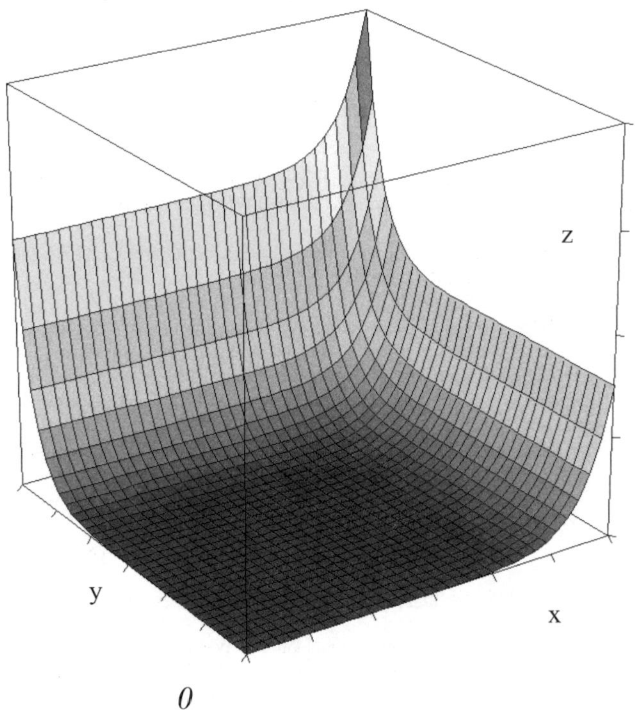

Figure 9. Example of a function which estimates the value of a dependent variable z (vertical axis: concentration of a liver enzyme as indicator of liver damage) in dependence of the two variables x and y (horizontal axes: dosages of two medicaments). It is visible that z grows strongly when x or y exceeds a toxic threshold. Data from the VRDs' feature vectors can be used for calculation of such a function (mathematical modeling).

Of course the data for such modeling could be also fetched from special databases. This requires extra programming. The standardized VRD structure, however, can be used generally by one and the same *evaluation engine* which allows to select VSIs and the numbers of the feature vectors' dimensions for specification of independent and dependent variables.

At last a possibility for anonymization should be mentioned: The patient can select the option that his VRDs can be used for decision support, but only statistically over more than e.g. 5 patients without showing the individual values. It would be possible to calculate and show the VRDs' average (about the therapeutic result) of minimal n (e.g. n=5) patients with similar diagnosis in dependence of therapy.

5. Conclusion

Vectorial representations are precise, directly comparable, and they allow advanced analysis, e.g. similarity calculation using well defined distance functions. Due to the shown advantages of vectorial representation the usage of standardized Vectorial Resource Descriptors (VRDs) is proposed for representation of medical data in patient records.

References

[1] HL7. Standards for electronic interchange of clinical, financial, and administrative information among health care oriented computer systems. [Online]. Available from: URL: http://www.hl7.org/. (viewed 2010-02-09)

[2] International Health Terminology Standards Development Organisation. SNOMED CT (Systematized Nomenclature of Medicine – Clinical Terms). [Online]. Available from: URL: http://www.ihtsdo.org/snomed-ct/. (viewed 2010-02-09)

[3] Pratt I, Lemon O. Logical and Diagrammatic Reasoning: the Complexity of Conceptual Space. Proceedings of the Nineteenth Annual Conference of the Cognitive Science; 1997; Stanford. p. 430-5

[4] Gärdenfors P. Conceptual Spaces - The Geometry of Thought. MIT Press; 2000.

[5] Gärdenfors P. How to make the semantic Web more semantic. In: Vieu AC, Varzi L, editors. Formal Ontology in Information Systems. IOS Press; 2004. p. 19–36.

[6] Dietze S, Domingue J, Orthuber W. Blending the Physical and the Digital through Conceptual Spaces, Workshop: OneSpace 2009 at Future Internet Symposium (FIS). 2009; Berlin, Germany.

[7] Guyon I, Gunn S, Nikravesh M, Zadeh L, editors. Feature Extraction, Foundations and Applications. Berlin, Heidelberg: Springer; 2006. (Studies in Fuzziness and Soft Computing; vol 207)

[8] Wikipedia. [Online]. Available from: URL: http://en.wikipedia.org/wiki/Normed_vector_space. (viewed 2010-02-09)

[9] Wikipedia. [Online]. Available from: URL: http://en.wikipedia.org/wiki/Metric_space. (viewed 2010-02-09)

[10] Bizer C, Cyganiak R, Heath T. How to Publish Linked Data on the Web. [Online]. Available from: URL: http://www4.wiwiss.fu-berlin.de/bizer/pub/LinkedDataTutorial/20070727/. (viewed 2010-02-09)

[11] Linked Data. Connect Distributed Data across the Web. [Online]. Available from: URL: http://linkeddata.org/. (viewed 2010-02-10)

[12] Daubechies I. The wavelet transform, time-frequency localization and signal analysis. IEEE Trans. Inform. Theory 1990;36:961-1005.

[13] El-Asir B, Khadra L, Al-Abbasi AH, Mohammed MMJ. Time frequency analysis of heart sounds. Proc IEEE 1996;2:553-8.

[14] Faloutsos C, Ranganathan M, ManolopoulosY. Fast Subsequence Matching in Time-Series Databases. ACM SIGMOD Int.Conf. on Management of Data 1994;419-29.

[15] Berchtold S, Böhm C, Kriegel H-P. The Pyramid-Tree: Breaking the Curse of Dimensionality. SIGMOD Conference; 1998. p. 142-53.

[16] Indyk P, Motwani R. Approximate Nearest Neighbors: Towards Removing the Curse of Dimensionality. In: Proc. of the 30th Symposium on the Theory of Computing; 1998. p. 604-13.

[17] Kattan MW, Leung DHY, Brennan MF. Postoperative Nomogram for 12-Year Sarcoma-Specific Death. Journal of Clinical Oncology 2002;20(3):791-6.

[18] Fang L, Gossard DC. Multidimensional curve fitting to unorganized data points by nonlinear minimization. Computer-Aided Design 1995;27(1):48–58.

[19] LOINC®. Logical Observation Identifiers Names and Codes. [Online]. Available from: URL: http://loinc.org/. (viewed 2010-02-10)

Medical and Care Compunetics 6
L. Bos et al. (Eds.)
IOS Press, 2010

doi:10.3233/978-1-60750-565-5-167

Clinical Events Classification for Using the EHR to Provide Better Patient Care

Tatyana LUGOVKINA[1], Bernard RICHARDS[2]
[1] *City Hospital N40, Clinical Pharmacology Department, Yekaterinburg, Russian Federation*
[2] *Medical Informatics, University of Manchester, United Kingdom*

Abstract. The Healthcare Record has been used in a "Before and After" situation to improve patient care. The main paradigm of the modern Health Care is changing towards pervasive person-centric care including prevention and home care. Medical compunetics is a very important applicative field for improving the interoperability and the quality of the healthcare information system, especially in the current climate with the empowerment patients. The success depends on the choice of the Clinical Events Classification for structuring the span of clinical information. For the purposes of universalizing medical electronic data-bases, it is very important to organize the data regarding Clinical Events in such manner that it would be possible to use this information-structure in different fields of Clinical Practice: e.g., for the creation of the diagnostic and drug-assistance protocols, for the evaluation of the quality of drug prescribing, and for communication with patients as well. For this purpose all Clinical Events were divided to 5 classes. This Paper will describe a "Before and After" situation consequent upon the introduction of the Clinical Events Classification and the introduction of Protocols for drug-prescribing. Use of the Protocol brought about a 50% reduction in mortality.

Keywords. Electronic Health Record, Antibiotic Prescribing, Decision Support System, Clinical Events Classification, Intensive Care Patients.

Introduction

The important relevance of the Clinical Events Classification within the Electronic Health Record (EHR) comes from the aim of the National Health System, namely maximizing the quality of care given to the patient, and in particular, the saving of patient-lives. Within this activity, drug-prescribing plays an important role. The 5-level protocols for prescribing the drugs (Antibiotics in our case) both allowed one to improve the quality of the decisions made in the process of drug choice in clinical practice, thereby saving the lives of the patients, and to reduce the consumption of the Antibiotics (AB) and hence, very importantly, to reduce the expenditure for drugs.

Materials and Methods

The Healthcare Record has been used in a "Before and After" situation to improve patient care. The Records of 100 newborn babies were analyzed and the AB treatments were recorded. After the introduction of the new restricted Protocols of AB prescribing, made on the basis of the Clinical Events Classification, a further 100 babies were studied.

Likewise, 36 patients suffering from Pneumonia in the Intensive Care Unit were studied under the old regime of AB prescribing in the years 2003 to 2005, and a further 40 after the introduction of the new Protocols in the years 2006 to 2008.

The Universal Events Classification System has five levels of Severity of the clinical status of a patient, viz 1, 2, 3, 4, 5. International Classification of the Diseases (ICD - 10) gives the main code of the event and the severity of the disease is marked by the code that corresponds with one of the five levels of the severity of patient's status at the moment of making a decision for the choice of diagnostic procedures or drug assistance.

In the case of infection-connected diseases, the Class of Clinical Status is the result of evaluation of the inflammatory reaction, together with the consideration of the additional factors that have the influence on the decision-making process. The criteria for determining the Inflammatory Reaction to Infection (IRI) were based on the criteria reflected in International Guidelines and National Recommendations for sepsis. The rules for Drug Prescribing were constructed by the Clinical Pharmacologist and the specialists in anti-microbial therapy according to the Evidence Based Medicine data, or the consensus decisions of the specialists. The Decision-tree algorithm IF…THEN was used in the process of constructing the rules for diagnostic assessment, drug assistance, and health care logistics.

All Clinical Events were classified into 5 discrete classes. This five-way split is quite adequate to reflect the most typical clinical situations and is optimal for the clinicians to make the operative decisions. This way corresponds with the "non-linear causal model of the organization of information in the field of physics knowledge": 1-mechanical, 2- thermal, 3-electric, 4-magnetic, 5-electromagnetic (including optical), phenomenon [1], as well as with the thesis about the most effective size of the mental space and the size of a unit in short-term storage [2,3,4].

According to the methodology described in this Paper, the Clinical Event includes: "A" - the formalized clinical diagnosis and "B" - the concordance Protocol of the recommended diagnostic procedures and drug assistance. (The protocols for the support of decision-making).

The formalized diagnosis ("A") consists of two parts:

1. ICD -10 (International Classification of Diseases) – constant part, and
2. CCS (Class of Clinical Status) – flexible part of the formalized diagnosis. It allows one to fix in code-format the image of a definite clinical situation at the moment of making an important decision.

In the cases of the infectious diseases, CCS depends on the severity of the inflammatory reaction and the existence of the additional factors which have influence on the AB choice for that specific case.

Thus, **CCS = f (IRI + AF)**; where IRI – Inflammatory Reaction to Infection; and AF – are Additional Factors with influence on the process of decision-making for ABP.

The severity of IRI (as a part of CCS) was also assigned to 5 levels. The Classification of the Agreement Conference of The American College of the Pulmonologists, and of the Society of the Specialists in Critical Care Medicine (ACC/SCCM -1992) was the starting point for the IRI ranges.

IRI - Inflammatory Reaction to Infection

(5 levels of severity)

1. site infection + local inflammatory reaction (tumour, rubour, colour, dolour, functio laesa).
2. site infection + local inflammatory reaction + general inflammatory reaction (Temperature t° is more than 36°C, but less 38.5°C , HR less than 90 per min, RR less than 30 per min; Blood Leucocytes are less than $12x10^9$ /l, but more than $4x10^9$ /l)
3. site infection + local inflammatory reaction + general inflammatory reaction (t° is less than 36°C or more than 38.5°C , HR more than 90 per min, RR more than 30 per min, Blood Leucocytes are less than $4x10^9$ /l or more than $12x10^9$ /l) Needs 2 from the four (T, HR, RR, BL) [ACC/SCCM -1992]
4. site infection + local inflammatory reaction + general inflammatory reaction (t° is less than 36°C or more than 38.5°C , HR more than 90 per min, RR more than 30 per min, Blood Leucocytes are less than $4x10^9$ /l or more than $12x10^9$ /l) + multi-organ insufficiency. [ACC/SCCM -1992]
5. site infection + local inflammatory reaction + general inflammatory reaction (t° is less than 36°C or more than 38.5°C , HR more than 90 per min, RR more than 30 per min, Blood Leucocytes less than $4x10^9$ /l or more than $12x10^9$ /l) + septic shock [ACC/SCCM -1992]

AF – Additional Factors,

The Additional Factors which have an influence on the process of decision-making for AB prescribing, include such things as:-

- Allergy (foods, previous drugs, other)
- Previous (during previous 3 months) AB usage
- Age (1-st year infants; patients over 65 y)
- Weight more than 90 kg
- COPD, smoking
- Diabetes Mellitus
- Haemorrhage 1500 ml and more, anemia
- Immunocompromised status (Splenectomy, AIDS, EID, Oncology, Postpartum)
- And so on - according to the significance for a definite disease.

The type of AF determines the choice of the rule for making the decision.

The seven new protocols for AB prescribing were created and implemented at the Clinical Hospital N40 over a 5 year period (for adults with severe pneumonia or bacterial meningitis; and for the newborns with risk of, or with the signs of, infection; and others).

The model for calculating the drug cost for the treatment of patients with the Swine-flu Virus H1N1, or with infection complications as AIDS patients, were based on the discussed Classification of Clinical Events.

Results

1. The percentage of the mortality among the patients with severe Pneumonia in the Intensive Care Units was reduced from 15.4% (before the implementation of the Protocol) to 7.2% (after the first 2 years of implementation of the Protocol), i.e. the implementation of the Protocol gave a substantial saving (50%) in the lives of the adult patients with severe pneumonia.
2. Microbiological monitoring in the newborn's stool-samples before the year 2005, and during the first year's implementation of the new restricted AB Protocols (1st, 2nd, 3rd quarters of 2006), gave a reduction in contamination of the stool samples by Candida Albicans by a factor of 6 .
3. By using the Protocol, the percentage of the AB prescribing mistakes, made by the physicians in the Intensive Care Units, was reduced from 30% (2004y) to 5% (2008y).

Conclusions

1. During the years 2005-2008, the implementation of the AB prescribing Protocols (Levels 1, 2, 3, 4, 5) brought an improvement in the quality of Clinical Practice and Clinical Results.
2. This research showed the applicability of such approach for constructing the Protocols for AB prescribing and for evaluation of the compliance with those protocols.
3. Through using the EHR, this research confirms the applicability of the Clinical Events Classification according to the five universal classes, and it thus forms an adaptive platform for personalized health services for communication with the physicians as well as with the patients. Further it enables the Hospital Authorities to control the quality of the healthcare and to regulate the drug assistance in a trustworthy environment on the basis of information technology.

References

[1] Novik IB, Abdullaev AS. Introduction to the Information World. Moscow: Science; 1991.
[2] Bukalov AV. About structures and quantation of the psycho-informational space. Synchronica. – Presentation at the XIV International Conference of Socionic. Kiev. 1998 Sep 19-26.
[3] Glancer M., Razel M. The size of a unit in short-term storage. J.Verb.Learn 1974;13.
[4[Miller G. The magical Number Seven, Plus Or Minus Two: Some Limits on Our Capacity for Information Processing. The Psychology Review 1956;63(2)
[5] Davis E. Attitudes to Electronic Prescribing // Current Perspectives in Healthcare Computing 2000. Weybridge (UK): BJHC; 2000. p. 211-219.

Medical and Care Compunetics 6
L. Bos et al. (Eds.)
IOS Press, 2010

doi:10.3233/978-1-60750-565-5-171

Patient Opportunities in the Estonian Electronic Health Record System

Madis TIIK, MD[a,1] Peeter ROSS, MD[b]
[a]*Tartu University, Estonian eHealth Foundation*
[b]*Tallinn University of Technology, East Tallinn Central Hospital*

Abstract. Estonia is the first country which has implemented a nationwide electronic health record system and gives full access to its citizens. This provides new opportunities to citizens, healthcare providers and e-health developers. Combining health data, citizens' self added health and welfare data, decision support and possibilities of service oriented architecture of the Estonian Electronic Health Record System – a new era of e-health services can begin.

Keywords. Nationwide electronic health record system, access rights, integrated EHR, patient's rights, health portal, patient's portal, patient empowerment.

Introduction

The Estonian Electronic Health Record System (hereafter EHR) is a globally unique EHR system as it encompasses the whole country, registers virtually all residents' medical history from birth to death, and is based on the comprehensive state-developed basic IT infrastructure [1,2,3]. The Estonian nationwide EHR was launched on 17th of December 2008. Since 1st of January 2009 all healthcare providers have an obligation to send agreed number of standardized medical documents to the EHR. The content of the information stored centrally is indicated by the legislation. Electronic documents are formalized as standard HL7 CDA documents that are stored in a central database (i.e. archived electronically). The person compiling the medical document has to be identifiable: documents containing medical information or a physician's decision must have the physician's digital signature, or it must be date-stamped by health care service provider's information system. Regardless of more than ten years history of digital collection of medical data by doctors, the medical data collected prior to 1st of January 2009was not transferred to the EHR due to its poor quality and insufficient standardization.

The purpose of this article is to give an overview of the Estonian EHR system, and based on the first year's experience of full deployment of the system analyse the initial results for citizens.

[1]Corresponding Author: Madis Tiik, Estonian eHealth Foundation, Lastekodu 6a, 10113, Estonia; E-mail: madis@e-tervis.ee

1. Materials and Methods

1.1. EHR– Overview of the System

The EHR is a database that is a part of the state information system. The health care related data is processed in this database in order to conclude and execute the health care services provision contract, ensure patients' rights, protect public health and quality of health care services, to maintain the registers of health conditions as well as to manage health care [4].

To secure the access to the EHR, the Estonian countrywide data exchange platform X-Road is used [5]. X-Road is based on a principle of using one integral set of user interfaces for organizing communication with databases (see Figure 1). The system ensures sufficient security for the treatment of inquiries made to databases and responses received. It is suitable for managing a dialogue between the consumer (citizen, civil servant and entrepreneur) and numerous databases as well as for realizing cooperation between application programs and databases. The technical solution of the project does not lie in the transition of all databases to some larger data management system, but in the creation of unified user interfaces for different databases. Citizens and institutions can join and use the X-Road free of charge. Identification of the person is based on the compulsory ID-card issued by the state. ID-card is used both for identification of the user and for digital signing of documents, e.g. discharge letters, radiology reports, etc. According to the Health Information System Statute, the processor of the EHR is the Ministry of Social Affairs, and the authorized processor of the EHR is the Estonian eHealth Foundation [4].

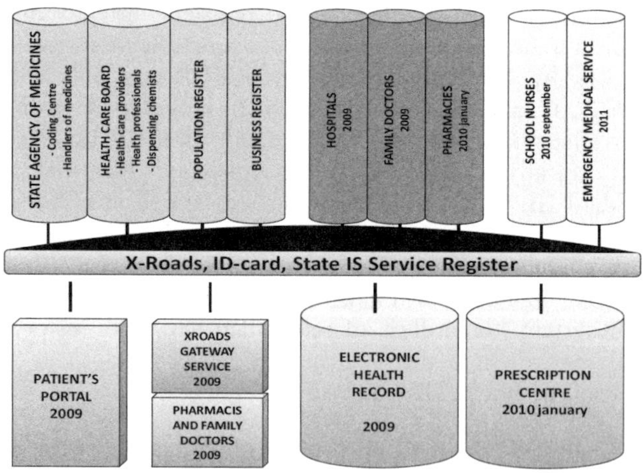

Figure 1. EHR partners and integration through secure data layer X-Road

1.2. Access Rights

- All healthcare providers must send agreed data to EHR.
- All access rights and data usage is regulated by the law.
- ID-card for authentication and digital signature for both, doctors and citizens.
- Access is enabled only to licensed medical professionals.
- The attending doctor concept – an attending physician is a health care employee currently associated with patient's treatment and registered with the Health Care Board.
- Citizens can access their own data through Patient's Portal, where they can also declare their intentions and preferences. Patient has a right to set access restrictions to documents, cases of illness, and to all his/her information in the EHR. The access ban can be set to one specific document or applied to the complete data in the EHR.
- The EHR will record information about when, how, and why the data was used (logging information), enabling citizens to monitor who has viewed their health data.

1.3. Services of EHR

The EHR is built according to the best practices of Service Orientation. Services of the system are based on standards that Estonian eHealth Foundation publishes openly on its website.

Interaction with end users is established via alternative channels. Also, there are portals that are served by the Estonian eHealth Foundation (e.g., Patient's Portal). There are also various information systems that are connected to the central EHR messaging services. The messaging standard is openly available for healthcare institutions, specialized healthcare registries and others, and they have taken advantage of this possibility to connect to EHR for message exchange.

The EHR processes messages according to regulated validation and security requirements.

Authorized messaging client of the EHR can benefit from the following services (Figure 2):

- Health event service enables to browse and search for health related events of patient treatment history. Health related events are for example diagnosis, visit, prescription, operation, diagnostic image, etc.
- Health status service enables to fetch information about certain health related parameters of a patient. These parameters are for example blood type, pregnancy, allergy, height, weight, smoking, etc.
- Booking service enables healthcare service providers to publish information about their healthcare services and available resources, so that doctors of other institutions and patients can book for appointments at these providers. Booking service keeps track of referrals and appointments.
- Reporting service provides users with prebuilt reports about patient health status. Here one can find so-called Time Critical Report that summarizes information about patient's health events and health status in a way most useful for emergency treatment.

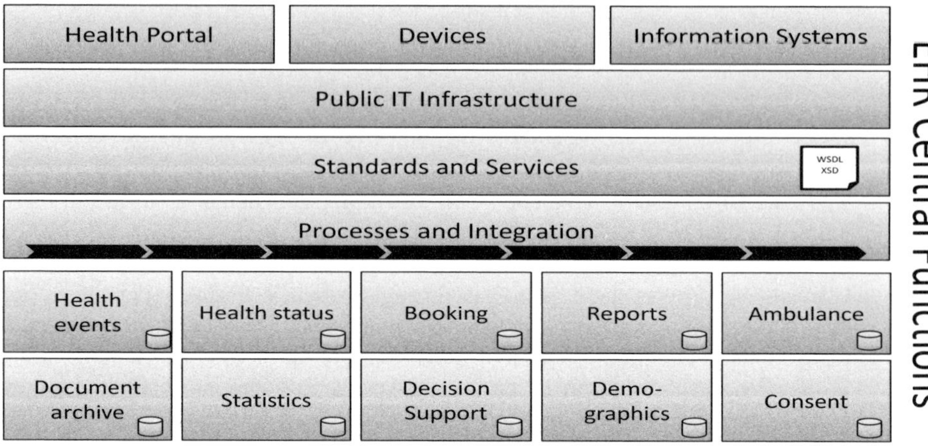

Figure 2. Functional Architecture of EHR

- Document archive service organizes all digital documents that are submitted to the central system. One can fetch a document by ID from a document archive.
- Statistics service reorganizes facts from patient health related documents for further statistical processing.
- Demographics service collects and reports general information about patient identity, locations, and relationships. The information is based on the data of the Estonian Population Registry, registration documents from healthcare institutions, and information submitted via Patient's Portal.
- Consent service maintains data about patients' will expressed in digital documents. Currently there are trustee access rights, healthcare service options, and health record access rights related consents implemented.

Patient's Portal (Figure 3) allows patient representatives (adult patient, parent of an underage, legal representative, trustee) to browse patient's health record, download documents, submit consents, update demographics data, book an appointment, and review patient health record usage logs via Web.

2. Results

More than350 000 medical documents, including about 10% of patient summaries, were sent to the EHR during 2009. Altogether 953 general practitioners (GP), private health care specialists, and hospitals have connected to EHR during the first year, and this number represents 90% of all health care institutions in Estonia. By the end of 2009, 143360 citizens had a medical document in the EHR. As of January 1st of 2010, this number has rapidly increased with additional 114 012 citizens due to the launch of the digital prescription. The population of Estonia is 1,304,021, meaning that by the

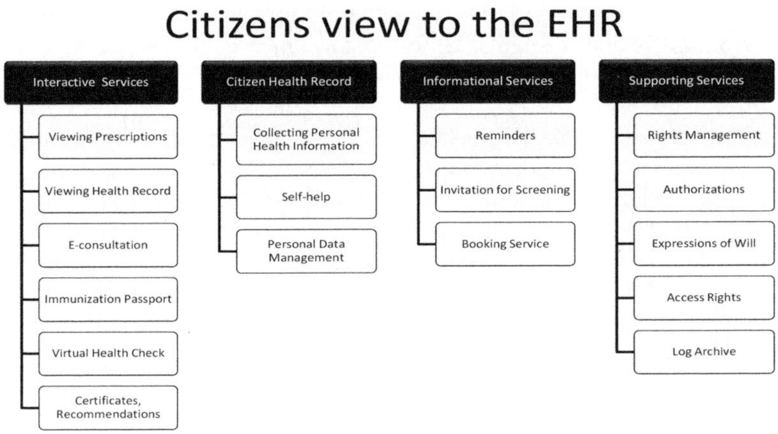

Figure 3. Health Portal functionalities.

end of January 2010twenty percent of citizens had some type of medical record in the EHR [6].

According to the law, all citizens have full access to data collected in the EHR [4]. For that function a Web-based Patient's Portal was launched on October 26 of 2009. During the first five months the portal was visited by 12993 citizens. This accounts for 1% of the Estonian population as of January 1st of 2010. There has not been any public campaign for citizens on how to use the Patient's Portal, and so far the information has been given by the doctors.

3. Discussion

Creating secure and easy internet access to patients' health data will increase patients' awareness of their health. Citizens can get an overview of their recent doctor's appointments, laboratory tests, and medical reports, etc. This allows patients to make more informed decisions about their health behaviour or prepare more thoroughly for the appointment with the health care professional. Citizens can also record their expressions of will (e.g., donation of organs, permit blood transfusion) or choose preferences which increases their involvement in decision making process related to their health condition.

The experience of implementation of EHR in Estonia has shown that technically and organisationally the task is achievable in a relatively short period. However, realising concrete benefits for patients, health care personnel, and society depend on the completeness and quality of the data in the central system. In our experience this is achievable only in the case when the common standards are used, and the majority of health care institutions connect to the EHR in a relatively short period. In Estonia the health care providers were obligated to interface with the EHR because of the recent amendments to the Health Services Organization Act. Despite this fact, there has been a considerable amount of reluctance among the health care providers to interface with the EHR. According to the feedback from the health care managers, it was mainly because interfacing with the EHR demanded additional information technology investments from GP's and hospitals. Unfortunately, the benefit of this investment is not realised in a short term, and thus hardly acceptable from an economical point of view.

The implementation of the EHR has increased the use of information technology in health care institutions. To overcome the potential problems caused by the inefficacious knowledge of computer skills among the personnel, several training programs for the health care professionals were carried out during the first year. Programs included training in computer skills, gave an overview of security regulations, and taught participants how to use the EHR. However, there still seems to be a quite large number of health professionals who are not fully satisfied with the design and functionality of the EHR.

The number of citizens who have used the Patient's Portal to view their own health data during the first four months is relatively low. This is not surprising, because the launch of this new service was not accompanied by wide public campaign. The information about the Patient's Portal is given to citizens by health care professionals. The reason for discreet introduction of the Patient's Portal is the unawareness of the influence of this service to patient behaviour and physician-patient relation. Also, there are different opinions among the health care professionals about the usefulness of sharing the health data openly with patients. However, the first experience is that citizens are accepting the Web-based access to their health data, and there have been no remarkable drawbacks.

The EHR can also provide a number of different services using decision support engine, existing medical documents, and citizen's added information. As an example, certificate for driver's license could be one of those. Another possible new intelligent service is a reminder service, which means sending an automatic SMS or e-mail remainder about the next visit to the doctor or to the lab to give a blood sample.

In further development the EHR can also provide data from the Estonian Genome Centre [7]. However, for that we need several new services. Firstly, consent on person's willingness to know their gene data. Secondly, we need a consent which allows the Genome Centre to send data to the EHR. The third possible service in this area could be an updating of personal health data for gene donors.

All these services with full access to the EHR give citizens more reliable information about their health status, and provide possibilities for an adequate care process. However, it also means more responsibility and commitments for citizens.

4. Conclusion

Electronic access to the shared health database increases the role of patient in the diagnostic and treatment processes. Health care providers should become more responsive to patients' needs and preferences and deliver better quality of care. Patients', having more adequate and related information about their health, can participate in the health care in many new ways. This includes communicating directly to healthcare professionals by using information on health and health care through internet channels, mobile devices, etc.

This might lead to a situation where patients start taking more control over their illnesses and treatments where possible.

Patients are given information in the belief that this will enable informed choices. Finally, this will lead to healthy behaviour and decrease cost of healthcare in the country.

Estonia has taken a big step in this direction and has potential to be the first country were patient is the main driving force of their personal health issues.

References

[1] [Online] Available from: URL: http://www.ehealth-era.org/documents/2007ehealth-era-countries.pdf.

[2] [Online] Available from: URL: http://www.epsos.eu/country-profile.html.

[3] [Online] Available from: URL: http://www.itif.org/files/2009-leadership-healthit.pdf.

[4] [Online] Health Services Organization Act and Associated Acts Amendment Act (available only in Estonian). Available from: URL: https://www.riigiteataja.ee/ert/act.jsp?id=12909773.

[5] [Online] Available from: URL: http://www.riso.ee/en/pub/2003it/p34.htm.

[6] [Online] Available from: URL: http://eng.e-tervis.ee/news/overview-2.html.

[7] [Online] Available from: URL: http://www.geenivaramu.ee/index.php?lang=eng.

Patient Empowerment

Medical and Care Compunetics 6
L. Bos et al. (Eds.)
IOS Press, 2010

doi:10.3233/978-1-60750-565-5-181

Holism, Health and Data – Managing the Person-centred Digital Haystack

Michael RIGBY[1]
School of Public Policy and Professional Practice; and Public Policy and Management Research Institute, Keele University, Keele, UK.

Abstract. There is currently very legitimate pressure to change the function of health information systems to more explicitly serve and support the individual. Concurrently other support services to health, including condition monitoring, social care and intelligent housing, add to the complexity of patient health related data. A paradigm shift is needed, to recognize that many agencies and systems outside as well as within the health sector all work to support the citizen's health, yet the essential integrated view is not being provided, even though much needed not least by the citizen and their agents. Broker technologies can enable this new paradigm. Moreover, a move to identifying the patient's appointments and support services would enable a daily life dimension to be given due weight, and would recognize the patient's viewpoint in wanting to live an ordered life, not one subservient and reactive to the delivery of care by providers.

Keywords. Health, integration, holistic care, broker technology, patient diary

Introduction

The focus of this conference of the ICMCC on considering the patient (or citizen) as the focus of health data, with integration and ontology as the refocused enablers, is clearly logical as being how the patient sees the situation. Instead of record systems or informatics driving, the citizen view prevails – technology is to be harnessed for the service of the citizen, and not the citizen adjusting to suit the information system. This is as commendable and logical as it is unusual.

However, it does raise a range of challenges which appear daunting – but not impossible. This paper argues that addressing the radical change in viewpoint is necessary in order to seek to develop alternative solutions, and the solutions are attainable.

1. A Holistic View of Health

It is clear both from the citizen's viewpoint, and from the WHO constitutional definition, that "health" is not solely about medical treatment, but is "a state of physical, mental, and social wellbeing and not merely the absence of disease or infirmity" [1]. It

[1]Professor Michael Rigby, Emeritus Professor of Health Information Strategy, School of Public Policy and Professional Practice, Chancellor's Building, Keele University, Keele, Staffordshire, ST5 5BG, United Kingdom, e-mail: m.j.rigby@keele.ac.uk

is important to appreciate that maintaining health involves far more than the services of formal health agencies. As pointed out in a recent paper to the Medical Informatics Europe conference advocated the closer working of social care services and their records with health systems, where a person suffers from a long-term or chronic illness, or where aspects of impaired daily living affect health, supporting services are needed to complement health care in order to maintain the health of the individual [2].

It is illogical, disadvantageous for individual citizens and inefficient for services, to consider healthcare as the only service domain to support health. The logical extension to this is that where other agencies are also keeping electronic records or using other automated information processing support such as automated monitoring, then these must be linked round the patient as a part of citizen-orientated informatics to support health.

2. The Panoply of Partners

Though social care services have been highlighted as a key partner in supporting person health, it is by no means the only one. Figure 1 below shows the range of services which can be involved in supporting the individual.

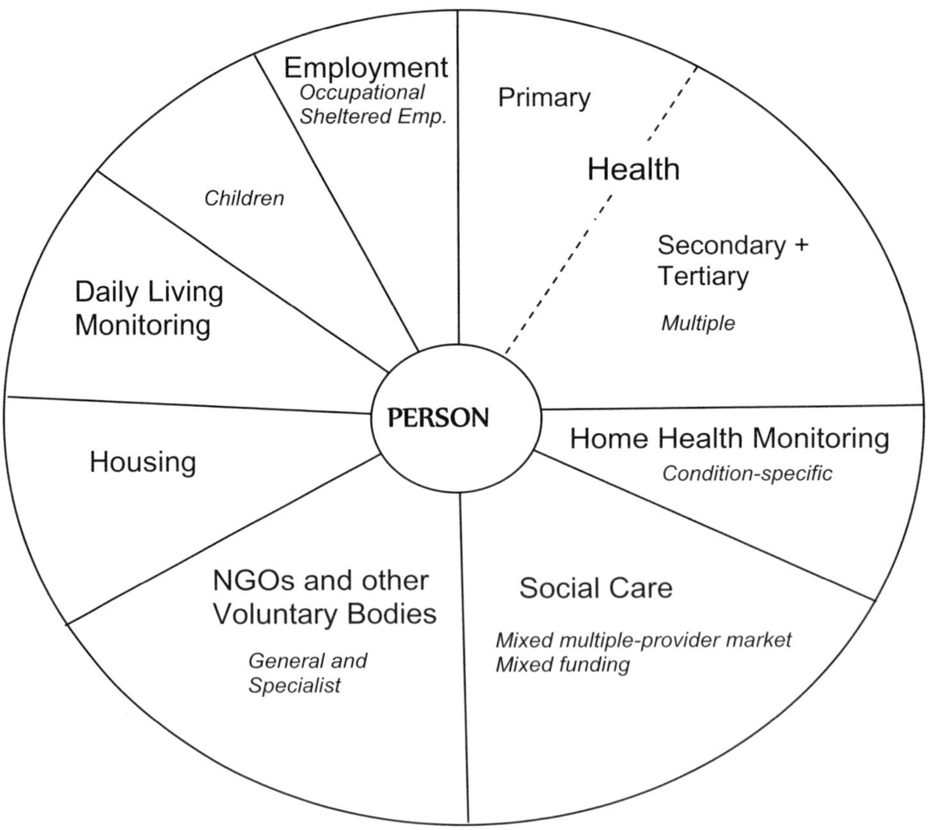

Figure 1. Potential Providers and Users of Individuals' Health Data

In theory almost all of these could be involved in supporting one individual. Indeed, this is increasingly likely to be the case with the increase in frail elderly, and in persons with chronic diseases able to be supported at home.

However, the nature and characteristics of the records and data sets about the citizen generated and used by these services vary widely. The major differences between health and social care data sets have been already elaborated [2, 3, 4]. Other services' data are equally different. In particular, automated monitoring data are large in volume, low in explicit confidentially, but of no use unless rapidly monitored and interpreted, with appropriate action being taken. By contrast, social care data are organizationally complex, with a mixed economy of providers, and with both central (public sector or insurance) and personal commissioning. Some records may lack technical detail, but the attitudinal and aspirational information contained is vital to healthy and fulfilling life.

Table 1 below summarizes the principle differences between the data characteristics of the eight different services shown in Figure 1.

Table 1. Mixed Characteristics of Health Support Services' Data

Data Source/Type	**Data Characteristics**
Health	Highly confidential Single data subject Mixed types
Home Health Monitoring	Vital signs or similar Usually disease/condition specific. High volumes of quantitative data Needs critical threshold rapid analysis
Social Care	Shallower and simple Largely text and terms Multiple data subjects Multiple providers to an individual
NGOs and other Voluntary Bodies	Need appropriate records for delivering services Increasingly important for social and caring activities Autonomous
Housing	Provide shelter or support functions Warden needs to know limitations, risks, referral signs
Daily Living Monitoring	Data driven Mixed data, different meanings and sensitivities Near-real time interpretation important Algorithm (or human monitoring) based May include video.
Education	Primarily for children Need to know for case management, limitations, risks, action needed
Employment	Need to know to know limitations, risks, referral signs Separate occupational health records Independent of the health sector

2.1. The Consequent Data Linkage and Sharing Challenge

Viewed from the viewpoint of an individual service, the issues of automation and electronic records are challenging because of the variety and complexity of human conditions and circumstances, but not impossible. However, putting them into an integrated format is seriously challenging – but essential to support the citizen holistically and seamlessly.

Challenges include:

- Patient identifier
- Meaning, terms, and mutual understanding
- Multiple data subjects (in different combinations)
- Trust (of content accuracy)
- Motivation; conflicts of interest
- Liability (for actions taken on external data)
- Data volumes
- Relative decay; retention needs and policies
- Resolving conflicts and inconsistencies.

The relative difficulty in resolving these will depend on the integration solutions, and in the relationships between the organizations, and of their staff. But the over-riding wake-up call when all seems difficult must be that the patient-citizen has one integrated life, and that if agencies have conflicts then these directly impact on the citizen who is worried and dependent.

3. The Potential of Broker Technology

Too often, one of only four options are considered - full integration (likely to be organizationally and practically impossible); separate data stores (compromising the integration objective); some form of distillation or summary (but who knows what will be important to whom ahead of the unanticipated crisis event?); or full interoperability (likely to be unacceptable across domains due to lack of control).

A broker system – as increasingly used in commercial systems used by consumers, such as travel booking and price comparisons – looks highly attractive, but seems to be little pursued due to lack of organizational 'ownership'. This technology enables each type of record to be kept and acted upon by its own agents and users. However, any authorized care delivery user can have role-specific access to a broker service (requiring only a browser as the core service is web-based) through which they can call up specific data subsets from specified partner systems; if necessary taxonomy mapping can be built in to come closer to a common language. The core data are undisturbed, the user acts and records their action solely in their own system, but by definition the results can be viewed by other partners using the broker themselves.

This solution has been researched in the UK and the results presented [5-7]. These findings look promising, but funding of a pilot is compromised because of the cross-domain nature. Perversely, no single agency is responsible for the citizen's overall health support.

The advantages of a broker include the fact that local systems are undisturbed, monolithic systems are avoided, and levels of access and viewing can be determined by each professional user, data-holding organization, and the data subject themselves. This leads to a double win – services can continue to manage their own data, yet a truly patient-centric picture is obtained when and where needed. Moreover, the difficult challenges of external interoperability can be avoided. [8].

Above all, though, the broker solution exemplifies and reinforces the person-centered philosophy, as well as the person-centric view of the health-related data. This solution recognizes the special needs of individual service providers, the different nature of each data set, but supersedes their storage formats by enabling the patient-based view.

3.1. The Patient-centric Paradigm

Moving to put the patient at the centre requires first and foremost a change in philosophy.

Figure 2 below shows the traditional paradigm, in which the organization serves the patient, but the composite group of patients is seen as secondary to the organization that acts as a pivot. The individual is peripheral to several organizations; their data (and their care) are small – indeed insignificant - parts of each provider' activity.

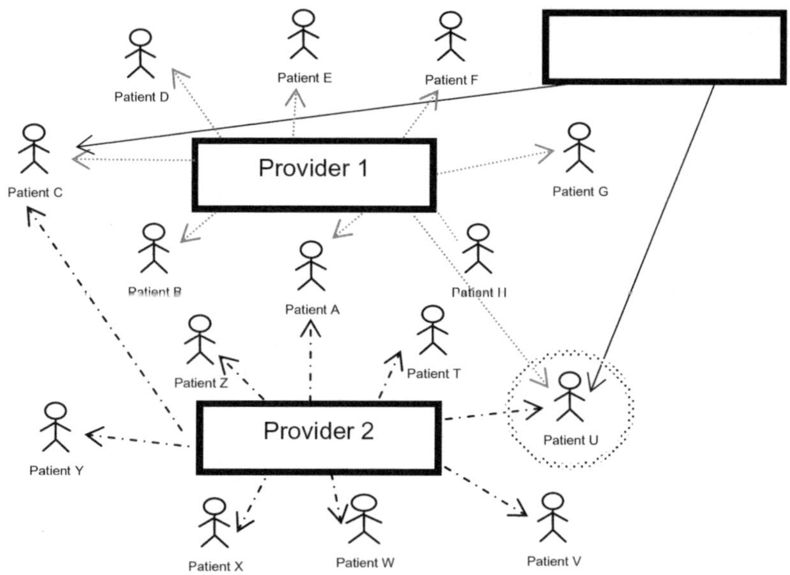

Figure 2. Providers' Traditional Views of Patients

However, the broker can achieve a radical change in this philosophy, without in any way changing the core organizational record systems. Using a broker enables a patient-oriented view to be obtained by the professional or patient's agent, within whichever organization they are located. This is shown in Figure 3; the patient is now central, and the organizations contribute respective parts of the care and support.

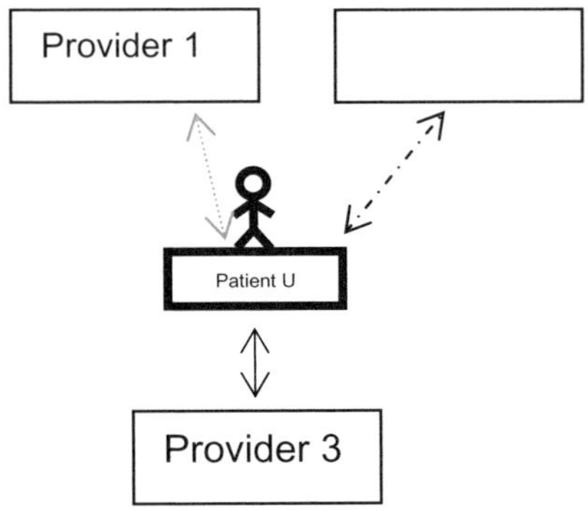

Figure 3. The Patient-centric View of Care Data

This uses exactly the same data as in Figure 2, from the same organizations, but it is drawn into a single need-specified integrated view. The organizations' systems, and their data recording, are not in any way changed, except that they have permitted controlled access to a trusted broker, and the access control is a composite of that of each contributing organization and that of the broker service – the most important of which are authentication, authority, and role at point of use.

4. A Patient Diary as a Potential Valuable Tool

While bringing together all the health and health support data round the patient brings challenges as described, it could also bring one important patient view solution – the schedule or diary. For each of the services described in Figure 1 and Table 1, and portrayed in Figures 2 and 3, there is a schedule of activity. This is currently predominantly organization-driven – the patient is given an appointment for the service of that provider (including domiciliary services), with only limited patient choice. Organizations manage their resources autonomously, and thus the patient is the only one who can seek to coordinate the different providers – with limited influence and success. Domiciliary appointments may cluster, hospital appointments may clash with other desirable activities, and the patient has no one overall schedule of what is planned for them. Frail, confused, or young patients may feel particularly confused and overwhelmed. Patient moderation of this is limited, thus wasting resources when a person knows that they will be away, have visitors, or when they are ill.

A patient diary, visible to all providers with a need to know, but also to the citizen and to family and informal cares of their choice, would be a major gain. Patients should also be able to input key events, which would feed to care providers if there was an impact. This would be a major improvement in quality of care, and would go a long way to making services user-friendly by understanding and fitting into their lives. The complexity of detailed record data would be at a different level, and the patient would simply see a manifestation of what was happening with and for them – true integration of care in terms clear and useful to the service user. The ideas have been previously expounded, but it is the linking of different services round the patient which could bring it to life with significant added value [9-11].

5. The Issues of Access

The bringing together of data from different sources in a patient-friendly format and with user-grounded ontologies will raise issues of access. Clearly it will be essential for the patient to be able to view most if not all of their data, though means of simplifying this and enabling interpretation will be important (without creating the potential to provide a smokescreen). But many patients will be frail, or for other reasons seek to share their problems with supportive carers. Two types of issue must be resolved – but the solution is common.

5.1. Carer Access

Members of the care team, including neighbors and informal carers, should be able to access parts of the record(s), and diary, in order to optimize their caring and their advice. But it should be the prerogative of the data subject citizen to decide who can see what, according to personal patterns of trust.

5.2. Family and Relative Access

Many family members will be anxious to support their loved ones, particularly elderly parents, by seeing what is happening to them. Not least, remote access to monitoring results may be helpful. However, it must not be assumed that all relatives are either benevolent or caring, nor should the autonomy of the individual be eroded just because they are older. Thus, unless there is an approved power of attorney order in place for someone who is known to be mentally compromised, relatives should be treated no differently to other third parties. It should be the citizen's unfettered right to decide who can see what.

Thus, for either aspect of third party access, the patient's wishes must prevail. A broker system front-end could facilitate this by being able to record, and then apply, the patient's wishes.

6. New View, New Paradigm

Many commentators see the bringing together of data of different types and different agencies into one holistic health support picture round the individual as impossible technically, and impractical. Indeed, if data pooling is considered the only solution, or indeed full interoperability across sectors, this is likely to be true. But it is essential to see health and care from a citizen viewpoint, as a part of their daily lives, articulated at least in part in vernacular terms. Therefore, if progress is to be made in the medium and long term, a complete new paradigm must be established which puts the citizen, and the planning of their care, at the center. All views should come from this, and should be expressed in plans and schedules as much as in historical analyses. Moreover, the technologies for this exist already – the challenge is changing traditional organizational-based view points to patient-centered ones, and concurrently changing the technology focus from data capture and recording into one of data re-assembly on demand to meet specific viewpoint needs.

7. Conclusion

The future vision for sensitive, personalized patient care is usually expressed in terms of individual organization's approached to their relationship with patients, enabled by informatics system interoperability. At the same time, there is a realization expressed by those familiar with patient needs to encourage patient involvement, including access to their records. But most of this activity is related to the health domain, while the issues of other supporters of the health of the citizen are not considered. The true goal should be to see holistically the full range of services which support citizen health, and to see these as the citizen does. A broker approach can achieve this, using technologies already familiar to many citizens. Moreover, a diary-based element would enable a transition from treating illness and problems, to interweaving support for health into daily life and future thinking.

References

[1] World Health Organization. Constitution of the World Health Organization Basic Documents. 45th ed; Supplement. Geneva; Oct 2006
[2] Rigby M, Hill P, Koch S, Kärki J. Social Care Informatics – the Missing Partner in eHealth. Proceedings of Medinfo; 2009.
[3] Hill P, Allman A, Rigby M, Wilson R. Social Care Informatics: Beginning to Face up to the Reality of the Mixed Services Economy? In: Cunningham P, Cunningham M, editors. Collaboration and the Knowledge Economy. Amsterdam: IOS Press; 2008. p. 14-21.
[4] Rigby M, Hill P, Allman A. Ensuring Trust and Governance in E-Social Care. In: Cunningham P, Cunningham M, editors. Collaboration and the Knowledge Economy. Amsterdam: IOS Press; 2008. p. 22-28.
[5] Budgen D, Rigby MJ, Brereton O, Turner M. A Data Integration Broker for Healthcare Systems. IEEE Computer 2007 Apr;40(4):34-41.
[6] Rigby M, Budgen D, Brereton P, Bennett K, Russell MJ, Turner M, Kotsiopoulos I, Layzell P, Keane J, Zhu F. The Data-Gathering Broker as a Future-Oriented Approach to Supporting EPR Users, Int J Med Inform 2007;76:137-44.
[7] Budgen D, Turner M, Kotsiopoulos I, Zhu F, Russell M, Rigby M, Bennett KL, Brereton P, Keane J, Layzell P. Managing healthcare information: the role of the broker. In: From Grid to Healthgrid. Proceedings of Healthgrid; 2005 Apr; Oxford, United Kingdom. Amsterdam: IOS Press; 2005. p. 3-16
[8] Rigby M. Citizens, Seamlessness, and Care - Inter-relationships and Inter-operability. Submission to EFMI STC Special Conference; Reykjavik; 2010.
[9] Rigby M. A Patient Care Electronic Diary to Empower the Patient and their Virtual Care Team. In: Cunningham P, Cunningham M, editors. Collaboration and the Knowledge Economy: Issues, Applications, Case Studies; Amsterdam: IOS Press; 2008. p. 57-63.
[10] Rigby M, Robins S. Practical Success of an Electronic Patient Record System in Community Care - A Manifestation of the Vision and Discussion of the Issues. Int J Biomed Comput 1996;42:117-22.
[11] Robins SC, Rigby MJ. Opportunities for community services provided by integrated electronic patient records and critical success factors for achieving this in practice. In: Van der Lei J, Beckers WPA, editors. Strategic Alliances between Patient Documentation and Medical Informatics. Proceedings AMICE 95 Conference; 2005. Rotterdam: VMBI/TMI Bureau; 1995.

Medical and Care Compunetics 6
L. Bos et al. (Eds.)
IOS Press, 2010

doi:10.3233/978-1-60750-565-5-189

The Mixed Management of Patients' Medical Records: Responsibility Sharing Between the Patient and the Physician

Catherine QUANTIN[a,b1], Maniane FASSA[b], Eric BENZENINE[b], David-Olivier JAQUET-CHIFFELLE[c], Gouenou COATRIEUX[d], François-André ALLAERT[b,e]

[a] *Inserm, U866, Dijon, F-21000, Univ de Bourgogne, Dijon, F-21000, France*
[b] *CHRU, Service de Biostatistique et d'Informatique Médicale, Dijon, France*
[c] *Bern University of Applied Sciences et Université de Lausanne, Suisse*
[d] *Institut TELECOM ; TELECOM Bretagne ; Unité INSERM 650 LaTIM*
[e] *Ceren Esc Dijon & Dpt biostat Ecole de Santé Publique Liège Belgique*

Abstract: Through this article, we propose a mixed management of patients' medical records, so as to share responsibilities between the patient and the Medical Practitioner by making Patients responsible for the validation of their administrative information, and MPs responsible for the validation of their Patients' medical information. Our proposal can be considered a solution to the main problem faced by patients, health practitioners and the authorities, namely the gathering and updating of administrative and medical data belonging to the patient in order to accurately reconstitute a patient's medical history. This method is based on two processes. The aim of the first process is to provide a patient's administrative data, in order to know where and when the patient received care (name of the health structure or health practitioner, type of care: out patient or inpatient). The aim of the second process is to provide a patient's medical information and to validate it under the accountability of the Medical Practitioner with the help of the patient if needed. During these two processes, the patient's privacy will be ensured through cryptographic hash functions like the Secure Hash Algorithm, which allows pseudonymisation of a patient's identity. The proposed Medical Record Search Engines will be able to retrieve and to provide upon a request formulated by the Medical Practitioner all the available information concerning a patient who has received care in different health structures without divulging the patient's identity. Our method can lead to improved efficiency of personal medical record management under the mixed responsibilities of the patient and the MP.

Keywords: medical record, patient identifier, direct access, data security, privacy, E-health

Introduction

The challenges of gathering and updating patients' administrative and medical data so as to reconstitute patients' medical histories, in order to improve their health care and ensure the success of public health strategies, are being discussed and analysed by

[1] Correspondance: Catherine.quantin@chu-dijon.fr

national, European and international health authorities. However, the main problem faced by patients, health practitioners and the authorities is to gather and update the correct administrative and medical data belonging to the right patient, and not anybody else, so as to reconstitute the patient's medical history accurately. Today it is technically possible worldwide to reconstitute almost automatically any patient's health care history if at least three conditions are met:

- The existence of appropriate tools for requests
- Guarantees of the interoperability of patient identification data through health structures and guarantees that the patient's health information relates to the patient [1].
- The possibility of correcting and updating patients' health information.

Thus, the administrative and medical data that have been requested must be validated to avoid errors. The first error type concerns the impossibility to gain access to some patient data due to modifications in identifying information because of a marriage (marital name) or a divorce (own family name), for example. The second error type concerns requests for data that belong to another patient, when there are collisions between the identification data of two different patients, which should be very rare if identifiers have been chosen carefully.

Thus, to avoid ethical problems such as consequences related to providing information that relates to another patient, this validation cannot be provided by the Medical Practitioner (MP) acting alone. Patients can confirm where and when they have benefited from health care. Patients who are in good mental health, can reconstitute, verify and update their administrative information more authentically, accurately, and precisely than anybody else. Of course, patients can seek help from the MP if needed. Furthermore, the MP is the only person who can verify the medical coherence of the requested data. MPs know better than anybody else about the disease and medical information of a patient they have cared for for many years.

This is why we propose to rely on the patient for administrative data and on the MP for medical data. As a consequence, we propose in this article the mixed management of patients' medical records, sharing responsibilities between the patient and the MP by making:

- the patient or the patient's legal representative responsible for the validation and updating of a patient's administrative information
- the MP (with the collaboration of the patient if needed) accountable for the validation and updating of a patient's medical information

Of course, in the case of mental handicap, an emergency or a new MP, through our proposed methodology, we suggest appropriate solutions made possible thanks to the existing medical history, current and former health structures and practitioners and the patient's family members, as shown in some recent studies.

The main objective, of this paper is then to propose a new method to reconstitute, update and provide the correct administrative and medical data belonging to a certain patient through the mixed management of patients' medical records. This will empower patients with regard to the management of their health data by increasing their responsibility [2-3], and increase the accountability of MPs concerning the medical data. The second objective, which is no less important, is to avoid ethical problems resulting from giving a patient access to the data of another patient (mistaking patients). We aim to correct and update patients' health information, so as to reconstitute the data efficiently with little if any increase in MPs' workload and with maximum authenticity and precision in the patient's medical history.

1. Methods

Patients can be considered key elements in the validation of their first and second names, date of birth, the health structures visited and dates of visits. MPs should also be considered core elements in the processes of medical data validation. It means that patients and MPs should be made responsible for the successful validation of the reconstitution and updating of medical history (administrative and medical information) of the patient. The division of responsibilities between doctors and patients is very timely for decision making [4-10], but has not been extensively investigated regarding the management of patients' medical records.

This proposed methodology relies on two processes:
The first process aims to provide patients' administrative data, in order to know where and when patients have received care (name of the health structure or health practitioner, type of care: outpatient or inpatient).

Patients will be responsible for the validation of this information [11-12]. The first objective of this validation is to obtain the right information for the right patient at any time and anywhere and to be sure that the information concerns only the patient and to avoid providing information on another patient. Secondly, the validation of this information retrieval will provide the patient's medical history. During this validation process, the MP may confer with the patient.

The validation of this administrative information will be the exclusive responsibility of the patient, with the help of the MP if needed.

The main objective of the second process is to provide patients' medical information. The MP will be accountable for the validation of these medical data,, with the help of the patient, if needed. For the validation process to be successful and efficient, it will be useful to take into account the help patients are able to provide in terms of their thorough knowledge of their administrative and medical information. In fact, patients who have all their mental faculties know the history of the care they have received better than anybody else. Patients could regularly update administrative and medical data, for example, once or twice a year depending on the national public health strategies with regard to periodic citizen health check-ups initiated by national health authorities or employers, who offer a minimum package of services for prevention and the follow up of workers regarding transmissible and non-transmissible diseases, for example.

During these two processes, of course, patients' privacy has to be ensured
Patients' privacy is one of the main concerns in the storing, sharing or transmission of personal medical data and it is comprehensively covered by legal acts like the HIPAA in the United States or Directive 95/46/EC in Europe. Many companies including employers Insurers or Banks are very interested in gaining access to such data. Recently, attempts to gain illegal access to such data have been reported in the network. Thus, systems to share medical data through open networks like the Internet

need to prevent access to the identity of the patient. Pseudonymization is one of the solutions that have been suggested for this purpose. It provides a trade-off between patients' privacy requirements and society's needs in order to improve health care systems by linking the patient's identity to a pseudonym from which it is not possible to get back to the patient's identity [13].

Cryptographic hash functions like the Secure Hash Algorithm can be used to reach this goal [14]. However, sharing this pseudonym or code without introducing secrecy in its calculation may lead to specific attacks, in particular when the total number of possible messages that could have been hashed (pre-image) is too small. In this case, the authorized receiver as well as a pirate eavesdropping on the communication could retrieve private information. A pirate, who obtains lists of patients' pseudonyms, by illegal access or simply by listening to the Internet network, may be able to retrieve the real identity of the patients.

The solution we have proposed in [15] of using a medical record search engine procedure, which is illustrated in figure 1 and in the appendix, would counter such risks. In the first step, it encrypts the patient's pseudonym (H(PI)) and the secret key to be used for its decryption and, in the second step, sends them through two different channels. If gaining access to private information becomes more difficult for someone who is spying on the network, such as MRSE intruders, it will be almost as difficult for the MRSE and Aggregator entities involved in information gathering, and which may be tempted to obtain information illegally. Any attackers will face a set of patient pseudonyms without being able to identify those associated with the same patient. In fact, a one-time pseudonym will correspond to each request. This is the main interest of using pseudonyms in our proposal.

1.1. FIRST PROCESS: reconstitution of a patient's history

First step: Pseudonymisation of the patient's identity and generation of several pseudonymous codes.

During a consultation between an MP and a patient, the MP enters all the components of that patient's identification such as his first and last names and his date of birth. Of course, the choice of these components will depend on their availability (exhaustiveness) and their quality.

To optimize the request concerning the patient's data, several identifiers can be generated, based on the different combinations of first names, last names and date of birth of a patient as follows:

- If a patient has two last names such as in the case of a married woman or a child whose parents are divorced, one can create two identifiers (one for each last name).
- It is also possible to do the same for one patient who has two first names (like David Olivier or François André).

Thus, if a patient has, for example, two second names and two first names, the 4 combinations of these names can be used to create 4 identifiers.

This information related to the patient's identity will be rendered anonymous (Figure 1 and appendix), using a robust cryptographic hash function with a specific pad to provide 4 hashed patient identities called $H\ (PI)_1$, $H\ (PI)_2$, $H\ (PI)_3$ and $H\ (PI)_4$. To improve patient's privacy, the pad used for hash coding is not the same for each request. A specific pad S is generated by the first Medical Record Search Engine (MRS E 1) and sent to the MP, after being encrypted with the MP public key. The MP can then hash the patient's identifiers with this pad. As a consequence the MP sends not only one pseudonymous identifier per patient but a list of pseudonymous partial identifiers for each patient. The aim of this first step is then to obtain several pseudonymous codes, but, hopefully, always the same ones for a given individual in order to link all of the information concerning any given patient.

Second step: Searching for a patient's administrative data.
The Medical Record Search Engine Procedure [15] is used to provide a patient's administrative data (Figure 1 and appendix).

MRSE1 will send the pad S, once the pad had been encrypted with the health structure public key, to all health structures. Each health structure can then search for administrative information corresponding to these pseudonymous codes (by comparing them with hashed identities of the patients cared for in the structure). All the pseudonymous codes created from the different possible combinations of each possible first name, each possible last name and each possible date of birth are considered.

This administrative information will be sent to the MP, through the aggregator, according to Figure 1.

Third step: validation of a patient's administrative data by the patient
Any patient of sound mind is the only person who can confirm, where, when and for what reasons she/he has consulted for health problems: which health structure? At what time, time, day, month and year.

In case of patients with mental handicap, the MPs will help patients to confirm or not the doubtful administrative information, thanks to their experience with these patients and their diseases.

The doubtful administrative information may relate to:

- a long distance between the patient's residence and the health structure the patient supposedly visited,
- discordance between the type of health care provided by that hospital or clinic and the patient's disease. For example, a health structure that cares only for cancers and the patient's disease which is certainly not cancer!

An automatic check for the coherence of a patient's administrative information can be implemented so as to identify, for example, a patient who received care at the same moment (time, day, month year) in two different health structures. It can also check for the coherence of the distance between the patient residence and that health structure.

The main objective of this automatic check for coherence is not to exclude any information automatically, but to help the MP and the patient to highlight potential errors and correct them if necessary

At the end of this validation, the list of administrative information (pseudonymous codes, dates and health structures) to be conserved is transmitted to MRSE 2.

1.2. SECOND PROCESS: access to relevant medical data for patient care.

First step: searching for a patient's medical data.

The Medical Record Search Engine procedure is used to provide a patient's medical data (Figure 1 and appendix).

Each health structure selected by the first process can then search for medical information corresponding to the pseudonymous codes and the dates also selected by the first process.

This medical information will be sent to the MP, through the aggregator, according to Figure 1.

Second step: validation of patient's medical information by the MP

The MP is accountable for the validation of the medical information, with the close collaboration of the patient.

To validate the information, the MP can also rely on an automatic check for coherence of medical data so as to identify:

- Serious events happening simultaneously with less than two weeks interval between them, for example, myocardial infarction (heart attack), strokes (cerebral vascular accidents), and cancers
- Care in a health structure which does not provide care related to the patient's disease.

These events, situations, and doubtful information which have been identified must be confirmed or not by the MP, always with the close collaboration of the patient.

2. Discussion

Some medical practitioners may complain that this procedure will increase their workload because they will be obliged to read all of the information to detect possibly false or missing information. The burden is not as heavy as they may think for many reasons. First, this enquiry on the patient's past history will not be necessary for all patients and generally the contents of their local records are sufficient to treat the patient. Secondly, few patients (but it should be verified by a survey on a real situation) have been hospitalised in many different hospitals and therefore, the number of different medical records that MPs will have to summarise will more frequently be one or two (or eventually three) rather than ten or twenty. Third, it is important to take into account that this work has to be done in collaboration with the patient, who could provide great help in the management of his own records. For example, concerning the doubloon risk (if the patient was registered with different identities than those requested) and the subsequent risk of losing information, it is easy to ask patients if they have been hospitalised in hospitals other than those that answered the requests and provided information. This doubloon risk is reduced thanks to the use of several combinations of the different possible names of the patient. However, the risk of collision, (the amalgamation of two or more MRs from different patients) is then increased. It is usually easy, except in emergency situations, to ask patients if they have in fact been hospitalised in all the hospitals that provided parts of their medical records. This potential collision error could then be largely avoided during the 1st process. As a consequence, this will avoid providing the MP with medical information regarding another patient, which is very important from an ethical point of view. Moreover, the MP's workload would then be reduced in terms of the number of medical records to be analysed. The situation is less easy if the records provided come from the same hospitals, but here again the patient should be able to confirm, during the 1st process, if the date of the stay is plausible. During the 2nd process, the MP and the patient could verify that the disease recorded corresponds to the patient. Of course, sometimes the patient is not conscious and cannot answer the questions. This case is not frequent, and we must not build a rule to solve an exceptional problem, and secondly, it is in such a case when the patient cannot give any information that it would be useful to have information on his past history quickly even if it is incomplete or insufficiently precise. Fourth, concerning the amount of gathered data, one may think that it could be useful to reduce this amount in order to make it easier to handle. Therefore, we may imagine adding a selection criteria tool to the basic request as in any kind of search engine. The criteria could concern the selection of a time period, a list of hospitals, a clinical department or event, the pathology about which the medical practitioner requests precise information. However, the information, even when reduced in quantity, will still need to be analysed and reorganized by the practitioner.

To facilitate the MP's work and to limit the duration of the patient's medical visit, the 1st process could also be done by the patient alone before meeting the MP, if the patient agrees and has the skills to do it. The feasibility and the consequences of giving patients direct access to their administrative information or their health care records have to be assessed. It would also be interesting to know the proportion of information patients may delete in their health record if they were able to modify it. One important risk is linked to the fact that some patients will voluntarily erase information they do not want to communicate. It is their right, but in such situations, the resulting medical record cannot be considered reliable and will have no legal value to bring evidence in the case of medical litigation. The main drawback in this case would be the loss of confidence between the patient and the physician, which may be prejudicial to the quality of care. Moreover, would a medical practitioner accept to treat patients on the basis of documents that contain potentially incomplete information? In France, for example, the possibility for the patient to erase or dissimulate some information has been widely discussed, but no consensus was found between health practitioners and patients' associations. Some patients' associations want very sensitive data to be masked so that a patient's medical history will not influence the quality of his or her current care. They consider that patients should have the right to mask sensitive health data (HIV/AIDS, Abortion, Psychiatry….) when they are not necessary to treat the current disease. Their request regarding masking data could then be granted. However, health practitioners do not agree as they think that they need all of the information not only to make the right decision, but also to avoid drug interactions and to take due precautions. Health practitioners consider that, at least, they have to be informed that some information was masked.

Moreover, in France, a patient's medical history, in terms of administrative data (when and where the care was given) is already available to every MP in the private health sector. The 1st process, therefore, has already been implemented, without the risk of losing any information if the patient has received care only in France.

On the other hand, the impact of a patient's collaboration with the MP to identify potential errors in his/her records should also be evaluated. For some diseases, the understanding of the natural history is fundamental [16]. Of course the history taking [17] requires the patient's help. A study concerning patients' access [18] reported that a substantial proportion of patients identified factual errors in their records, but concluded that it was difficult to assess the rate of finding clinically important errors. In this procedure, we have to find a balance between the potential increase in the overall quality of the information induced by patients' management of data collection from all sources and the risk of altering the accuracy of the data when there is the possibility that some information has been erased.

One peculiar point concerns the contribution of the patient to his medical record. Some people may worry that patients can record incorrect information or deliberately falsify their own data. This situation may happen independently of the management of the medical record, in the daily practice of any kind of medical consultation.

It is an unavoidable aspect of the relationship between the patient and the medical practitioner, which is based on reciprocal trust. In cases of medical litigation, which could be induced by a medical error resulting from an erroneous information, it will be fundamental to identify who recorded the information (traceability and signature) to identify who may be liable. Then the judge will eventually investigate whether these incorrect data were introduced by mistake or deliberately.

Of course, appropriate modifications to our methodology have to be proposed in the case of mental handicap, emergency care or even in the case of a patient meeting a new MP. In the case of mental disabilities, the patient's task could be performed by a trusted party that could be chosen by the patient among family members. When the patient meets a new MP, the main question is to know if the new MP will be able to communicate with the previous one. The answer to this question will depend on the patient's willingness. Of course, further work is needed to define more precisely the limits of patients' responsibilities, taking into account their age, mental faculties and disabilities. In the case of emergency care, family members are not always present to provide help. We can imagine that either the emergency physician can be given access to the medical synthesis previously constituted by the MP or apply the methodology proposed in this paper. In the case of an emergency, a physician could exceptionally be authorized to gain access to all of the data requested, even if the patient has not validated the administrative data as planned in the 1st process. Above all, whatever the amount of lost or false information, the situation (from the point of view of professionals and patients) will be better than the great lack of information we have now. Moreover, one last but by no means minor advantage is that these Medical Record Search Engines using Pseudonymisation of patient's identity will make it possible to retrieve the past histories of all patients without the need to reformat the data and above all without the need to build an additional specific structure. Therefore it could be implemented rapidly at a much lower cost than a central medical record structure.

3. Conclusion

The advantage of our methodology lies in the fact that it gives more responsibility to the patients regarding the management of their personal medical records. Increasing the efficiency of this management under the mixed responsibilities of the patient and the MP can help to provide better health care by two means. First, the MP would obtain more reliable information, which would provide a better basis for decision making and lead to more appropriate treatment. Second, the patient would be more involved in his health care. Moreover, the sharing of these responsibilities would enhance the doctor/patient relationship and hopefully mutual trust.

The disadvantages of our proposition are the possible temptations of patients to erase health information. This has triggered a major debate on ethical and medical aspects which has not yet led to a consensus at either the National or European level.

References

[1] Quantin C, Allaert FA, Fassa M, Avillach P, Fieschi M, Cohen O. Interoperability issues regarding patient identification in Europe. Conf Proc IEEE Eng Med Biol Soc du 23 au 26 août 2007; Lyon; France. 2007;1:6160.

[2] Jones PS, Meleis AI. Health is empowerment. ANS Adv Nurs Sci 1993;15:1-14.

[3] Lau DH. Patient empowerment—a patient-centred approach to improve care. Hong Kong Med J 2002;8(5):372-4.

[4] Visse MA, Teunissen T, Peters A, Widdershoven GA, Abma TA. Dialogue for Air, Air for Dialogue: Towards Shared Responsibilities in COPD. Practice. Health Care Anal 2010 Jan 10. (epub ahead of print).

[5] Lopez JE, Orell M, Morgan L, Warner J. Empowerment in older psychiatric inpatients: development of the empowerment questionnaire for inpatients (EQuIP). Am J Geriatr Psychiatry. 2010 Jan;18(1):21-32.

[6] Baars JE, Markus T, Kuipers EJ, Van der Woude CJ. Patients' Preferences regarding Shared Decision-Making in the Treatment of Inflammatory Bowel Disease: Results from a Patient-Empowerment Study. Digestion. 2010;81(2):113-9.

[7] Gerris J, de Sutter P. Self-operated endovaginal telemonitoring (SOET): a step towards more patient-centred ART? Hum Reprod 2010;25(3):562-8

[8] Larkin GL, Beautrais AL, Spirito A, Kirrane BM, Lippmann MJ, Milzmann DP. Mental health and emergency medicine: a research agenda. Acad Emerg Med 2009;16(11):1110-9.

[9] Burton DA, Blundell N, Jones M, Fraser AG, Elwyn G. Shared decision-making in cardiology: Do patients want it and do doctors provide it? Patient Educ Couns 2009 Nov 27. (epub ahead of print)

[10] Tariman JD, Berry DL, Cochrane B, Doorenbos A, Schepp K. Preferred and actual participation roles during health care decision making in persons with cancer: a systematic review. Ann Oncol 2009 Nov 25. (epub ahead of print)

[11] Mandl KD, Szolovits P, Kohane IS. Public standards and patients' control: how to keep electronic medical records accessible but private commentary: Open approaches to electronic patient records commentary: A patient's viewpoint. BMJ 2001;322(7281):283–7.

[12] Røstad L. An Initial Model and a Discussion of Access Control in Patient Controlled Health Records The Third International Conference on Availability, Reliability and Security. IEEE 2008;935-42.

[13] Neubauer T, Riedl B. Improving Patients Privacy with Pseudonymization. In: Andersen SK et al, editors. eHealth Beyond the Horizon – Get IT There. IOS Press; 2008. p. 691-6.

[14] Schneier B. Applied cryptography, 2nd edition. Wiley-India; 2007.

[15] Quantin C, Jaquet-Chiffelle DO, Coatrieux G, Fassa M, Allaert FA. Medical record search engines, using pseudonymised patient identity: an alternative to centralised medical records. In: Collaborative meetings on Health Informatics (CoMHI 2009); IMIA WG4(SiHIS), Hiroshima. 2009. p. 5.

[16] Mehta AB. Anderson-Fabry disease: developments in diagnosis and treatment. Int J Clin Pharmacol Ther 2009;47(Suppl 1):S66-74.

[17] Clauser BE, Balog K, Harik P, Mee J, Kahraman N. A multivariate generalizability analysis of history-taking and physical examination scores from the USMLE step 2 clinical skills examination. Acad Med 200;84(10 Suppl):S86-9.

[18] Ross SE, Lin CT. The Effects of Promoting Patient Access to Medical Records: A Review. J Am Med Inform Assoc 2003;(10):129-38

Legend

Figure 1: Gathering patient's data through Medical Records Search Engines
All cryptographic keys are in index.
All abbreviations are defined in the appendix.

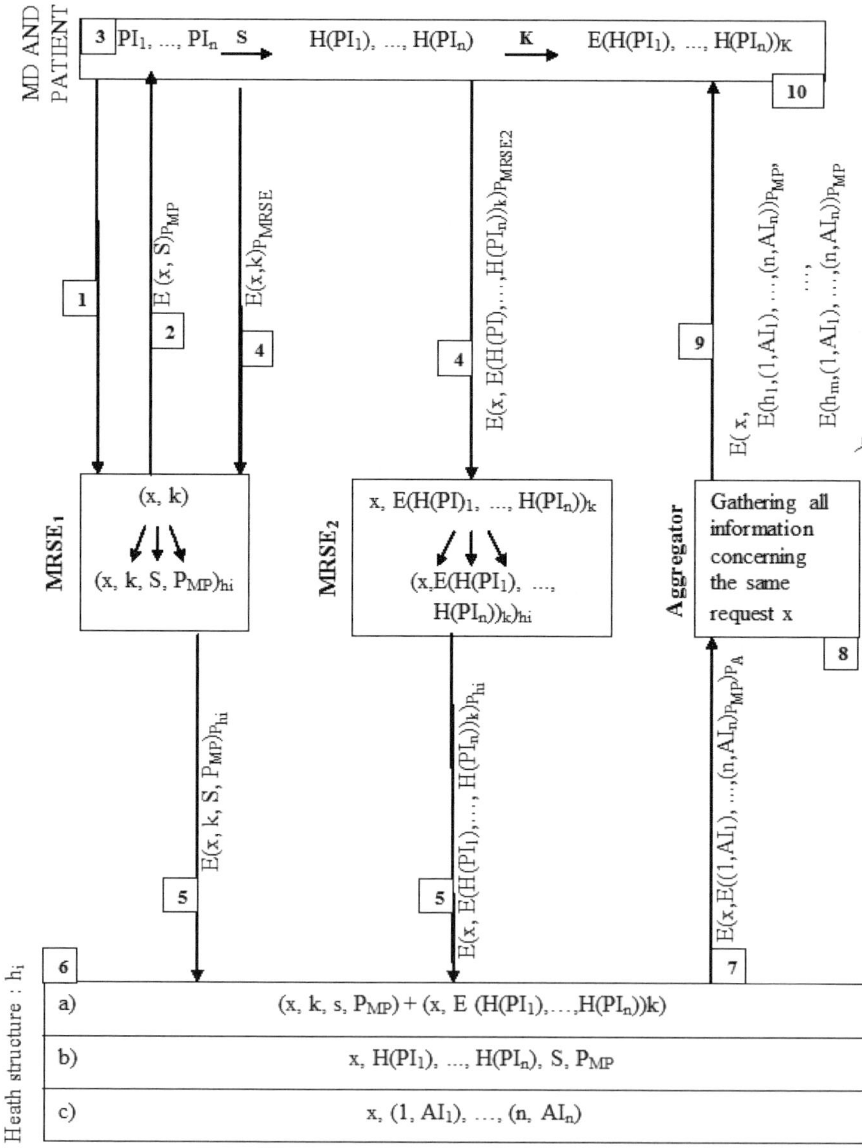

Appendix

It is assumed that participants in these processes know the public keys of the other participants with whom they have to communicate. All data exchanged are encrypted with the receiver's public key before transmission and decrypted with the receiver's private key.

First process:

1) The MP asks MSRE1 for a specific pad.
2) A request number x, and the specific pad S are sent by MSRE1 to the MP
3) Several (n) identifiers are generated using different components of patient identification: PI_1 , … , PI_n
   - Every identifier is hashed using S: $H(PI_1)$, … ,$H(PI_n)$
4) Sending the request to the two MRSEs
   - MRSE1 receives
     a) X, the number of the request
     b) K, a session key
   - MRSE2 receives
     a) X, the number of the request
     b) $E(H(PI_1), \ldots ,H(PI_n))_k$, an encrypted list, using K, of hashed identifiers
5) Transmitting the request
   - MRSEs consult a health structure directory
   - MRSE1 sends X, K, S, and P_{MP} the public key of the MP to each of the m health structures
   - MRSE2 sends X, $E(H(PI_1), \ldots ,H(PI_n))_k$ to each of the m health structures
6) Inside each health structure hi:
   - $E(H(PI_1), \ldots ,H(PI_n))_k$ is decrypted using K
   - The health structure is able to hash (using S) its own database identities and search for administrative information (AI) corresponding to the patient's pseudonyms (comparing its own hashed identities with the patient's hashed identities $H(PI_1)$ … $H(PI_n)$).
   - The health structure generates a list of AI for each identifier sent by the MP: $((1,Ai_1),..,(n,AI_n))$, and encrypts the list with P_{MP}.
7) Transfer of results to the aggregator

   Each health structure sends to the aggregator the number of the request and the list encrypted with the MP's public key: $E((1,Ai_1),..,(n,AI_n))_{P_{MP}}$
8) Gathering all patient information at the aggregator level

   The aggregator collects and gathers together all the information received from all health structures (h_1 … h_m).

   $X, (h_1,\ E((1,Ai_1),..,(n,AI_n))_{P_{MP}}), \ldots , (h_m,\ E((1,Ai_1),..,(n,AI_n))_{P_{MP}})$
9) These results are sent to the MP
10) The MP will then be able to decrypt these results with is own private key.

The patient can then check and validate the AI corresponding to his/her medical history.

Second process:

The second process relies on the same flow as the first one except that:

- when sending the request, the MP only sends the AI validated by the patient: only the selected health structures with the corresponding selected H(PI) are contacted.
- the results transferred by the health structures to the aggregator and or by the aggregator to the MP include the medical records (MR).

Medical and Care Compunetics 6
L. Bos et al. (Eds.)
IOS Press, 2010

doi:10.3233/978-1-60750-565-5-201

A Context-Aware Approach to Process-based PHR System Security

Eleni MYTILINAIOU, Vassiliki KOUFI[1], Flora MALAMATENIOU, and George VASSILACOPOULOS
Department of Digital Systems, University of Piraeus, Piraeus 185 34, Greece

Abstract. Healthcare delivery is a highly complex process involving a broad range of healthcare services, typically performed by a number of geographically distributed and organizationally disparate healthcare providers requiring increased collaboration and coordination of their activities in order to provide shared and integrated care. Under an IT-enabled, patient-centric model, health systems can integrate care delivery across the continuum of services, from prevention to follow-up, and also coordinate care across all settings. In particular, much potential can be realized if cooperation among disparate healthcare organizations is expressed in terms of cross-organizational healthcare processes, where information support is provided by means of PHR systems. This paper assumes a process-oriented PHR system and presents a security framework that addresses the authorization and access control issues arisen in these systems. The proposed framework ensures provision of tight, just-in-time permissions so that authorized users get access to specific objects according to the current context. These permissions are subject to continuous adjustments triggered by the changing context. Thus, the risk of compromising information integrity during task executions is reduced.

Keywords. Personal Health Record, process, agent, role-based authorization, least privilege principle, context-aware access control

Introduction

Healthcare delivery is a highly complex process involving a broad range of healthcare services (e.g. in-patient, out-patient, emergency), typically performed by a number of geographically distributed and organizationally disparate healthcare providers, requiring increased collaboration and coordination of their activities in order to provide shared and integrated care [1]. As healthcare providers are mostly hosting diverse and disparate information systems, it is difficult to obtain a complete picture of a person's healthcare record at the point of care when needed.

Recently, there has been a remarkable upsurge in activity surrounding the adoption of personal health record (PHR) systems [2]. A PHR is a consumer-centric approach to making comprehensive electronic health records (EHRs) available at the point of care while protecting patient privacy [3]. In particular, a PHR can be defined as a set of tools that allow patients to access and coordinate their lifelong health information and make appropriate parts of it available to those who need it. PHR data can come from EHRs or directly from the patient – including non-clinical information (e.g. exercise

[1] Corresponding author. vassok@unipi.gr

habits, diet, etc) [4]. The key difference between PHRs and EHRs is that, unlike traditional EHRs which are based on the 'fetch and show' model, PHR architectures are based on the fundamental assumptions that the complete records are held on a central repository and that each patient retains authority over access to any portion of his/her record [3][5]. Hence, quality and safety of patient care is enhanced by providing patients and health professionals with relevant and timely information when and where needed, while ensuring protection and confidentiality of personal data.

Providing patients with access to their electronic health records offers great promise not only for improving patient health and satisfaction with their care but also for enhancing professional and organizational approaches to health care [5]. In particular, much potential can be realized if cooperation among disparate healthcare organizations is expressed in terms of cross-organizational healthcare processes, where information support is provided by means of PHR systems. However, due to concerns regarding the validity of patient-entered information, clinical decisions should only be based on clinical information included in a patient's PHR.

Healthcare processes are fundamentally different from those of other domains for a number of reasons including: (a) patient care requires availability of an extensive amount of medical data (medical images and free texts, XML documents, medical charts, etc), (b) ad hoc collaborative work and high degree of communication between healthcare professionals is an integral part of activities surrounding patient care, (c) each healthcare professional is involved in the care of several patients in parallel and (d) healthcare professionals are working in a mobile environment where their availability status is subject to rapid change due to the constant interruptions anytime, anywhere. Moreover, the computing environment in healthcare organizations is becoming increasingly complex as multiple heterogeneous technologies are employed and highly interactive user applications are supported. In such an environment, privacy and security of personal health information are considered critical factors in advancing the interests of both healthcare providers and consumers [6][7]. Thus, one important consideration in the development of process-oriented PHR systems is to secure personal information against unauthorized access, collection, use, disclosure or disposal by ensuring a tight matching of permissions to actual usage and need. To this end, the least privilege principle should be enforced which, in turn, requires continuous adjustments of the sets of user permissions to ensure that, at any time, users (e.g. healthcare professionals) assume the minimum sets of permissions required for the execution of each task of a healthcare process.

In healthcare processes, however, certain user permissions depend on the process execution context. That is, contextual information available at access time, such as user-to-patient proximity, location of attempted access and time of attempted access, can influence the authorization decision regarding task execution. This enables a more flexible and precise access control policy specification that satisfies the least privilege principle.

This paper assumes a PHR-based architecture whereby healthcare processes are automated using the Web Services Business Process Execution Language (WS-BPEL, or BPEL for short) and presents an agent-based security framework that addresses authorization and access control issues arisen in process-based PHR systems. In particular, a context-aware authorization model and mechanism is presented that incorporates the advantages of broad, role-based permission assignment and administration across object types, as in role-based access control (RBAC) [8], and yet provides the flexibility for adjusting role permissions on individual objects at BPEL process enactment according to the current context. Thus, during the execution of a process instance, changes in contextual information are sensed to adapt user permissions to the minimum required for completing a job.

1. Related Work

Ensuring adequate security of information has always been an issue of growing concern in the healthcare sector. Hence, the need for suitable access control mechanisms preventing abuses and ensuring appropriate use of resources becomes imperative. RBAC constitutes a very attractive solution for providing security features in several computing infrastructures [9]. Although RBAC models vary from very simple to pretty complex, they all share the same basic structure of subject, role and privilege [8][10]. Other factors such as time and location, which may be part of an access decision, are not considered in access control decision making [10].

During the last few years, research efforts regarding the development of highly adaptive security systems to achieve real-time, accurate and effective access control have been on the rise. Some involve the extension of the RBAC model, in order to enable the enforcement of more complex rules and the inclusion of context information in access control decisions. Zhang and Parashar have proposed a Dynamic RBAC model that extends the role based access control model and dynamically adjusts static Role Assignments and Permission Assignments based on context information [10]. In [11] a context-aware access control architecture is presented, in order to support fine-grained authorizations for the provision of secure e-services. The proposed architecture is based on a Role-Based Access Control (RBAC) model, which incorporates dynamic context information in the form of context constraints. The latter involve the evaluation of both simple and composite context conditions. In [12] access control relies on the well-known RBAC model as well as the notion of conditional role which is based on the notions of role attribute and system attribute. The role attributes can be viewed as cached user information that is relevant to the specific roles, and the role attribute values of a user should be updated if the user information changes. In [13] a framework of RBAC with privacy-based extensions is proposed. This framework aims at tackling the need for confidentiality of personal identifiable information and protected health information such as Electronic Health Records in e-Healthcare services. In [14] a context-aware RBAC (CARBAC) model for pervasive computing applications is presented. In this access control model, dynamic context information is used in role admission policies, in policies related to permission executions by role members, and in policies related to access of dynamically interfaced services by role members. In [15] a group-based RBAC model (GB-RBAC) is proposed for secure collaborations. This model is based on RBAC96 and extended with the group concept to capture dynamic users and permissions. Thus, global or system level management by system administrators is supported as well as local or group level management by group administrators.

In this paper, a security framework is proposed which addresses access control issues in the context of a process-oriented PHR system. The proposed framework allows for the definition of flexible and precise security policies that reflect real-time access control requirements. To this end, the traditional role-based model is enhanced by adding context-awareness features thus leading to an individualized security system for the regulation of access over tasks and data objects.

2. Motivating Scenario

To illustrate the main principles of the proposed system architecture and implementation, a sample integration project is described which is concerned with the automation and remote access to cross-organizational healthcare processes. As patient referrals are usually made among various healthcare providers (e.g. for hospitalization, for inpatient/outpatient consultation or for performing specialized medical procedures), there is a need to ensure that automated healthcare processes can be executed remotely and integrated patient information can be accessed through the execution of these processes by authorized users where and when needed. Thus, the sample process considered here is concerned with patient referrals issued by healthcare professionals to a clinical department of the same or another hospital.

Suppose a healthcare delivery situation where a hospital's physician, while on a ward round, visits one of his/her patients. While assessing the patient's condition, at the point of care, the physician needs to access the patient's medical record and to request a medical consultation from a cardiologist. After receiving the request, the consulting physician assesses the patient's condition by taking into account the relevant portions of his medical record. In order to inform the referring physician of his medical findings, he sends him a consultation report. In turn, the referring physician forms a suitable treatment plan for his patient.

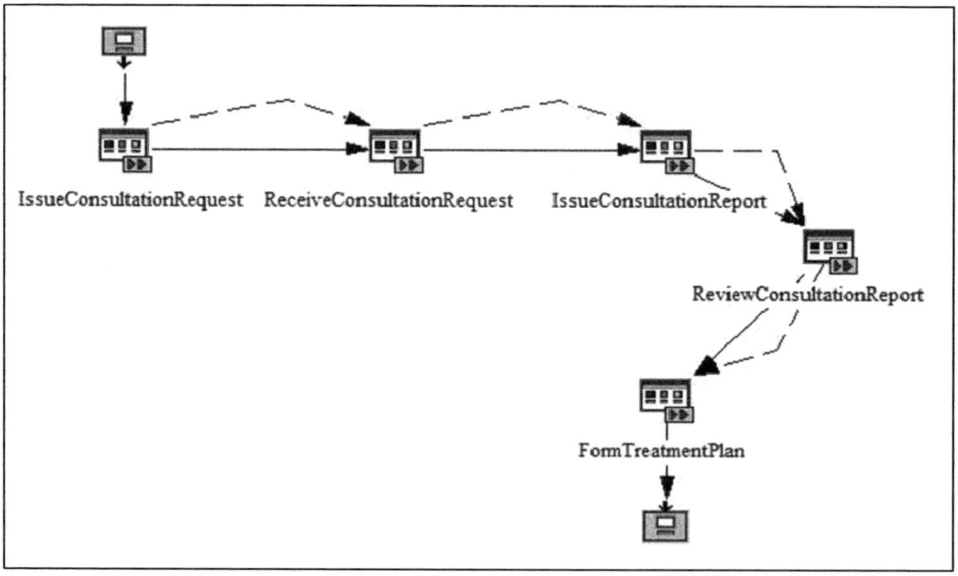

Figure 1. Consultation process model using IBM WebSphere Workflow

Figure 1 shows a high-level view of the healthcare process pertaining to consultation management using the IBM WebSphere Workflow build-time tool [16]. In the sample healthcare process, two hospital departments are involved: Department of General Medicine and Department of Cardiology. Two of the participating roles in the healthcare process are: Physician (PH) and Cardiologist (CR). Table 1 shows an extract of authorization requirements regarding task execution and related data access privileges.

Table 1. Extract of authorization requirements or the healthcare process of Figure 1.

	Authorization Requirement
1.	PHs may issue consultation requests for their patients only (IssueConsultationRequest).
1.1	PHs may write consultation requests for their current patients.
1.2	PHs may edit consultation requests for their current patients before sent.
1.3	PHs may send consultation requests for their current patients to doctors who hold the relevant specialty/sub-specialty.
1.4	PHs may cancel consultation requests for their current patients after sent.
1.5	PHs may write and read PHRs of their current patients but they may read-only past PHR versions of their patients.
2.	CRs may issue patient consultation reports on request by PHs (IssueConsultationReport).
2.1	CRs may read patient consultation requests issued by PHs
2.2	CRs may read-only certain portion of the PHRs of patients they are requested to issue consultation reports for.
2.3	CRs may write patient consultation reports for their current patients.
2.4	CRs may edit patient consultation reports for their current patients before sent.
2.5	CRs may send patient consultation reports for their current patients to the requesting PHs only.
2.6	CRs may cancel patient consultation reports issued by them after sent.
2.7	CRs may read past patient consultation reports prepared by them.
3.	PHs may form treatment plans for their patients after having received the consultation reports issued by CRs on request by them (FormTreatmentPlan).
3.1	PHs may read-only consultation reports issued by CRs only if requested by them.
3.2	PHs may form a treatment plan for their current patients.
3.3	PHs may alter a treatment plans for their current patients before putting it on the patient.
3.4	PHs may write and read PHRs of their current patients.

From an authorization perspective, the healthcare process of Figure 1 surfaces several requirements with regard to task execution and related data access privileges. These requirements include the following:

- **Task execution** - In certain circumstances the candidates for a task instance execution should be dynamically determined and be either a sub-group of the authorized users or only one, specific authorized user. For example, the request for a consultation from a cardiologist (issued by a physician) should be routed only to the sub-group of cardiologists who hold the relevant sub-specialty (e.g. interventional or echocardiography) and the consultation report (issued by a cardiologist) should be routed only to the requesting physician.
- **Data access** - Given that a role holder can execute a specific task, he/she should be allowed to exercise a dynamically determined set of permissions on certain data objects only. For example, during the execution of the “IssueConsultationRequest” task, a physician is allowed to read patient record data and to issue (write, edit and send) consultation requests only for his/her patients while on duty and within the hospital premises.

- **Permission propagation** - Some role holders should receive additional permissions on certain data objects in order to effectively execute a task but these permissions should be revoked upon successful execution of the task. For example, for an effective execution of the "IssueConsultationReport" task with regard to a patient, in response to a request submitted by a physician, a consulting physician (e.g. the cardiologist) should receive the permission to read the patient's record but he/she should not be allowed to retain this permission after successful task execution.

The above requirements suggest that certain data access permissions of the healthcare process participants depend on the process execution context. In particular, contextual information available at access time, such as user-to-patient proximity, location of attempted access and time of attempted access, can influence the authorization decision regarding task execution and, given this permission, associated web service invocation to access the relevant data objects. This enables a more flexible and precise access control policy specification that satisfies the least privilege principle by incorporating the advantages of having broad, role-based permissions across process tasks and data object types, like RBAC, yet enhanced with the ability to simultaneously support the following features: (a) predicate-based access control, limiting user access to specific data objects, (b) a permission propagation function from one role holder to another in certain circumstances, and (c) determining qualified task performers during a process instance based not only on the role-to-task permission policy, specified at process build time, but also on application data processed during the process instance. In addition, the model should not incur any significant administrative overhead and should be self-administering to a great extent.

3. System Architecture

The prototype system described here facilitates remote execution of automated healthcare processes and, in turn, access to comprehensive patient information which is stored in a central repository. In this environment, a robust security framework is in place in order to ensure that health information follows patients throughout their care in a secure manner and that comprehensive information is made available to appropriate people anywhere, anytime.

Figure 2 illustrates a high-level view of the system architecture, which consists of three subsystems, namely the business process subsystem, the PHR subsystem and the security subsystem.

3.1. Business Process Subsystem

The Business Process Subsystem is responsible for managing healthcare processes. Apart from the process modeling tools, a core component of this subsystem is the Process Engine, a robust platform for executing process-based applications. Interactions with the Process Engine are performed by means of a customized web portal which has been developed in order to establish secure access to healthcare processes and the web services invoked by them. To this end, digital signatures are utilized for certain parts of the messages exchanged during a BPEL process enactment. For example, each request for a task execution results at a request for a web service invocation. This request is performed by means of a SOAP message, parts of which

(SOAP body and/or header) are digitally signed using the private key of the user's X.509 certificate. Thus, integrity of information exchanged in each transaction is ensured. Likewise, the web service response is digitally signed to ensure data integrity.

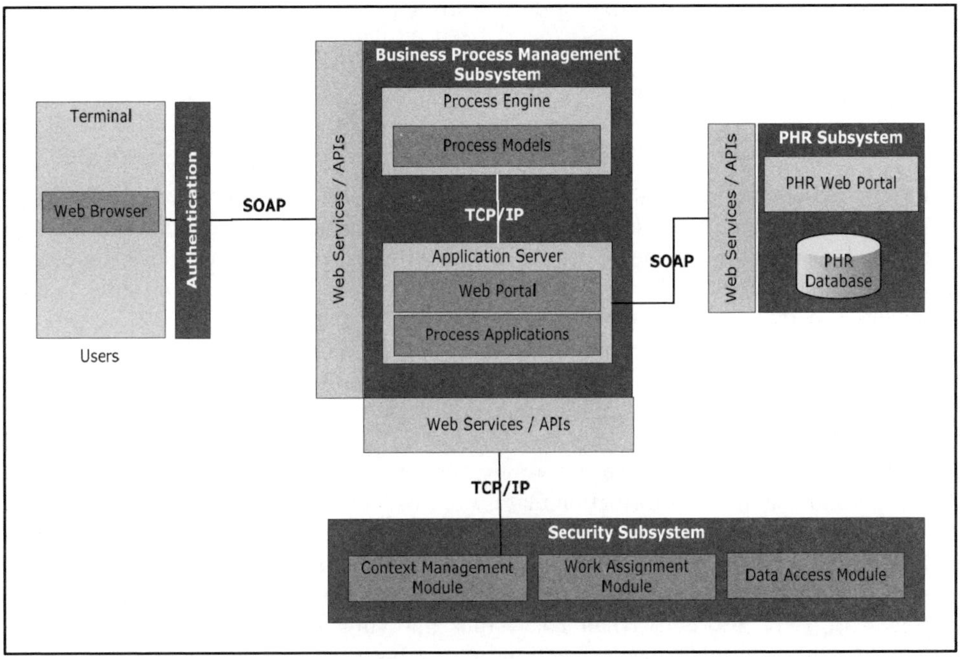

Figure 2. System Architecture

3.2. PHR Subsystem

The PHR subsystem supports both patients by enabling them to actively manage their own health and authorized healthcare professionals by ensuring quick and secure availability of patients' health data. The PHR subsystem comprises:

- A central repository where the complete patient records are held,
- A web portal through which a patient can access and manage his/her lifelong health information and make appropriate parts of it available to those who need it, and
- A number of web services which comprise a uniform interface to the central repository.

In a typical PHR system, authorization for access to medical information contained in the patient's PHR is exclusively granted either by the record owner (consumer or patient) or by an assigned "gatekeeper" (e.g. next of kin) [17][18].

3.3. Security Subsystem

The Security Subsystem is responsible for regulating access to BPEL process tasks and associated web services. There is one Security Subsystem installed in each healthcare institution. Each one of these subsystems consists of three modules that cooperate to ensure the security policies are faithfully and consistently enforced. These modules are the Context Management Module (CMM), the Work Assignment Module (WAM) and the Data Access Module (DAM). The CMM acquires contextual information influencing authorization decisions and communicates it to WAM and DAM which are responsible for regulating access over BPEL process tasks and PHR data objects respectively. A more detailed description of this subsystem will be provided in the next two sections.

4. Access Control Model

User interactions are currently not covered by WS-BPEL which is primarily designed to support automated business processes that orchestrate activities exposed as web services [18]. However, the spectrum of activities that make up general purpose processes, including healthcare processes, is broader than this, because people participate in the execution of business processes. In particular, a healthcare process comprises disparate and distributed pieces of logic performed by a large number of personnel. For each piece of logic (i.e. task) authorization decisions cannot be made during design time as there is not enough information about the context on which the decision should be based. More specifically, in a healthcare process, role-based authorization is often based on a combination of contextual constraints imposed on each task and user roles, information that is not available during process modeling.

Within a process-oriented PHR system there is a need to address authorization in a centralized manner in order to enforce the least privilege principle. In turn, this requires ensuring that access permissions with regard to process tasks and associated web services are only awarded dynamically, thus allowing users to assume the absolute minimum role required for task executions and web service invocations. Hence, there is a need to enforce context-aware authorization constraints regarding BPEL task executions and associated web service invocations that result in accesses to PHR information.

4.1. Process Execution Context

Context can be defined as any information which is available at run time and is considered relevant to the resource accesses considered [20]. Thus, it may be assumed that a context is defined by an evaluation of a relevant set of context types that may be divided into two main classes: static and dynamic. Static context types are those whose values are known at design time and are not subject to change during a BPEL process execution (e.g. physician's identity and specialty). Dynamic context types are those whose values are determined at runtime and are subject to constant change during a BPEL process execution. For example, information related to the environment (e.g. spatio-temporal) and the "proximity" relationship between a physician and a patient (i.e. physician X is an attending physician to patient Y).

In a typical RBAC environment, roles are often defined as named collections of capabilities and privileges intended to perform healthcare functions and are assigned to users at design time through a many-to-many relationship. Users acting on a role are automatically assigned all the access permissions encapsulated in that role [21]. However, these permissions may be more or wider than those required for process task executions and web service invocations. Hence, to enforce the least privilege principle, context-based derivative roles are defined which, at any time, encapsulate the minimum sets of permissions that are tailored to run time access needs of users, so that users are provided with tight, just-in-time permissions when needed [22].

On these grounds, in addition to the role concept of the typical RBAC model, a new concept is introduced, namely subrole. Roles correspond to existing organizational structures and define the division of work and the lines of authority based on job functions and seniority (e.g. "physician" and "cardiologist"); they are specified during process design and may be taken on by users at run time, possibly subject to a number of contextual constraints such as spatio-temporal [23]. On the other hand, subroles are derived from one or more roles based on certain contextual constraints (e.g. "attending physician" and "consulting physician") and may be assigned to and revoked from individuals at run time on the occurrence of specific events. For example, the subrole "consulting cardiologist" for a patient is derived from the roles "cardiologist" and "patient" and is taken on by a cardiologist when he/she is assigned to provide consultation in response to a request issued by the "attending physician" of that patient. In addition, it may be perfectly acceptable for a user holding the subrole "attending physician" for a patient to modify or cancel a submitted request for consultation before the latter is performed by a user holding the subrole "consulting cardiologist" for that patient, but certainly not after it has been performed. Hence, the subrole "consulting cardiologist" for a patient is revoked on the occurrence of the event that earmarks the performance of the consultation procedure.

Within the proposed system, the context information influencing authorization decisions is related to the users, the objects (i.e. tasks and associated web services) and the environment. In particular:

- The user context consists of static attributes (e.g. identity, specialty) and dynamic attributes (e.g. doctor's location, workload and availability)
- The object context consists of static attributes (e.g. patient-determined policies on PHR data) and dynamic attributes (e.g. object status)
- The environmental context consists of dynamic attributes (e.g. time of attempted access)

4.2. Context-Aware Permission Assignment

In the proposed system, context based subroles are used for controlling access to process tasks (execution) and associated web services (invocation). Hence, a subrole is translated into task execution permissions and given these permissions into web service invocation permissions (i.e. data access permissions). In particular:

(a) Upon request for a task execution, the relevant context is evaluated and if certain conditions are met the user is assigned a subrole which he holds throughout task execution.

(b) Given that the user has been assigned a subrole (i.e. has received the permission to execute a task), the corresponding permissions for invoking the associated web service (i.e. to access the relevant portion of the patient's PHR) are also assigned to him provided that certain conditions are met.

In both cases, whether required conditions are met is determined through the evaluation of relevant contextual constraints. For example, in the healthcare process of Figure 1, an authorization requirement may specify that "A physician can issue requests for consultation from within a hospital, between 8am to 5pm and for his/her patients only". This requirement contains three contextual constraints: (a) "for his/her patients only" which describes a physician-to-patient "proximity" relationship between a physician and a patient that can be expressed by the subrole "attending physician", (b) "from within a hospital" (location), and (c) "between 8am to 5pm" (temporal). All these constraints are taken into account in deciding whether an attempted access by a user can be permitted or denied. Hence, the above requirement can be expressed as follows: "An attending physician to a patient can execute the "IssueConsultationReport" process task and invoke the associated web service from within a hospital and between 8am to 5pm".

5. Access Control Mechanism

As shown in Figure 2, the three modules of the security subsystem cooperate upon each request for BPEL task execution and associated web services invocation in order to determine the relevant permissions. All three modules are agent-based. In particular, each module implements the core functionality of a corresponding agent which is responsible for performing a certain task. In our prototype system, three types of agents have been defined, namely Context Acquisition Agent (CAA), Work Assignment Agent (WAA) and Data Access Agent (DAA).

- **Context Acquisition Agent (CAA)** - it is responsible for capturing the runtime context and communicating it to the relevant agents handling permission assignments (either for a task execution or for web service invocation).
- **Work Assignment Agent (WAA)** - it is responsible for assigning to each user the required permissions for a task execution. In particular, upon creation (initiation) of a process instance a WAA is automatically created. WAA tracks task initiations and terminations by receiving relevant messages by the process instance that created it. When WAA receives a task initiation message, it evaluates the context recorded by the CAA against the security policies it implements and identifies the subgroup of users who are eligible to execute the task. For each one of these users, the list of pending tasks is updated so as to include the new task. When a member of the subgroup accepts to undertake the execution of a task, the WAA is informed and alters the state of the task to unavailable in the work lists of the rest of the members of the subgroup. When the WAA receives a task termination message, it revokes all permissions assigned earlier.
- **Data Access Agent (DAA)** - it is responsible for assigning to each user the required permissions for a web service invocation that results in data access. After a user picks a task for a execution, the DAA is invoked. This agent evaluates the runtime user context, that is, time of access, location of the user and other environmental variables and according to the policy rules it implements it determines the permissions the user should acquire in order to invoke the relevant web service. When a task is terminated the DAA revokes all permissions granted to the user.

6. Prototype Implementation

To illustrate the functionality of the proposed security model a prototype consultation request management system was implemented in a laboratory environment. The system was developed as a web application using the Apache/Tomcat as Web/Application Server. The platform used for the generation of sample patient PHRs is Care2X

Integrated Healthcare Environment. Care2X can store patient's complete medical information in one convenient and secure location [24]. In addition, it supports the definition of static authorizations on each PHR. In particular, a patient can authorize healthcare providers to access his/her record and assigns to them specific access privileges [24]. Access to data stored in Care2X repository is achieved by means of web services which make use of the Care2X Application Programming Interface (API).

The Security Subsystem was implemented as a multi-agent system using the Java Agent Development framework (JADE) as a construction and execution environment [25][26]. JADE is an open-source software framework, aiming at assisting the development and execution of agent-based applications in compliance with the Foundation for Intelligent Physical Agents (FIPA) specifications for interoperable multi-agent systems [27].

Agents execute tasks periodically or stimulated by an event or a message. These tasks are carried out within operations called behaviours. Several behaviours are executed concurrently by each agent. When there are no tasks available for execution, the agent's thread goes to sleep in order not to consume CPU time. The thread is woken up again once a task becomes available for execution after a stimulus. Agents communicate with each other using FIPA Agent Communication Language (ACL) [28] over a specific protocol based on asynchronous message passing. Each agent has a 'mailbox' (the agent message queue) where the JADE run-time posts messages sent by other agents. Whenever a message is posted in the mailbox, the receiving agent is notified. The communication of the agents with the BPEL process is accomplished in two steps:

- WSIF (Web Services Invocation Framework) enables the connectivity of BPEL processes with resources other than web services by describing each resource in WSDL even if it is not a web service. In the case of Java Classes, WSIF provides bindings for BPEL processes. The data exchange between BPEL and the Java classes requires data transformation. Because BPEL variables are XML and Java variables are not, a mapping between XML and Java is required. For that reason XML façades are utilized. XML façades are a set of Java interfaces and classes through which data stored in BPEL variables can be accessed using get/set methods [29].
- JADE agents can be started from an external application. The JADE runtime is created to host them. These external applications are Java classes that can communicate with the BPEL process with the help of WSIF. Data is transferred in the Java class, and an agent is created in order to send a message containing the data and the requested operation, to the mailbox of the appropriate agent. Depending on the message, the right operation is executed.

In achieving the robust security framework envisaged, additional security features have been incorporated. In particular, physicians authenticate themselves by using X.509 certificates and all subsequent web transactions are executed under the Secure Socket Layer (SSL) via HTTPS. In addition, security in the communication among the agents of the agent platform is ensured by setting up a secure, confidential and mutually authenticated, connection amongst containers of the agent platform by leveraging TLS/SSL support provided by Java [26].

7. Concluding Remarks and Future Work

Process-oriented PHRs offer significant potential to stimulate transformational changes in healthcare delivery as they can meet collaboration requirements among health professionals and address healthcare information needs by providing a complete copy of each patient's medical record. In such environments, new challenges and new opportunities with respect to protecting the privacy and security of health information are created. Hence, it is essential to provide an effective access control mechanism that meets the requirements imposed by the least privilege principle. In turn, adherence to the least privilege principle requires continuous adjustments of user permissions in order to adapt to the current situation. This paper presents a process-oriented PHR system that facilitates authorized access to healthcare processes. To this end, agent technology is used for the implementation of a fine-grained access control mechanism which regulates user access to BPEL process tasks and associated web services resulting is PHR data accesses. Thus, a tight matching of permissions to actual usage and need is ensured.

References

[1] Koufi V, Vassilacopoulos G. HDGPortal: A Grid Portal Application for Pervasive Access to Process-Based Healthcare Systems. Proceedings of the 2nd International Conference in Pervasive Computing Technologies in Healthcare; 2008 Jan 31-Feb 2; Tampere, Finland.

[2] Tang PC, Ash JS, Bates DW, Overhage JM, Sands DZ. Personal Health Records: Definitions, Benefits, and Strategies for Overcoming Barriers to Adoption. J Am Med Inform Assoc 2006:13(2):121-6.

[3] Lauer G. Health Record Banks Gaining Traction in Regional Projects. 2009. [Online]. Available from: URL: http://www.ihealthbeat.org/features/2009/health-record-banks-gaining-traction-in-regional-projects.aspx.

[4] Alberta Health Services, Engaging the patient in healthcare: An overview of Personal Health Record Systems and Implications for Alberta. White Paper. 2009.

[5] Wiljer D, Urowitz S, Apatu E, DeLenardo C, Eysenbach G, Harth T, Pai H, Leonard KJ. Patient accessible electronic health records: exploring recommendations for successful implementation strategies. J. Med. Internet Res 2008;10(4):e34.

[6] Atluri V, Huang W. An Authorization Model for Workflows. Proceedings of the 4th European Symposium on Research in Computer Security. LNCS, 1146. 1996. p. 44–64.

[7] Wu S, Sheth A, Miller J, Luo Z. Authorization and Access Control of Application Data in Workflow Systems. J Intell Inf Syst 2002;18(1):71-94.

[8] National Institute of Standards and Technology (NIST), Role Based Access Control (RBAC) and Role Based Security. [Online]. Available from: URL: http://csrc.nist.gov/groups/SNS/rbac/.

[9] Feinstein H, Sandhu R, Coyne E, Youman C. Role-based access control models. IEEE Computer 1996;29(2):38-47.

[10] Zhang G, Parashar M. Context-Aware Dynamic Access Control for Pervasive Applications. Proceedings of the Communication Networks and Distributed Systems Modeling and Simulation Conference (CNDS 2004); 2004 Jan 18-21; San Diego (CA), USA.

[11] Kapsalis V, Hadellis L, Karelis D, Koubias S. A dynamic context-aware access control architecture for e-services. J Comput Secur 2006;25:507-21.

[12] Byun JW, Bertino E, Li N. Purpose Based Access Control of Complex Data for Privacy Protection. Proceedings of the 10th ACM Symposium on Access Control Models and Technologies (SACMAT'05); 2005 Jun 1-3; Stockholm, Sweden.

[13] Hung PCK, New Brunswick, Canada, Proceedings.

[14] Kulkarni D, Tripathi A. Context-Aware Role-based Access Control in Pervasive Computing Systems. Proceedings of the 13th ACM Symposium on Access Control Models and Technologies (SACMAT'08), 2008 Jun 11-13; Estes Park (CO), USA.

[15] Lia Q, Zhangb X, Xua M, Wu J. Towards secure dynamic collaborations with group-based RBAC model. J Comput Secur 2009;28:260-75.

[16] IBM Corporation. IBM Websphere Workflow – Getting Started with Buildtime V. 3.6, 2005.

[17] ICW eHealth Framework. Lifesensor. [Online]. Available from: URL: http://idn.icw-global.com/solutions/lifesensor/lifesensor.html.
[18] Power K, Global Mobile Healthcare An Electronic Framework for Portability of Health Records. Medical Tourism Magazine 2009.
[19] Kloppmann M, Koenig D, Leymann F, Pfau G, Rickayzen A, von Riegen C, et al. WS-BPEL Extension for People – BPEL4People, White Paper. 2005.
[20] Emig C, Schandua H, Abeck S. SOA-aware authorization control. Proceedings of the International Conference on Software Engineering Advances; 2006 Oct 28-Nov 2; Papeete, Tahiti, French Polynesia.
[21] Casati F, Castano S, Fugini M. Managing workflow authorization constraints through active database technology. Inform Syst Front 2001;3(3):319-38.
[22] Liu DR, Shen M. Workflow modeling for virtual processes: An order-preserving process - view approach. Inform Syst 2003;28(6):505-32.
[23] Marjanovic O. Towards IS supported coordination in emergent business processes. Bus Proc Manag J 2005;11(5):476-87.
[24] Care2X Integrated Healthcare Environment. [Online]. Available from: ULR: http://www.care2x.org/
[25] Bellifemine F, Caire G, Greenwood D. Developing Multi-Agent Systems with JADE. Wiley Series in Agent Technology; John Wiley & Sons; 2007.
[26] JADE, Java Agent DEvelopment Framework. [Online].Available from: URL: http://jade.tilab.com.
[27] The Foundation for Intelligent Physical Agents (FIPA). [Online]. Available from: URL: http://www.fipa.org/
[28] The Foundation for Intelligent Physical Agents (FIPA), Agent Communication Language Specifications. [Online]. Available from: URL: http://www.fipa.org/repository/aclspecs.html
[29] Juric MB, Mathew B, Sarang P. Business Process Execution Language for Web Services. Packt Publishing Ltd; 2006.

Medical and Care Compunetics 6
L. Bos et al. (Eds.)
IOS Press, 2010

doi:10.3233/978-1-60750-565-5-214

Patient Empowerment by the Means of Citizen-managed Electronic Health Records: Web 2.0 Health Digital Identity scenarios

Filipa FALCÃO-REIS [ab1] and Manuel E. CORREIA [ab]
[a] *Computer Science Department, Faculty of Science, University of Porto, Portugal*
[b] *CRACS - Center for Research in Advanced Computing Systems*

Abstract. With the advent of more sophisticated and comprehensive healthcare information systems, system builders are becoming more interested in patient interaction and what he can do to help to improve his own health care. Information systems play nowadays a crucial and fundamental role in hospital work-flows, thus providing great opportunities to introduce and improve upon "patient empowerment" processes for the personalization and management of Electronic Health Records (EHRs). In this paper, we present a patient's privacy generic control mechanisms scenarios based on the Extended OpenID (eOID), a user centric digital identity provider previously developed by our group, which leverages a secured OpenID 2.0 infrastructure with the recently released Portuguese Citizen Card (CC) for secure authentication in a distributed health information environment. eOID also takes advantage of Oauth assertion based mechanisms to implement patient controlled secure qualified role based access to his EHR, by third parties.

Keywords: Digital Identity, Electronic Health Records, Patient Empowerment, Smart Cards, Privacy, OpenID, Distributed Health Information environments

1. Introduction

Throughout the modern world, healthcare systems are in a crisis, as an ageing population and sky-rocketing costs are putting unprecedented financial and organizational pressure on state and private healthcare providers (1). In response to this crisis, health systems are suffering major changes: focusing more on the patient and what the patient can do to help to improve his own health care. The shift from a paper-based to an electronic media-based society is opening new opportunities that were not conceivable just a few years ago. Cost is no longer a major barrier to the recollection, storage and processing of huge amounts of information. This became common practice for critical businesses processes, major industry sectors and in the health sector, where we are witnessing a large increase on the deployment of Health Information Systems (HISs) and consequentially Electronic Health Records (EHRs) (2).

[1] Corresponding author. falcaoreis@dcc.fc.up.pt

Market forces and societal pressures are also colluding to improve citizen's health, which is further acerbating the need for more patient-centric systems. Governments all around the world are currently engaging with their agendas on reforming health care systems, despite great economic constraints. This health care reform is focusing more and more on the patient and encouraging him to assume the role of a pro-active consumer, with the ability to make his own choices and be held accountable for them. One can say that these reforms are making this patient empowerment processes inevitable. Numerous studies can also be found in the literature defining what 'patient empowerment' is. According to its very nature and underlying philosophy one can denote the existence of two 'patient empowerment' distinct dimensions, one inter-personal and another intra-personal. Therefore, 'patient empowerment' may be perceived either from a provider–patient interaction point of view (considered as a process of communication and education in which knowledge, values and power are shared, i.e. an interactive process where power is 'given' by someone to the patient) or from a patient inner point of view (considered as a process of personal transformation, i.e. empowerment occurs within the patient), or even both. Although the objectives are the same, i.e. to gain more power over one's life, the nature of the two processes is rather different. Nevertheless both processes must be actively promoted in today's society (3).

2. The Patient's role in the 21st century

To be a patient in the 21st century is to be a 'patient 2.0', deeply connected with emergent new technologies and highly motivated to assume control and responsibility over his own health care. However, all this enthusiastic feeling around the 'patient empowerment' process must be put into perspective. There are not many studies related to this issue and it is fundamentally important to conduct more studies in order to assess real patient's desires and motivations for further empowerment: do they wish to be empowered using an EHR? What level of 'patient empowerment' will the EHR achieve (4)? What are the main advantages and disadvantages concerning the patient within this approach? How are patients going to be able to express their intentions within Health Information Systems?

All of these issues lead to important questions that need to be answered. Focus group interviews are a good tool to gather patient's opinions about these matters. In our opinion these interviews could be first steps towards kick starting the 'patient empowerment' process. As soon as these proceedings are done, it would become much easier to elaborate a plan to effectively help to establish the patient's real needs for self-empowerment. Moreover, to help them to understand and accept their role (just like in the self-service industries, such as fast food chains where the consumers know what is expected of them) and to achieve knowledge about their options (an informed choice will improve patient's performance and commitment to his healthcare). In order to achieve this plan, some recommendations must be taken in consideration, such as (5):

- **Target health conditions for 'patient empowerment' where there exists a significant potential** (patients faced with an acute and urgent medical crisis are less able to gather information and to deliberate than those with chronic conditions).

- **Analyze the treatment process** (conditions should be analyzed to identify the steps in the treatment process where greater patient power would have the largest impact on improving efficient health outcomes).
- **Remove barriers to empowerment** (this may involve redefining and communicating the patient's role, enhancing both their knowledge about their options, health condition and personal health status as well as their skills to carry out the required proceedings competently by improving their self-efficacy and health literacy).
- **Create a facilitating environment for patient empowerment** (this might include the promulgation of patients rights, a number of choices that are consistent with patients' needs, easy access to valid information about the choices available, as well as helping patients with information-processing and decision-making by doctors that must be trained to perform different roles, complementing each patient's preferred role).
- **Ensure equity** (because patients are different, empowerment efforts must be customized to different patient groups, the need to target efforts applies particularly to health literacy, due to the fact that those with better education, better health insurance and higher incomes are in a better position to make choices than those who lack these benefits).
- **Motivate the empowered patient to achieve more efficient health outcomes** (empowering patients may or may not result in improved efficient health outcomes because of lack of patient motivation, so incentives to patient's commitment to his/her healthcare would result in better and more efficient outcomes).

One should add that these actions must involve both patients and health professionals with interactive health information systems, which must be developed to provide appropriate tools to allow patients to effectively take control of their EHRs at the level they desire and are capable of. Nevertheless, little has been done to involve the patient in the process of designing these tools, although quite a few studies have demonstrated that if the patient is involved in his own healthcare, not only their health will improve, but also fewer patients end up attending hospital emergencies unnecessarily (5). This involvement could be the result of being able to participate in decision-making, being educated regarding health problems and promoting a close relationship with healthcare providers, one that can potentially lead to a reduction in operational costs.

3. Extended OpenID for increasing Patient Empowerment

Nowadays, there are many platforms that are specially designed to help patients to build their own Personal Health Record (PHR) such as Google Health and Microsoft Health Vault or web sites that promote discussions on matters related to patients chronic diseases, for example social networking web sites such as Facebook have more than 500 groups where discussions primarily focusing on diabetes are taking place. Even YouTube is part of this global trend, with 36,000 pages devoted to some aspects of surgery. These occurrences characterize the popular phenomenon of Health 2.0 that is based on the use of social software and its ability to promote a partnership between patients, their caregivers and health professionals in health (6).

Yet, with the continuing growth of the number of such health web sites and services, patients end up registering personal data into multiple systems throughout the Internet, scattering their identity, duplicating their data and increasing in a most dramatic way the difficulty of managing this data. Eventually users end up losing track of their passwords and account settings if they do not use these web sites on a regular basis. Under this context it is only inevitable that sooner or later users end up compromising their security by using the same set of credentials for the different health related web sites. Such dangerous behavior is one direct result of the lack of user's knowledge and service provider's willingness to acknowledge the existence of mechanisms that can help users manage their own accounts and passwords. The continuous growth of privacy incidents involving personal health data, such as profiling and mining an individual's health history on profile sites by human resource departments or insurance companies, is demonstrating the fragile awareness of the general public for these matters. It is equally important to raise awareness among patients, caregivers, and health professionals, so that the concern over the privacy and security of EHRs becomes a priority. It is thus important to develop systems and processes that can help manage and control the access, and even the discloser and finality of these resources. These systems should provide identity management tools for the patient to secure for themselves their own privacy. As an example for these potential mechanisms we present a digital identity framework based on the OpenID protocol that could be used to mitigate these problems.

3.1. OpenID contextualization

One could start employing OpenID 2.0 and several of its extensions. OpenID is a decentralized system protocol for user-centric identification and digital identity management in the Internet. It is a "*single sign on*" (SSO) system, thus it eliminates the need for multiple user names and passwords across different security domains, i.e. in the OpenID universe relying parties. A relying party, sometimes designated as "*service provider*", is a site that wants to determine the end-user's identity. OpenID allows for the simplification of the user online experience. Indeed it constitutes a very good approximation of real life identity brought to the digital world. It allows users to add as much attributes as they believe that best describes them and assume profiles, also called *Personas*. Patients could easily create their *Health Persona* with attributes they consider to fit, thus preventing duplication of data across the Internet in an active and built-in way. It is this dynamics of creating and changing one's character that best defines the essence of the OpenID protocol. The following list outlines the most important features of OpenID (12):

- ***Open***: it is based on a community-driven development effort, with many components proposed as IETF (Internet Engineering Task Force) projects.
- ***Decentralization:*** users may reuse identifiers at any *OpenID*-enabled website, or provide a list of identifiers or switch in case one provider is unavailable, or even run their own identity provider.
- ***Free***: fostering interoperability between multiple vendors' identity technologies.
- ***User-centricity***: the end-user has absolute control over the use and dissemination of his identity information.
- ***Ubiquity***: easy to remember, pervasive, with a single password.

- User authentication flexibility.
- ***HTTP session protection*:** SSL/TLS, client certificates.
- ***Identifiers delegation***.

The OpenID Authentication process is very simple: when a user wants to sign into a website, which as a "*Relying Party*" would like to verify the user's identity, he has to choose an OpenID Identity Provider that he trusts and best meets his operational and privacy needs to create and manage a digital identity. The OpenID Identity consists of a unique Uniform Resource Identifier (URI). These URIs can be used by the owner to identify him at a website that has implemented OpenID and acts as an OpenID relay (13). During normal usage, the user submits his URI to the relying party, who uses the identifier to determine the identity provider's home address. The relying party optionally associates and establishes a shared secret with the identity provider (both shared secret and session should be encrypted). The relying party then redirects the user's browser to the identity provider site. The user then logs in with the identity provider with his actual credentials, which are then verified. If the user does not trust the relying party after all, they may choose to reject the login (12). The verification between the Relying Party and the Identity Provider is processed by using a mechanism that verifies the assertion: the check_authentication message. The check_authentication is a direct, out of band, communication that uses HTTP POST method between the Relying Party and the Identity Provider. Once the Identity provider has received this message, it will determine the validity of the assertion and reply back with a "yes" or "no" answer. The "is_valid" parameter present in the message shows the success or failure of an assertion. Once the Relying Party has received this success message, the authentication process is complete and can then allow the End User to login to the Relying Party web site. The Relying Party can also take other actions: if the Identity Provider did not return all of the requested parameters, it may grant a lesser level of access to data or if it is the first time that a user has logged in the web site, the Relying Party may also go through his own complementary registration process. Nevertheless, the Relying Party actions after the completion of authentication process are out of the scope of the OpenID protocol (14).

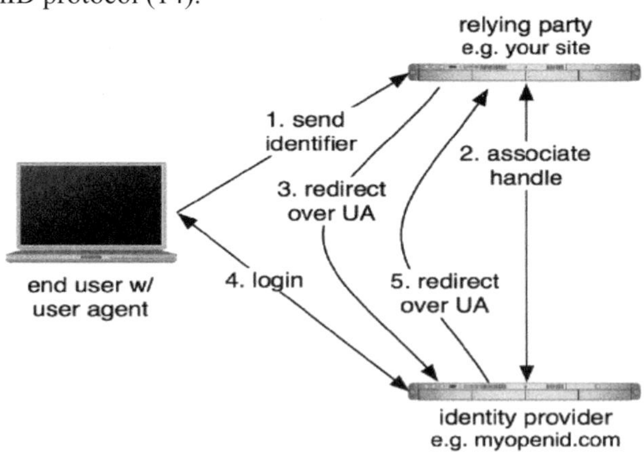

Figure 1. OpenID authentication process (13)

The advantage of such a system is that the user does not need to register for any OpenID enabled website once he owns an OpenID identity, he just has to select or even pre-select the attributes he wishes to share in different web sites for registration purposes. These attributes are "*attached*" to his digital *OpenID* personas, thus eliminating the need for memorizing passwords or even usernames for the different web sites he registers, thus minimizing the problem of too many multiple identities. There are however some security limitations (12):

- ***Trust*:** once authenticated the relying party can only *assume* the user owns the identifier, but not whether both the user *and* the identity provider are trustworthy enough.
- ***Security:*** OpenID can be susceptible to Phishing/Spoofing attacks, where (users are tricked into entering their password in a forged identity provider webpage or vulnerable to man-in-the-middle attacks via cross-site scripting requests).
- **Spamming:** spammers can register a large number of throwaway identities.

The OpenID community is developing solutions to mitigate these problems: the development of Firefox plugins that allow users to authenticate themselves in their OpenID identity provider is one solution for combating phishing and spoofing. Another useful security mechanism is also being developed: OpenID Provider Authentication Policy Extension (PAPE). This extension to the OpenID Authentication protocol provides a mechanism by which a Relying Party can request that particular authentication policies be applied by the OpenID Provider when authenticating an End User (13). This extension also provides a mechanism by which an OpenID Provider may inform a Relying Party which authentication policies were used, thus a Relying Party can request that the End User authenticate, for example, using a phishing-resistant or multi-factor authentication method, such as the use of security tokens, smart cards or biometrics (12). Also the use of certificates for both the End User and the Identity Provider confers a more trustworthy characterization to both and increases the level of security of the authentication process.

3.2. Improving Patient Empowerment with smart cards, the use of the Portuguese Citizen's Card in healthcare

Today's 'patient empowerment' process is becoming a central issue for healthcare providers worldwide as they face new challenges in achieving better and personalized health outcomes. Therefore, they need to adopt a patient-centered approach if they want to effectively incorporate empowerment into their clinical processes. This requires more personal involvement with their patients and implies a shift in the representation of their roles, moving away from the role of skilled technicians towards roles which underline the importance of people skills, and from knower to facilitator, thus reducing the existing gap between doctors and patients. As a result of their empowerment process, patients are expected not only to better self-manage their illness, by better understanding their choices, but also to be able to share their EHRs with the health professionals they wish or need to, thus allowing a much more distributed approach regarding health care providers. Information systems play a decisive role in empowering patients by providing them with the appropriate tools to help them secure and manage their EHRs.

Keeping this in mind and in order to achieve this desirable goal, one must efficiently translate real world infrastructures to the virtual world starting with patient's identification. Smart cards enable people's identities to be securely authenticated and communications to be secured, providing mechanisms for implementing strong security, differential access to data, and definitive audit trails, thus providing the mechanisms to enable trust in healthcare communications and business processes. They contain an embedded microprocessor chip that has the capability of running applications and can also carry data, such as personal details, that can only be accessed with the user's permission by entering a PIN code settled at the time of issuance. As this information is encrypted, it ensures that only authorized personal have access to the stored data in case the card is lost or stolen. Smart cards can additionally increase the level of identity verification by storing other identity information as qualified digital signature and biometric fields moving healthcare towards information management as a public utility rather than a personal millstone (7).

Smart cards are exploding worldwide and are a solid proven technology. In 2008, 5.045 billion smart cards were shipped worldwide — an impressive 13.2% increase over the 2007 figure of 4.455 billion. Because of their size, flexible form factors, and relatively low cost, smart cards are ideal for applications in healthcare where personal identity, privacy, security, convenience, and mobility are key factors (9). Some countries already have smartcard-based healthcare technology, such as USA (since the late 70's), Germany (since 1989), France (1998), Slovenia (since 2001) and more recently England. It is important to denote the Taiwan health care smart card project, which is one of the largest health care smart card solutions (since 2001) (19).

Most agree that the use of this type of technology is essential to achieving many critical milestones for healthcare reform, such as:

- The need to lower costs and create administrative efficiencies
- The need to improve patient outcomes and enhance physician and patient relations
- The need to meet increasing privacy, security and identity concerns, as a result of governments directives mandating increased control over private information

An identity and authentication solution based on smart card technology currently provides a best of breed foundation for improving HISs in a secure, private and sensitive way.

Many governments worldwide are currently making huge efforts for technological modernization and innovation. This is also becoming a reality in Portugal, where the Portuguese government has also realized the strategic need to innovate and modernize public administration infrastructures. One key ingredient is the new national identity card, the "citizen card" (Cartão de Cidadão – CC), which is basically a smart card that provides identification (ID number, Tax payers number, Elector's ID number, National Health System number and Social Security number) to all Portuguese as well as support for strong PKI X509 digital signatures and authentication certificates. This technology creates a perfect opportunity for the government to review public administration information, processes and applications architecture, both locally and centrally, especially in the area of user provisioning, authentication procedures, role based authorization and digital signatures of documents and associated processes (8). Briefly, to translate real world national authentication mechanisms to the digital world, in a well elaborated and secure way, which creates an opportunity window to leverage the OpenID framework with a strong PKI national infrastructure supported by smart cards, in this case the Portuguese CC. For healthcare providers, the challenge is not only to secure the funding for new technology, but also to weigh the potential benefits of new and emerging technology against the costs. Thus to embrace the Portuguese CC in healthcare is to exploit a new opportunity to simplify and provide secure access to patients' EHRs simultaneously reducing costs and budgets.

The Extended OpenID project is a conceptualization of this opportunity and the idea is to provide every Portuguese citizen with the possibility to enjoy Internet services in a secure, user centric and accessible way, by using their CCs to provision and strongly authenticate an OpenID digital identity. To walk towards this goal we have adapted and deployed an OpenID IP server, in which the authentication process makes use of the CC as a verifiable nationally deployed secure token (16).

3.3. Identity Services for Healthcare

Digital identities can play a great role in assisting citizen's to manage EHRs. Digital identity can be defined has a set of characteristics that uniquely describes a digital subject and its relations with other digital subjects (17). These characteristics or attributes can eventually change over time or even be certified by third parties thus adding a trusting character to it. In the digital world we are building a virtual society based on these principles and concepts. Although, the principles and concepts may not be new, the means in which they are processed and used produce a distinctive impact on its application, thus conferring a whole new dimension to it. Therefore, it is not only important to understand the mechanisms and roles behind the creation of a digital identity based society, but also how much control individuals will be able to take – or will want to take – over their digital identities (17). As a result, we investigated several complex scenarios with an OpenID identity provider based on the eOID project (16). Our goal is to employ this Identity Provider (IP) in a healthcare context and to extend the OpenID protocol to meet several healthcare challenging scenarios related to role delegation and authorization.

We thus consider the following attributes as critical and in need of being integrated into a patient Health Digital Identity (HDI):

Table 1. Patient's Health Digital Identity basic attributes

Personal Data	Clinical Information	Special Attributes
Full Name, Date of birth and Gender	Preference hospital, preference health center (health unit designation, GP name)	Authentication and signature certificate
Home Address, Telephone, Cellphone, Email	Organ donor, blood donor	Extra attributes (Attribute Designation, Value)
Emergence Contacts (Name, Cellphone, Kinship)	Blood type	
	Known Alergies (Designation, Date)	
National ID number, Tax payers's number, Social Security number, National Health System number	Known Chronic illness (Designation, Date)	
	Imunizations (Designation, Date)	

The authentication process within the eOID server is made by using the digital authentication certificate stored in the Portuguese Citizen Card. First, the user needs to register a digital identity on the eOID identity provider. The system then checks the validation of the authentication's certificate and consults the list of revoked certificates provided by the Certificate Authority (CA) responsible for the issuing and managing of the Portuguese Citizen Card certificates. If the user certificate is valid the eOID's authentication system associates the received certificate with the user's internal credential (16).

In order to create this service one must denote that health computing environments need to be modular, secure, and web-enabled. Much of the current thinking on distributed computing environments in health is based on the excellent previous works of the (then) OMG Corbamed taskforce, and the Distributed Healthcare Environment (DHE) work done in Europe in EU-funded projects such as RICHE and EDITH, and the HANSA and PICNIC implementation projects (22). Nevertheless, our proposal does not intent to create a framework that can have a single EHR for every Portuguese citizen. Building such a system is an enormously challenging task, involving several major research and development challenges. Instead, our proposal is to maintain the different EHRs as they are, while provisioning identity and authorization through the means of digital identity services. Our approach is thus to help enable the development of a truly distributed, scalable, and reliable healthcare information system that can take advantage of a federation of Health Identity Providers for patients. The notion of a distributed health computing environment is a key part of our vision. Our intent is to develop a distributed modular system to provide each Portuguese citizen with a Health Digital Identity (HDI) that could enable them to securely access their EHRs, scattered throughout different heterogeneous healthcare institutions. This infrastructure would enable patients to use their health information in the most convenient way, at their own discretion and at the same time to share it with health professionals as needed, ultimately providing them with important health information that will certainly help them in achieving much better health outcomes.

It is essential to stress the importance of developing an appropriate architectural model for provisioning digital identities in healthcare information systems. It is vital to identify and define exactly each stakeholder's responsibilities, by providing guidelines by which the process must be conducted and thus producing a more productive cooperation between the parts.

We have identified relevant stakeholders among the different Portuguese Health organizations to start implementing the proposed system architecture. We consider that the patient Health Digital Identity (HDI) could start to be deployed by the Portuguese Regional Health Administration (ARS – Administração Regional de Saúde) within their five regional health administrations (ARS Norte, ARS Centro, ARS Lisboa e Vale do Tejo, ARS Alentejo and ARS Algarve).

Nowadays, relational database technology has grown to the level where systems can store hundreds of terabytes of data in a database cluster using Storage Area Networks. However, the centralization of all information in a single system leads to a central point of failure that needs to be remedied by the use of expensive high availability equipment supported by a very expensive system administration infrastructure. Our proposal is to partition data geographically (according to the locations of the different Portuguese ARSs), by using a user-specific identifier, so that user-specific data is located within the same administrative domain, thus preventing data queries that span multiple, geographically distributed partitions (21). Suitable database partitioning algorithms will have to be devised for geographical distribution of patients HDI, while ensuring that data access is efficient and within acceptable time limits.

The mains advantages in using distributed databases are that they are very economical and reflect organizational structure, while maintaining local autonomy, since a department can control the data about them. Also it provides protection of valuable data (in case of disaster, such as a fire, all of the data would not be in one place, but distributed in multiple locations) and improves performance, as the data is located near the site of greatest demand, and the database systems themselves are parallelized, allowing load on the databases to be balanced among servers (a high load on one module of the database won't affect other modules of the database in a distributed database). Moreover, these systems perform more reliable transactions due to the replication of the database and are modular, which allows for systems to be modified, added and removed from the distributed database without affecting other modules (systems).

As a result we have identified the requirements for our HDI Provider (20):

- high data availability even in the presence of faults in the network or computer hardware (eg due to power outages, environmental disasters and regional strife)
- high performance to ensure the system can function even under the high loads that may arise in emergency situations (such as a pandemic, large-scale accident or war)
- security to protect patient data and digital identity from misuse, unauthorized access or attacks.

As part of this distributed approach, it is our intention to develop data replication algorithms to ensure that security, performance and data availability requirements are met. Our replication algorithms must take into consideration Brewer's Conjecture: it is impossible for a data store in an asynchronous network to simultaneously provide (i) partition tolerance, (ii) availability and (iii) consistency. Typically, systems can be built that simultaneously provide two of these three properties and it is generally assumed that designers of new systems should pick the two properties that are most important to their requirements (21). Further developments in our work will include a model for implementing the presented HDI Provider and we will investigate the design of partially synchronous networks that can enable us to overcome this limitation.

3.4. MedID – Digital Identity for health professionals

The use of digital identity certificates and federated identity systems provides the means to assure health professionals the opportunity to use their credentials in multiple health environments from different health institutions (5). Simultaneously, this will allow certifying health professionals with the secure credentials to translate their physical world role to the digital world. Our proposal is to adapt the eOID Identity Provider to meet the requirements for providing health professionals with a Medical Digital Identity, which ultimately will allow them to access the data they require to provide the best quality care at any given time.

We thus considered the following attributes to integrate a health professional Medical Digital Identity (MedID):

Table 2. Physician's Digital Identity basic attributes

Personal Data	Academic Data	Occupational Data	Special Attributes
Full Name, Date of birth and Gender	Education (degree, institution), Date of conclusion	Name used in clinical practice	Authentication and signature certificate
Naturality, Nationality	Date of entry in the Medical Order	College of Specialty (Designation, Date)	Extra attributes (Attribute Designation, Value)
		Regional Health Section	

The authentication process within the eOID server is made by using the digital authentication certificate stored in the MedicalID Card. The MedicalID card is not deployed yet and is based on a proposal for a smart card to provide health professionals' with strong PKI X509 qualified digital signatures and authentication certificates.

To use this service, the health professional needs to register a medical digital identity on the eOID identity provider. The system then checks the validation of the authentication's certificate and consults the list of revoked certificates provided by the Certificate Authority (CA) responsible for the issuing and managing of the MedicalID Card certificates. If the user certificate is valid the eOID's authentication system associates the received certificate with the user's internal credential.

We suggest that the entity responsible for the deployment of both the Certificate Authority and the Identity Provider should be the Portuguese Medical Order (Ordem dos Médicos). Regarding the Identity Provider it should be federated among their three regional sub-sections (Secção Regional do Norte, Centro and Sul) for better management and reliability.

4. Granting secure access to EHRs – the patient's choice

In the Portuguese legislation the patient can access is health related data with the consent of his GP and upon his request. Regarding EHRs several efforts are being made so that the patient is entitled to have a copy of his own EHRs upon his request. This will permit patients to access their own EHRs scattered among the different healthcare institutions thus allowing them to share them with the health professionals they wish to. The key feature in our vision is to provide the patient with the tools to share his EHRs in a fast and secure way, without having to reveal his access credentials in the process. We thus present a simple and flexible solution that enables the patient to easily grant authorizations to his own EHRs that can be scattered among several different health information systems.

4.1. Using OAuth to secure access to EHRs

Current health-oriented websites offer innovative services integrating functionalities from very diverse systems. This interoperability among different applications is highly desirable, but the same cannot be said about some of the interoperability implementations available today in the way they handle patient sensitive data and credentials, like user name and passwords (15). When a patient inadvertently shares his secret credentials with someone else he gives him full access to his account and personal data. The OAuth security protocol allows the user (patient) to grant access to his private health data residing on one site or application, often called a Service Provider, via an API to another site or application, often called a Consumer (15). While OpenID can be used to allow a patient to sign on into many health web sites or applications with the same identity, OAuth can be used to grant conditional access to patient data without having to share his identity at all (or his credentials). Using this type of protocol is extremely important regarding users privacy in the matters of managing EHRs. More generally, OAuth creates a freely-implementable and generic methodology for API authentication. By combining the OpenID protocol with OAuth we can arrive at a simple solution, more centred on the individual that can effectively help patients to be empowered by gaining an easier, more flexible and secure control over the dissemination of their own personal health data.

Moreover, we want to explore new ideas in the use of 'valet key' authorization mechanisms for the issue and user-centric management of temporal automatic access authorizations for strongly identified entities on a federation of trusted identity providers. The 'valet key' concept is a specially issued credential the owner of the data gives to another entity, in order for this entity to have conditional access to his data. Regardless of what restrictions the valet key imposes, the idea is that the owner gives limited access to his data to the bearer of a certain 'valet key', while he continues to use his regular key to access everything (18). We are currently exploring the concept of 'valet key' with an implementation combining OpenID with the OAuth protocol (15).

5. Case studies

In order to better understand the numerous advantages provided by such a model, we present and discuss a simple scenario where this type of technology could be applied to improve healthcare outcomes.

5.1. Patient's authorization to access their EHRs in an Health Information system during consultation time

The Patient X has severe pains regarding his back. He has been treated in two different hospitals by two different doctors, but his problem has not yet been solved. Now he seeks another medical opinion for his problem and makes an appointment to another doctor, who has been referenced by a good friend, Doctor Y.

Doctor Y has no knowledge about Patient X medical history as it is his first time they met. Patient X does is best to explain all the treatments he has been subject to by the other 2 doctors. He describes is back pains the better as he can and even shows some X-rays he has in his possession. But the given information is not enough for Doctor Y to have a clear idea of the treatments and diagnoses Patient X has been submitted to. Doctor Y then asks for permission to access Patient X EHRs in those two different HISs by using an installed application in his desktop that allows the display of the requested information. Patient X accepts Doctor Y's request and grants him an authorization for one session to access his EHRs by both 'asked' HISs.

OAuth authorization for installed applications involves a sequence of interactions between the third-party application (which only purpose is to display EHRs information), the Health Digital Identity Provider, and the end user (the patient). This diagram illustrates the sequence where the doctor has previously logged in with his MedicalID card (11):

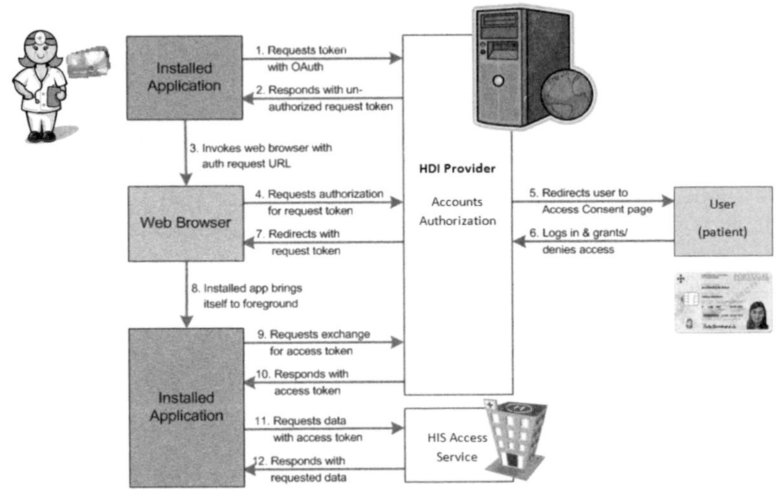

1. The installed application contacts the HDI Provider Authorization service, asking for a request token for one or more HISs. The request is signed using the "anonymous" consumer key/secret.
2. The HDI Provider verifies the request and responds with an unauthorized request token.
3. The installed application invokes a web browser.
4. In the browser, the installed application sends an OAuth request for token authorization, referencing the received request token.
5. HDI Provider displays an authorization page and prompts the user (the patient) to log into their account using his CC's card (for verification) and then either grant or deny limited access to his HIS service data by the third-party application that will allow the doctor to visualize the patient's EHRs.
6. The user (patient) decides whether to grant or deny access to the third-party application. If the user denies access, they are directed to the home page and not back to the application.
7. If the user (patient) grants access, the HDI Provider Authorization service redirects the user back to a web page designated by the third-party application. The redirect includes the now authorized request token.
8. The installed application auto-detects that an authorized token has been received, retrieves the token, and reclaims focus from the browser.
9. The installed application sends a request to the HDI Provider Authorization service to exchange the authorized request token for an access token.
10. The HDI Provider verifies the request and returns a valid access token.
11. The third-party application sends a request to the HIS service in question. The request includes the access token.
12. If the HIS service recognizes the token, it supplies the requested data.

Once the process is completed, Patient X removes is CC and the logout is automatically done. Now, Doctor Y is able to access important information on the two HISs his patient have granted access to and learn more about the patient's medical history. Accessing reports made by other doctors saved Doctor Y time and simplified his diagnoses decision. The information was available in the right time, to the right person and much more important in a secure way, thus preserving doctor-patient's confidentiality.

In an emergency situation there is no need for the patient to allow access. The information can be displayed at the doctor's request by using some "break the glass" mechanism with proper auditing activated for later investigation on the reasons that lead the doctor to act in this way (23).

6. Conclusions

Nowadays Electronic Health Records are seen as 'patient empowerment' process facilitators: by giving patients a source of information that is specific to them (4). Healthcare providers need to adopt a patient-centered approach if they want to effectively translate empowerment into their clinical practice: which requires that they get personally involved in the relationship with their patients and implies a shift in the representation of their roles, a shift that will place increased emphasis on improving the equity of the doctor-patient relationship, reducing the reliance on instruction and building more on partnership. As a result of their empowerment process, patients are expected to better self-manage their illness, by better pondering their choices: some patients may decide to delegate to their doctor the responsibility for some aspects of their treatment, while other patients under similar circumstances would prefer to learn to self-manage some if not all aspects of their illness and treatment (3). Although this behavior might be correlated with several different aspects of each patient, like age, gender, qualifications, education, as well as some aspects concerning today's society, every patient is an unique case and if well guided and motivated he can achieve a better self-manage of himself. However, this does not mean that patients should be left alone to decide what is best for them: it is the healthcare providers' responsibility to provide guidance and motivation for patients to learn how to manage effectively their illness and their lives (3).

Information technology plays a decisive role in empowering patients by providing them with the appropriate tools to help them to secure and manage the self disclosure of the data regarding their health, such as their PHRs or even their EHRs. Although there are a variety of solutions available to effectively help patients within their privacy, making extensive use of the OpenID protocol together with smart cards, 'valet keys' or even biometrics constitutes a tentative approach that should be further explored and promoted. Also, it is critical for doctors to have accurate and complete information about their patients' health in the right moment in order to provide more efficient health services. Therefore, time and access are indubitably key factors. Keeping this in mind, the solution we presented could effectively enabled patients to share their EHRs with the health professionals they desire in a secure and practical way. However, patients need time to adapt and adjust to these new emergent technological solutions. Patient empowerment is unquestionably a long process, which involves not only the collaboration of patients and health professionals, but also appropriate integrated and supporting digital health systems, thus promoting health to a whole new level.

7. References

[1] Patient-centric: the 21st century prescription for healthcare. IBM; 2006.

[2] Falcão-Reis F, Costa-Pereira A, Correia ME. Access and Privacy rights using web security standards to increase patient empowerment. In: Bos L, et al, editors. Medical and Care Compunetics 5. IOS Press; 2008. p.275-285.

[3] Aujoulat I, d'Hoore W, Deccache A. Patient empowerment in theory and practice: Polysemy or cacophony? Patient Educ Couns 2007;66(1):13-20. Epub 2006 Nov 2. Review.

[4] Munir S, Boaden R. Patient Empowerment and the Electronic Health Record. Patel V, et al, editors. Amsterdam: IOS Press; 2001.

[5] Angelmar R, Berman PC. Patient Empowerment and efficient health outcomes. 2007.

[6] Sarasohn-Kahn J. The wisdom of Patients: Health care meets online social media. California Health Foundation. 2008.

[7] Neame R. Smart Cards – the key to trustworthy health information systems. BMJ 1997;314:573.

[8] Cartão de Cidadão. Agência para a Modernização Administrativa, IP - Presidência do Conselho de Ministros, 2008. [Online]. Available from: URL: http://www.cartaodecidadao.pt/.

[9] A Healthcare CFO's Guide to smart card technology and applications. Smart Card Alliance. Feb 2009. [Online]. Available from: URL: http://www.smartcardalliance.org/download/pdf/Healthcare_CFO_Guide_to_Smart_Cards_FINAL_012809.pdf

[10] Falcão-Reis F, Correia ME. New trends on user centric web access control mechanisms and identity management for clinical settings. eHealth 2009 Second International ICST Conference on Electronic Healthcare for the 21st century. 2009 Sep 23-25; Istanbul, Turkey.

[11] [Online]. Available from: URL: http://code.google.com/intl/pt-PT/apis/accounts/docs/OAuthForInstalledApps.html

[12] Recordon D, Reed D. OpenID 2.0: A Platform for User-Centric Identity Management. 2007.

[13] OpenID. [Online]. Available from: URL: http://openid.net/.

[14] Rehman RU. The OpenID book. Conformix Technologies Inc.; 2008.

[15] OAuth. [Online]. Available from: URL: http://oauth.net/about.

[16] Falcão-Reis F, Almeida D. Correia ME. On the strengthening of OpenID authentication mecanisms with the portuguese citizen card. CISTI'2009 (4ª Conferência Ibérica de Sistemas e Tecnologias de Informação), Póvoa de Varzim; 2009 Jun 17-20.

[17] Windley PJ. Digital Identity. O'Reilly; 2005.

[18] International Organization for Standardization. ISO/TS 22600 - Health informatics – Privilege management and access control ISO TC 215. 2006.

[19] Hildebrand C. Currente state and future smart cards in Europe. Institute for Biomedical and Medical imaging, German Research Center for Envrionmental Health. [Online]. Available from: URL: http://www.hscf.net/029esemenyek/029_281007eugy_ea/Electronic_Health_Cards_in_Europe.pdf

[20] Dowling J, Haridi S. Developing a distributed electronic health record store for India. Oct 2008 ERCIM News.

[21] Technology development for building distributed, scalable, and reliable healthcare information store. Medical Informatics Group. Centre for development of advanced computing.

[22] [Online]. Available from: URL: http://dight.sics.se/files/docs/ehr-proposal.pdf.

[23] OpenEHR. [Online]. Available from: URL: http://www.openehr.org.

[24] Ferreira A, Cruz-Correia R, Antunes L, Farinha P, Oliveira-Palhares E, Chadwick D, Costa-Pereira A. How to break access control in a controlled manner. Proceedings of the 19th IEEE International Symposium on Computer-Based Medical Systems (CBMS); 2006; Los Alamitos (CA), USA. IEEE Computer Society;. 2006. p. 847–54.

Publication Only

Medical and Care Compunetics 6
L. Bos et al. (Eds.)
IOS Press, 2010

doi:10.3233/978-1-60750-565-5-231

A Neuro-Fuzzy Decision Support System for the Diagnosis of Heart Failure

Charles O. AKINYOKUN[1], Okure U. OBOT[2], Faith-Michael E. UZOKA[3] and [4]John J. ANDY
[1] *Dept of Computer Science, Federal University of Technology, Akure,, Nigeria*
[2] *Dept of Math, Statistics and Computer Science, University of Uyo, Uyo, Nigeria*
[3]*Dept of Comp Science and Info. Sys, Mount Royal University, Calgary, Canada*
[4]*College of Health Sciences, University of Uyo, Nigeria*

Abstract A neuro-fuzzy decision support system is proposed for the diagnosis of heart failure. The system comprises; knowledge base (database, neural networks and fuzzy logic) of both the quantitative and qualitative knowledge of the diagnosis of heart failure, neuro-fuzzy inference engine and decision support engine. The neural networks employ a multi-layers perception back propagation learning process while the fuzzy logic uses the root sum square inference procedure. The neuro-fuzzy inference engine uses a weighted average of the premise and consequent parameters with the fuzzy rules serving as the nodes and the fuzzy sets representing the weights of the nodes. The decision support engine carries out the cognitive and emotional filtering of the objective and subjective feelings of the medical practitioner. An experimental study of the decision support system was carried out using cases of some patients from three hospitals in Nigeria with the assistance of their medical personnel who collected patients' data over a period of six months. The results of the study show that the neuro-fuzzy system provides a highly reliable diagnosis, while the emotional and cognitive filters further refine the diagnosis results by taking care of the contextual elements of medical diagnosis.

Keywords: Dyspnea, Orthopnea, Palpitation, Tachycardia, Cyanosis, Oedema

1. INTRODUCTION

The limitations of the conventional methods for the diagnosis of diseases have been highlighted in [1,2]. There has been increasing needs to combine neural networks and fuzzy logic for a successful design of an expert system that would have a human-like reasoning capability [3]. Neural networks derive their strengths from the ability to generalize data relationship and the suitability to computations of data with non linear relationship such as found in medical records. They however suffer from inability to handle linguistic, vague, imprecise and noisy data, which are prevalent in medical records. A hybridization of fuzzy logic with neural network takes care of such shortcomings.

The normal function of the heart is the pumping of blood and circulating it through all parts of the body. When the heart's output cannot meet the normal work, a condition known as heart failure occurs. The general signs and symptoms of heart failure include; chest pain, dyspnea (shortness of breath), orthopnea, palpitation, cough, fatigue, tachycardia, cyanosis, oedema, nocturia, high blood pressure, low blood pressure, heart rate, rales, (crackles in lungs), elevated neck veins, hepamegaly, wheeze, heart sound, alteration in thought process, changes in level of consciousness, absence of emotion, heart murmur, pleural effusion, pulmonary oedema, cardio thoracic ratio, upper zone flow distribution and echocardiogram.

Researchers in medical expert systems in the past decade have attempted to find ways to manage uncertainty in medical diagnosis using soft computing methods [4, 5]. One of the earliest efforts in this direction attempted to develop heuristic methods for imposing structure on ill-structured components of medical diagnosis, resulting in the INTERNIST-1 diagnostic program [6, 7]. Evolutionary algorithms [8], case-based reasoning [9], and hypertext-based [10] systems, and knowledge base technology [1, 11] have been applied in the management of imprecise and unstructured medical knowledge. However, the utilization of neural networks and fuzzy logic became very popular in attempting to resolve the problems of imprecision and uncertainty in medical diagnosis. This is because of the ability of fuzzy logic to handle vague information and the training capability of neural networks [12]. Neural network based models for medical diagnosis are proposed [13, 14], while fuzzy models are discussed in [15, 16, 17].

In this paper, an expert system driven by neural networks and fuzzy logic for the diagnosis of cardiovascular diseases with emphasis on heart failure is developed. The architecture is composed of a knowledge base, neuro-fuzzy inference engine and a decision support engine. The knowledge base consists of quantitative knowledge of medical diagnosis of cardiovascular diseases, neural networks and fuzzy logic of both quantitative and qualitative knowledge of medical diagnosis of cardiovascular diseases. The neuro-fuzzy inference engine uses a weighted average of the premise and consequent parameters with the fuzzy rules serving as the nodes and the fuzzy sets representing the weights of the nodes. The decision support engine carries out the cognitive filter of the objective feelings and the emotional filter of the subjective feelings of the medical practitioner regarding the environmental and attitudinal contexts of diagnosis. The system is meant to be an adjunct to cardiologists by complementing their jobs. The design method employs back-propagation neural networks to train the neural networks. A measure of the significance of each input to the output is performed in order to eliminate the insignificant variables. The networks are then retrained to generate the outputs, which are then used to extract fuzzy rules from the data. The resultant neuro-fuzzy system is a network-like multilayered fuzzy rule based evaluation model. The fuzzy logic system employs the root sum square method of drawing inference. This paper attempts to report the results obtained from the case study of the patients of some Specialists Hospitals in Nigeria.

2. Materials and Methods

The architecture of the neuro-fuzzy expert system adopted in this study is proposed in [3] and presented in Figure 1. The detailed study of the architecture which is not presented in this paper in order to minimize its volume has been carried out and reported in [18]. The foci in this paper are the implementation details and a case study of heart failure. In order to implement the design of diagnosis of heart failure, the following activities have been undertaken:

a) Relevant data relating to the diagnosis and therapy of heart failure patients were obtained from the University of Calabar Teaching Hospital, Calabar, University of Uyo Teaching Hospital, Uyo and Ikot Ekpene Specialist Hospital, Ikot Ekpene, Nigeria over a period of six months.

b) NeuroSolutions 5.0 software, a neural network package, which models training and analysis, was used to train the neural networks on the data obtained using back propagation neural networks with supervised learning methodology.
c) The significant input variables were employed in retraining the neural network on the same set of data and the results obtained were compared with those trained using seventeen input variables.
d) Fuzzy rules were extracted from the trained datasets using the significant variables and used in developing linguistic labels and degree of membership for the fuzzy set for the diagnosis of heart failure. The fuzzy rules were also used to implement fuzzy logic diagnosis of heart failure using the Root Sum Square inference procedure.
e) A decision support engine was developed to assist in optimizing the final decision value. It consists of the cognitive and emotional filters that refine the objective and subjective feelings of the medical practitioner, thus assisting him to form preferences, make judgment and take final diagnosis decision.
f) The programming component of the system was carried out using Microsoft Visual basic.Net IDE

2.1. Data Collection and Analysis

The data for the research numbering one hundred and fifty items were collected from three hospitals, 70% of the datasets were used for training the neural networks, 20% were employed as testing datasets and the remaining 10% were used as cross validation datasets. The testing datasets for diagnosis are presented in Table 1. The value attached to the title of each column represents the maximum point that a patient can score on such sign, symptom or chest radiology. As a patient is examined for any of the signs or symptoms, a score that represents the feelings of the medical practitioner in respect of the sign or symptom is recorded for the patient. Based on all the recorded values, the patient is diagnosed. The degree of severity of diagnosis was considered to be ‘mild’, ‘moderate’ or ‘severe’.

2.2. Data Processing

NeuroSolutions 5.0 was employed in the training of the neural networks. In order to ensure optimal outputs, the datasets were divided into training dataset, testing dataset and cross validation dataset. The neural network was trained to ensure that it performs well on the data that it has not been trained on. The testing datasets provide a true indication of how the neural network will perform on a new dataset. It is used in establishing the performance and the efficiency of the connection strength of the neural network used during training. The cross validation dataset were used to elucidate the significant input variables and measure their contributions to the output variables.

Table 1: Testing Dataset for Diagnosis

Patient Number	Resdys (4)	Doe (1)	Clidys (1)	Orthop (4)	Pnd (4)	Palp (1)	Oed (1)	Hr (2)	Jvp (2)	Hepa (3)	Wheez (3)	S3S4 (3)	Luncrac (2)	Plefus (3)	Cadrat (3)	Zonflo (2)	Pulede (4)	Mil	Mode	Severe
UCTH28	0.8	1	0.5	0.8	0.9	1	0.2	0.5	0	0	0.4	0.8	0.5	0	0	1	0.9	0	0	1
UCTH29	0.4	0	1	0	0	0	0.2	0.6	0	0	0	0	0.5	0	0	0	0	0	0	1
UCTH30	0.3	0.1	0	0	0.3	0.3	0.3	0	0	0	0	0	0.5	0	0	0.3	0	0	1	0
UCTH31	0.6	1	1	0.9	0	1	0	0.5	.5	0	0.4	0.7	0.3	0	0.3	0	0	1	0	0
UCTH32	0.8	1	1	0.4	0.6	0	0.2	0.5	1	0.7	0	1	0	0	0.7	0	0.8	1	0	0
UCTH33	0.8	.1	1	0.5	0.8	1	1	1	0	0	0	1	0	0.7	0.7	0.3	0.8	0	1	0
UCTH34	0.4	1	1	0.8	0.4	0	0.2	1	0.5	0.7	0	0.7	0.5	0.4	0.4	0	0.8	0	1	0
UCTH35	0.4	1	0	1	1	1	1	1	1	0.7	0.4	0.7	0.3	0.4	0.4	0	0.5	1	0	0
UCTH36	0.8	1	1	0.4	.9	0	0.2	1	1	0.3	0	0.7	0.3	0.7	0.7	0	0.8	0	1	0
UCTH37	0.4	.2	0	0	.9	0.3	0.1	0.5	0.5	0.7	0.4	1	0.5	0.4	0.4	0.5	0.4	0	0	1
UUTH31	0.8	1	1	0.8	0.9	1	0.3	0.6	0.6	0.7	0.5	0.8	0.5	0.7	0	0.3	0.4	0	0	1
UUTH32	0.5	1	0	0.2	0.5	0.3	1	0.6	0.6	0.7	0.5	0.9	0.5	0.7	0.4	0	0	1	0	0
UUTH33	0.7	0.2	1	0.8	0.8	1	0.1	1	0.6	0.7	0.4	1	0	0	0	0.3	0.8	0	1	0
UUTH34	0.4	1	0.5	0.4	0.5	0.3	0.1	0.5	0.6	0.5	0.4	0.8	0	0	0.4	1	0.4	0	1	0
UUTH35	0.3	1	0	1	0.7	0.1	0.1	1	0	0.5	0.7	1	0.5	0	0.7	0	0.8	0	1	0
UUTH36	0.8	0.3	1	0.4	1	0.2	0.3	0	0	0.5	0	1	0	0	0.4	0.5	0.4	0	1	0
UUTH37	0.3	1	1	0.2	0	0	0.1	0	0.6	0.7	0	1	0	0	0	0	0.4	1	0	0
UUTH38	0.2	0	1	0.8	1	1	1	1	1	0.4	1.8	1	0	0.3	0.4	0	0.9	0	0	1
UUTH39	0	0	1	0	0	0	0	0.3	0	0	0	0	1	0.3	0	0.3	0	0	0	1
UUTH40	0.4	0.2	0	0	0.9	0.3	0.1	0.3	0.3	0.7	0.4	1	0.3	0.4	0.4	0.4	0.4	0	0	1
IKGH31	0	0	1	3	0	0	0	0.3	0	0.4	0.4	0.8	0.3	0.7	0.4	0	0.8	0	1	0
IKGH32	0.4	0	1	0	0	1	0.1	1	0.3	0.4	0	1	1	0.3	0.3	0.4	0.6	0	1	0
IKGH33	0.3	1	0	1	0.7	0.1	0.3	1	0	0.5	0.7	1	0.3	0	0.7	0	0.8	0	0	1
IKGH34	0.6	1	0.3	0.6	0	1	0	1	1	0	0	1	0	0	0.4	1	0	0	1	0
IKGH35	0.4	1	0	0.3	0.8	0	0.3	1	1	0	0	0.7	0	0	0.7	0	0.9	0	1	0
IKGH36	0.6	0	1	0	1	1	0	1	0	0.7	0.7	1	1	0.7	0.3	1	0.4	0	0	1
IKGH37	0.4	1	0	0.9	0.7	1	0.3	1	0.3	0.5	0	0.9	1	0.4	0.5	1	0	0	1	0
IKGH38	0.8	1	1	0	0.8	1	0	0	0	0.7	0.4	0	0	0	0.4	0	0.8	0	0	1
IKGH39	0.8	0.2	1	0	0.8	0	1	0	0	0.3	0.7	0.4	1	0.7	0.7	1	0.8	0	0	1
IKGH40	0.4	0.3	0.3	0.2	0.6	0	1	1	1	0.7	0.5	0.7	1	0.3	0.7	1	0.4	0	0	1

In order to extract fuzzy rules from the results of trained data of neural networks, a sensitivity analysis of the contributions of the input dataset to the output reports was carried out. The results show that six input variables are significant to the outputs of the diagnosis. The six input variables were used to retrain the neural networks. Table 2 shows the inputs contributions to the 'mild', 'moderate' and 'severe' outputs of diagnosing heart failure using the test dataset during the training process. A variable (signs and symptoms of heart failure) is considered significant if it has a minimum of 4% in at least two of the fuzzy sets.

The system is processed in a menu driven environment where the main menu as depicted in Figure 2 calls other sub menus.

The knowledge base submenu presents the user with the database, neural networks, and fuzzy logic processing options. The database option calls up a processing screen that gives access to and updates database elements such as patient's biodata, symptoms history, results of physical examination, and chest radiography. Presented in Figure 3 is a sample user interface for populating the database tables – symptoms history.

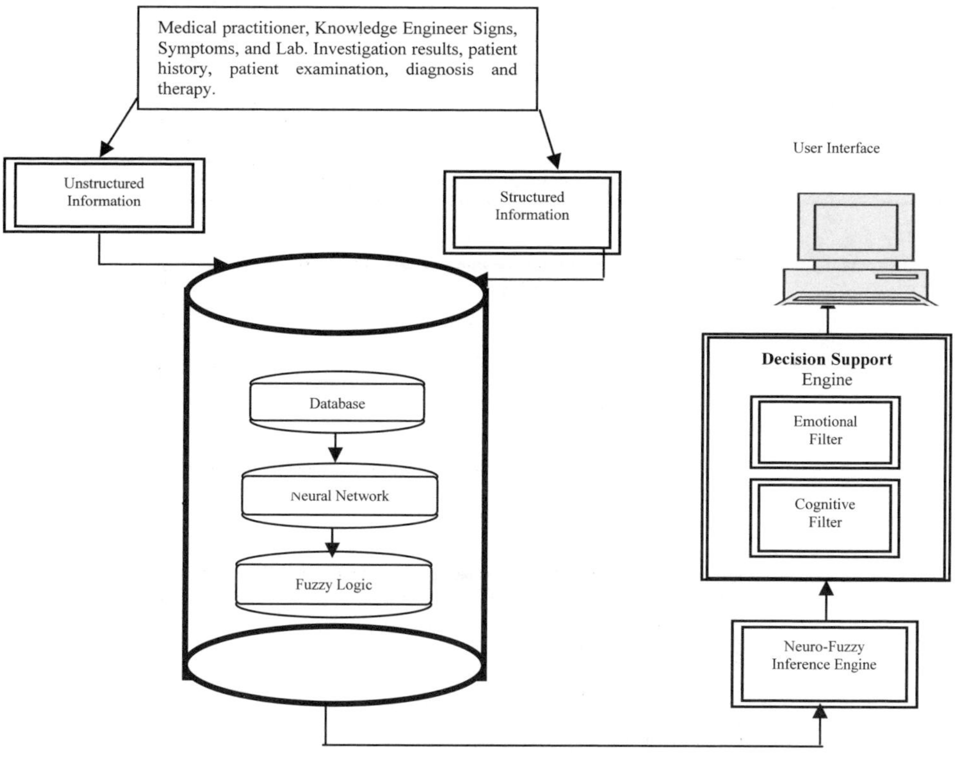

Figure 1: Architecture of Neuro-Fuzzy Expert System for Diagnosis of heart failure

Table 2: Inputs Contribution to Outputs

Variable	Mild	Moderate	Severe	Remarks
Resdys	0.041(4.1%)	0.019(1.9%)	0.027(2.7%)	Insignificant
Doe	0.020(2.0%)	0.040(4.0%)	0.027(2.7%)	Insignificant
Clidys	0.040(4.0%)	0.018(1.8%)	0.048(4.8%)	Significant
Orthop	0.047(4.7%)	0.121(12.1%)	0.150(1.5%)	Significant
Pnd	0.069(6.9%)	0.670(67.0%)	0.594(59.5%)	Significant
Palp	0.023(2.3%)	0.005(0.5%)	0.026(2.6%)	Insignificant
Oed	0.033(3.3%)	0.015(1.5%)	0.052(5.2%)	Insignificant
Hr	0.060(6.0%)	0.486(4.9%)	0.439(43.9%)	Significant
JVP	0.018(1.8%)	0.005(0.05%)	0.019(1.9%)	Insignificant
Hepa	0.057(5.7%)	0.066(6.6%	0.123(12.3%)	Significant
Whez	0.068(6.8%)	0.287(2.9%)	0.304(30.4%)	Significant
S3S4	0.022(2.2%)	0.004(0.04%)	0.028(2.8%)	Insignificant
Luncrac	0.031(3.1%)	0.008(0.08%)	0.041(4.1%)	Insignificant
BP	0.041(4.1%)	0.009(0.09%)	0.056(5.6%)	Significant
Cadrat	0.041(4.1%)	0.009(0.09%)	0.037(3.7%)	Insignificant
Zonflo	0.018(1.8%)	0.005(0.05%)	0.019(1.9%)	Insignificant
Pulede	0.027(2.7%)	0.009(0.09%)	0.027(2.7%)	Insignificant

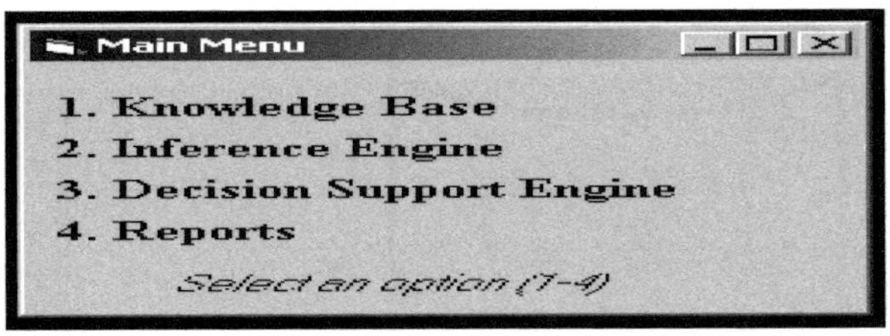

Figure 2: The Main Menu

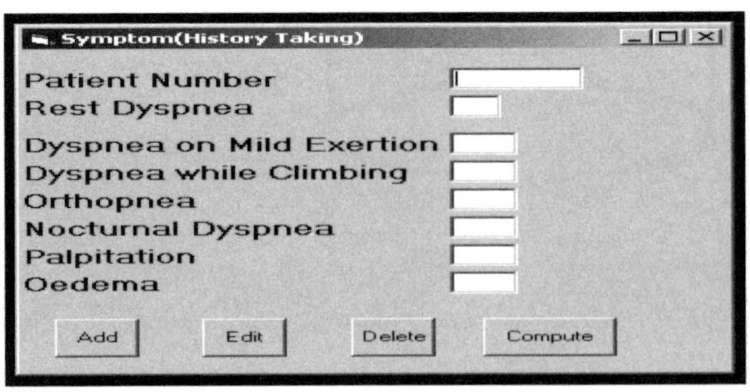

Figure 3: Symptoms (History) Taking Dialogue

The selection of the option 'Inference Engine' of the main menu causes a display of fuzzy logic inference, and subsequently the neuro-fuzzy inference engine activates the cognitive and emotional filter dialogs shown in Figures 4 and 5 respectively. This dialog enables the doctor to ask contextual questions related to the environment, habit, and history of the patient.

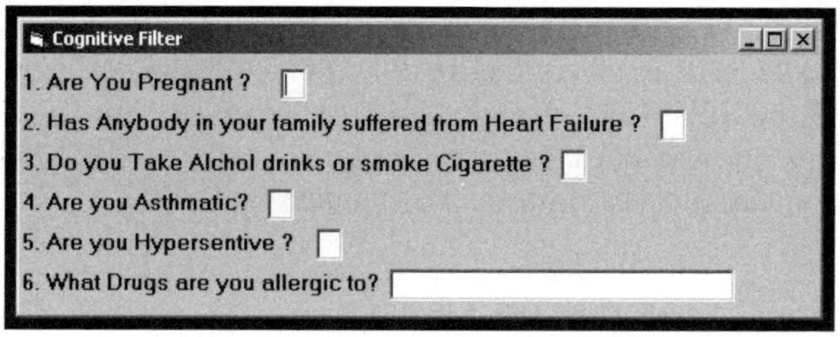

Figure 4: Cognitive Filter Menu

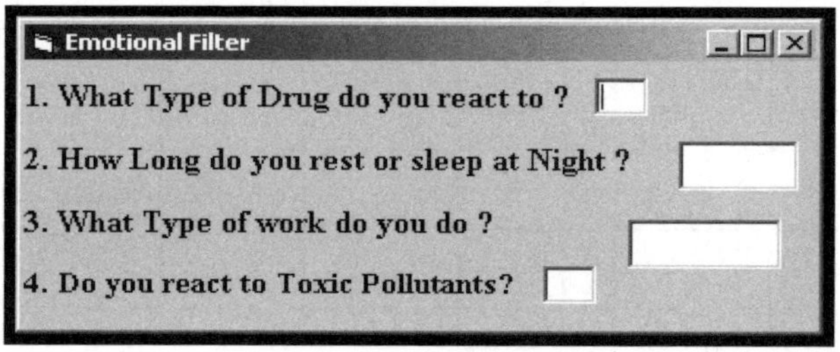

Figure 5: Emotional Filter Menu

3. RESULTS

In order to set alternative diagnoses and select the most appropriate model that best fits the *multilayer perceptron networks*, the hidden layers and *processing elements* of the hidden layers were varied. Performance was measured based on Mean Square Error, Normalized Mean Square Error and Correlation Coefficient (r) obtained during the training process. Three different performance runs were made on each model and the mean of each of the performance parameters was taken while learning curves were observed.

3.1. Analysis of Diagnosis Training

In Table 3, a summary of the models performance measures of trained diagnosis data is presented. The analysis of average Mean Square Error, High Standard Deviation, Normalized Mean Square Error and correlation coefficient obtained during the training process were carried out. Based on the results of the analysis, an optimal model was selected. Training was undertaken with varying parameters starting from two processing elements, incrementing by one step and stopping after four variations.

The best results were obtained from the neural networks with four hidden layers and five Processing Elements. This records Mean Square Error of 0.021, High Standard Deviation of 0.036, average minimum Normalized Mean Square Error of 0.026, a correlation coefficient of 0.988 and an overall percentage error of 1.24%, with a low Akaiike Information Criteria (AIC) of –171.288 and Minimum Description Length of –129.107. The networks with two hidden layer is the worst structure having a correlation coefficient of 0.74 and an overall error of 9.5% and average minimum Normalized Mean Square Error of 0.454. The networks structure of four hidden layers and five Processing Elements was selected as the optimal structure. In Table 4, the results of diagnosis training are presented for the testing dataset.

Table 3: Model Performance Measures for Diagnosis

Hidden Layer	PEs of Hidden layer	Average Min MSE of training	Average (SD+) of training	Average NMSE of training	R of training	AIC of training	MDL of training	%Error of training
1	2	0.216	0.279	0.151	0.920	15.412	57.592	3.697
	3	0.179	0.219					
	4	0.103	0.134					
	5	0.106	0.131					
2	2	0.167	0.178	0.454	0.742	10.379	32.940	9.495
	3	0.175	0.199					
	4	0.156	0.169					
	5	0.159	0.171					
3	2	0.167	0.175	0.086	0.960	-26.080	19.038	2.420
	3	0.096	0.126					
	4	0.077	0.106					
	5	0.042	0.054					
4	2	0.161	0.175	0.026	0.988	-171.28	-129.11	1.240
	3	0.090	0.114					
	4	0.064	0.075					
	5	0.021	0.036					
5	2	0.166	0.182	0.065	0.971	-73.35	-31.16	2.400
	3	0.106	0.115					
	4	0.057	0.066					
	5	0.036	0.061					

3.2. Fuzzy Logic Result

The inference procedure employs the Root Sum Square method of drawing inference. In this procedure, the degrees of truths of the rules are determined for each rule by finding the nonzero minimum value. The Root Sum Square is given by the formula:

$RSS = \sqrt{\sum r^2_i}$, where r = value of the firing rule.

Table 4: Test Dataset Results for Diagnosis Training

Patient ID	Mild	Moderate	Sever	Mild	Moderate	Severe	Output (Symbolic)
UCTH28	0	1	0	-	0.62135259	0.44059541	Moderate
UCTH29	0	0	1	0.105	0.96400315	0.03630702	Moderate
UCTH30	1	0	0	0.118	0.96834124	-0.0052607	Moderate
UCTH31	1	0	0	0.960	-0.0348036	0.1328989	Mild
UCTH32	1	0	0	0.136	0.00177469	0.88826805	Severe
UCTH33	0	1	0	0.088	0.99500418	-0.0114542	Moderate
UCTH34	0	1	0	0.630	0.23523769	-0.0333697	Mild
UCTH35	0	1	0	-	0.66534656	0.47596472	Moderate
UCTH36	0	0	1	0.750	0.1075849	-0.0173746	Mild
UCTH37	0	0	1	0.367	0.65005958	-0.0324285	Moderate
UUTH31	0	1	0	0.115	0.01102993	1.00016363	Severe
UUTH32	0	1	0	0.794	0.05708266	0.45884201	Mild
UUTH33	0	0	1	-	0.36877704	0.60726683	Severe
UUTH34	0	1	0	-	0.74296003	0.29355415	Moderate
UUTH35	0	1	0	0.094	0.01385562	0.9351429	Severe
UUTH36	0	1	0	0.138	-0.0016936	0.909376	Severe
UUTH37	0	1	0	0.109	0.0160907	0.85026475	Severe
UUTH38	0	1	0	0.115	0.00992398	0.99928294	Severe
UUTH39	1	0	0	0.065	1.01509173	-0.0222392	Moderate
UUTH40	0	1	0	-	0.97817649	0.11067308	Moderate
IKGH31	0	1	0	0.174	-0.0154493	0.962944	Severe
IKGH32	0	1	0	0.067	1.01409675	-0.0227827	Moderate
IKGH33	0	1	0	0.109	0.00600441	0.95189114	Severe
IKGH34	0	1	0	0.075	1.00891646	-0.0284992	Moderate
IKGH35	0	1	0	0.001	0.90121907	-0.0223443	Moderate
IKGH36	1	0	0	0.852	0.00741113	0.18788331	Mild
IKGH37	0	1	0	0.122	0.95948249	-0.0164853	Moderate
IKGH38	0	0	1	0.068	0.04096163	0.85652824	Severe
IKGH39	0	0	1	0.177	-0.0160873	0.96421255	Severe
IKGH40	0	1	0	-	0.68019072	0.39472856	Moderate

Fuzzy rules grow exponentially with the increase in the number of membership functions and the number of input variables [19]. The number of fuzzy rules denoted by 'x' is defined by: $x = M^{t}$; where M is the number of membership functions and t is the number of input variables. For six input variables and three membership functions, there are $3^6 = 726$ rules. Such a number makes the interaction between a model and the system designer practically impossible. Forty seven of these rules each of which is of the following have been extracted and presented in [18]. The results of the test dataset for the fuzzy logic of diagnosis computation are presented in Table 5.

3.3. Neuro-Fuzzy Inference Engine and Final Diagnosis

The implementation of the neuro-fuzzy inference engine uses the Adaptive Neural Fuzzy Inference System type-3 rule implementation [20] as modified and presented in [18]. The output report of the neuro-fuzzy inference engine serves as the input to the

Table 5: Fuzzy Logic Results for Diagnosis

Patient	Fuzzy Set	Linguistic
	0.82	Severe
	0.62	
	0.40	Mild
	0.38	Mild
	0.42	Mild
	0.63	
	0.58	
	0.64	
	0.43	Mild
	0.75	Severe
	0.84	Severe
	0.60	
	0.77	Severe
	0.85	Severe
	0.69	
	0.84	Severe
	0.55	
	0.94	Severe
	0.81	Severe
	0.62	
	0.82	Severe
	0.60	
	0.80	Severe
	0.56	
	0.41	Mild
	0.63	
	0.59	
	0.79	Severe
	0.81	Severe
	0.62	

decision support engine. Table 6 shows the diagnosis results. The cognitive filter average (CFA) plus the neuro-fuzzy value (NFV) gives the decision support intermediate value (DSIV), while the emotional filter average (EFA) value plus the DSIV gives the decision support final value (DSFV). Finally, linguistic variables are attached to the crisp output using the following function:

$$\text{Output} = \begin{cases} \text{Not Likely} & \text{if Output} < 0.2 \\ \text{Mild} & \text{if } 0.2 < \text{Output} <= 0.4 \\ \text{Moderate} & \text{if } 0.4 < \text{output} <= 0.7 \\ \text{Severe} & \text{if } 0.7 < \text{Output} <= 1.0 \\ \text{Very Severe} & \text{if Output} > 1.0 \end{cases}$$

Table 6: Neuro-Fuzzy Results for Diagnosis

Patient Number	NeuroFuzzy (NF) Value of the patient	Cognitive Filter (CF) Ave of the Doctor	Cognitive Rank (CR) = NF+CF	Emotional Filter (EF) Avg of the Doctor	Emotional Rank (ER) = CR+EF	Linguistic Variable
UCTH2	0.81	0.1	0.91	0.0	0.91	Severe
UCTH2	0.60	0.0	0.60	0.05	0.65	Moderate
UCTH3	0.41	0.05	0.46	0.05	0.51	Moderate
UCTH3	0.40	0.10	0.50	0.0	0.50	Moderate
UCTH3	0.42	0.10	0.52	0.0	0.52	Moderate
UCTH3	0.61	0.05	0.66	0.0	0.66	Moderate
UCTH3	0.59	0.05	0.64	0.0	0.64	Moderate
UCTH3	0.66	0.10	0.76	0.0	0.76	Severe
UCTH3	0.41	0.05	0.46	0.0	0.46	Moderate
UCTH3	0.78	0.10	0.88	0.05	0.93	Severe
UUTH3	0.82	0.10	0.92	0.0	0.92	Severe
UUTH3	0.63	0.15	0.78	0.0	0.78	Severe
UUTH3	0.71	0.15	0.86	0.05	0.91	Severe
UUTH3	0.81	-0.20	0.61	0.0	0.61	Moderate
UUTH3	0.66	0.0	0.66	0.0	0.66	Moderate
UUTH3	0.80	0.0	0.80	0.0	0.80	Severe
UUTH3	0.60	0.01	0.61	0.05	0.66	Moderate
UUTH3	0.90	0.05	0.95	0.05	1.00	Very
UUTH3	0.32	0.05	0.37	0.0	0.37	Mild
UUTH4	0.80	-0.05	0.75	0.0	0.75	Severe
IKGH31	0.83	0.05	0.88	0.05	0.93	Severe
IKGH32	0.63	0.05	0.68	0.0	0.68	Moderate
IKGH33	0.79	0.10	0.89	0.05	0.94	Severe
IKGH34	0.56	0.05	0.61	0.0	0.61	Moderate
IKGH35	0.43	0.10	0.53	0.05	0.58	Moderate
IKGH36	0.60	0.05	0.65	0.0	0.65	Moderate
IKGH37	0.56	0.10	0.66	0.0	0.66	Moderate
IKGH38	0.76	0.10	0.86	0.0	0.86	Severe
IKGH39	0.78	0.0	0.78	0.0	0.78	Severe
IKGH40	0.60	0.05	0.65	0.01	0.66	Moderate

4. DISCUSSION AND CONCLUSION

In the research presented in this paper, a multilayered feed-forward neural network with fuzzy rules extracted from trained data has been developed. Training of the networks was undertaken with NeuroSolutions 5.0 software package. In order to eliminate some insignificant variables of heart failure, inputs to outputs contributions measure was performed, then the significant variables were used to retrain the networks.

The hidden layers of the trained neural networks and processing elements were varied in order to obtain alternative diagnosis and select the most appropriate model that best fits the neural networks. Performance was measured based on mean square error, normalized mean square error and correlation coefficient. Fuzzy rules were extracted from the trained data. The rules represent the nodes of the networks while the weights are represented with fuzzy sets, resulting in a neuro-fuzzy model. Inference on the neuro-fuzzy system is performed on the weighted average of the rules firing strength, the premise and consequent parameters of the rules. The results of the neuro-fuzzy system are fed into the decision support engine to give the final diagnosis results. A strong correlation between the orthodox results and the neuro-fuzzy results was observed.

Thirty datasets (30 patients) were used as the testing datasets in the study. In the conventional diagnosis (Table 1), five cases were diagnosed as mild, thirteen as moderate, and twelve as severe. In the Neural Networks (NN) training subsystem (Table 4), five cases were diagnosed as mild, fourteen as moderate, and eleven as severe. Out of this number, two mild cases in the conventional diagnosis returned as severe cases after training the neural networks, while the remaining three mild cases maintained their status. Of the thirteen moderate cases in the conventional system, three returned as moderate while four returned as severe leaving six to maintain their status quo in the NN subsystem. One of the twelve severe cases in the conventional system returned as a mild case, while five returned as moderate, and six maintained their status as severe in the NN subsystem.

Three out of the five mild cases in the NN training subsystem, returned as moderate in the fuzzy logic subsystem (Table 5), the remaining cases remained as mild. Three moderate cases in the NN system changed to mild, while four cases changed from moderate to severe in the fuzzy logic subsystem, the other seven cases remained as moderate. Eleven severe cases in the NN subsystem have their status changed as follows in the fuzzy subsystem; one severe to mild, two severe to moderate while the other eight cases remained as severe.

In the hybrid (neuro-fuzzy) system (Table 6), there were one mild, sixteen moderate, twelve severe and one very severe case. These were obtained as follows from the NN subsystem; four cases changed from mild to moderate, one changed from mild to severe, four changed from moderate to severe, three changed from severe to moderate and one changed from moderate to severe. Three cases changed from severe to moderate and one from severe to very severe. In the fuzzy logic subsystem, all five mild cases changed to moderate; there were three moderate cases that changed to severe and one severe to moderate. Nine cases remained as severe and thirteen maintained their status quo as in the fuzzy logic subsystem.

Figure 6 shows the distribution of diagnosis for the fuzzy set, neuro-fuzzy set, cognitive ranking, and emotional ranking. From the graph, there is a visual evidence of relationship between the fuzzy diagnosis (FS) and neuro-fuzzy diagnosis (NF). A pairwise correlation analysis was carried out on the four diagnosis methodological components, namely fuzzy sets, neuro-fuzzy sets, cognitive ranking, and emotional ranking. The summary of the correlation analysis (Table 7) indicates that the highest correlation exists between the cognitive ranking and emotional ranking (0.990), while the least correlation exists between the Fuzzy set and emotional ranking (0.696).

A neuro-fuzzy expert system for the diagnosis of heart failure can function as an intermediary between a medical practitioner and a patient. The medical practitioner still has to examine his patient as he does in the orthodox practice. The neuro-fuzzy expert system enhances the medical practitioner's performance for quick, accurate, flexible and reliable diagnosis of heart failure, the features that are lacking in the orthodox or conventional practice. The system's strength is also found in its ability to assign some

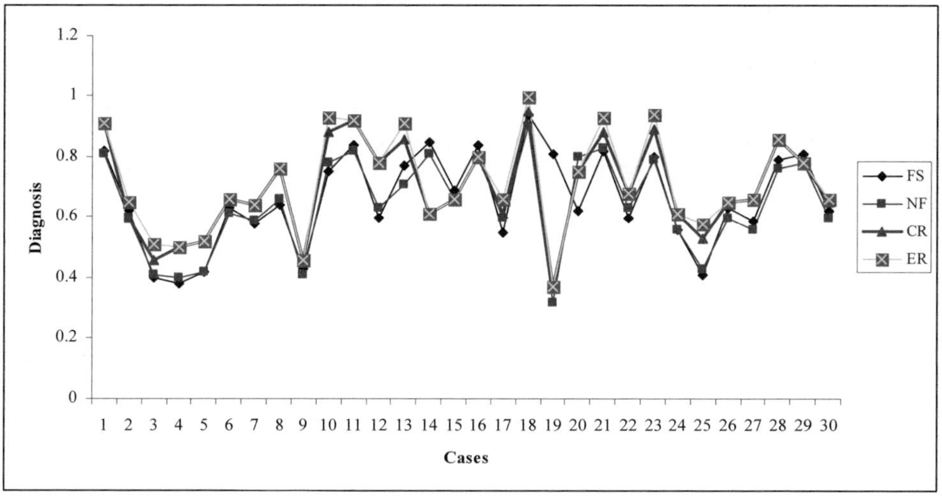

Figure 6: Diagnosis Graph

Table 7: Pairwise Correlation analysis

Method 1	FS	FS	FS	NF	NF	CR
Method 2	NF	CR	ER	CR	ER	ER
Correlation	0.798	0.714	0.696	0.909	0.894	0.990

degrees of severity, modesty and mildness to each diagnosed case. This can assist the medical doctor to assign therapies according and avoid the incessant cases of drug abuse. This study improves on previous medical diagnosis studies that applied fuzzy logic, neural networks, or neuro-fuzzy methodologies by introducing the decision support (cognitive and emotional) filters. In real life, the decision support filters (DSF) enhance the performance of the medical expert in the diagnosis of diseases. The filters aid in clarifying both the objective and subjective value judgments made when evaluating the possible consequence of alternative decisions. The DSF helps the medical practitioner to relate the diagnosis to emotional, environmental, and other conditions of the patient, which could produce symptoms akin to a particular disease.

In this paper, we have addressed the subject of heart failure diagnosis using a hybridization of fuzzy logic, neural networks and preference technology. We furthered the study by utilizing the same subjects in studying therapy of heart failure. A future paper would report the results of the study. We have also begun the application of multicriteria techniques (such as the analytic hierarchy process) in medical diagnosis and therapy. Recent literature has pointed to the potency of the AHP and its hybridization with other soft-computing tools in medical and health care decision making [21].

ACKNOWLEDGEMENTS

We thank the University of Uyo, Uyo, Akwa Ibom State, Nigeria that funded the research reported in this paper. We thank the medical personnel of University of Uyo Teaching Hospital, Uyo, Nigeria, University of Calabar Teaching Hospital, Calabar, Nigeria and Ikot Ekpene Specialist Hospital, Ikot Ekpene, Nigeria for their assistant and support.

REFERENCES

[1] Akinyokun OC, Adeniyi OA. Experimental Study of Intelligent Computer Aided Medical Diagnostics and Therapy. AMSE Journal of Modeling, Simulation and Control 1991;27(3):1-20
[2] Obot OU. Knowledge Based Server for Medical Diagnosis and Therapy of Tropical Diseases. M.Tech Thesis. Federal University of Technology. Akure, Nigeria. 1999.
[3] Akinyokun OC. Neuro-Fuzzy Expert System for Evaluation of Human Resource Performance. First Bank of Nigeria Plc Endowment Fund Public Lecture Series I. Federal University of Technology, Akure. 2002.
[4] Szolovits P. Uncertainty and Decisions in Medical Informatics. Methods Inf Med 1995;34:111-21
[5] Song Q, Kasabov N. (2003)., A Novel Generic Higher-order TSK Fuzzy Model for Prediction and Applications for Medical Decision Support. Proc. of The Eighth Australian and New Zealand Intelligence Information Systems Conference (ANZIIS2003); 2003 Dec 10-12; Sydney, Australia. 2003. p. 241-5.
[6] Pople HE. Heuristic Methods for Imposing Structure on Ill-Structured Problems: The Structuring of Medical Diagnostics In: Szolovits, editor. Artificial Intelligence in Medicine. Boulder (CO): Westview Press; 1982 (Chapter 5).
[7] Miller RA; Pople HE, Myers JD. INTERSIT-1: An Experimental Computer Based Diagnostic Consultant for General Internal Medicine. New England Journal of Medicine 1982;316:250-8
[8] Podgorelec V. Kokol P. (2001); Towards More Optimal Medical Diagnosing with Evolutionary Algorithms. J Med Syst 2001;25(3):195-219.
[9] Ochi-Okorie AS. Disease Diagnosis Validation in TROPIX using CBR. Artif Intell Med 1998;12:43-60.
[10] Timpka T; Padgham L; Hedblom P; Wallin S, Tibblin G. A Hypertext Knowledge Base for Primary Care. ACM (0-89791-321-3/89/0006/0221). 1989. p. 221-8
[11] Uzoka F-ME, Famuyiwa FO. A framework for the application of knowledge technology to the management of diseases. Int J Health Care Qual Assur 2004;17(4):194-204.
[12] Bonnisone PP; Geobel K; Khedkar PS. Hybrid Soft Computing Systems: Industrial and Commercial Applications. Proceedings of the IEEE; 1999 Sep. 1999;87:9.
[13] Economou GPK; Hallas JA; Mariatos EP, Goutis CE. Artificial Networks in Medical Decision Making Systems: An Application to Pulmonary Diseases' Diagnosis through VHDL Synthesis. Proceedings of the European Design and Testing Conference. 1995. p. 590.
[14] Gomez-Ruiz JA; Jerez-Aragones JM, Munoz-Perez J. (2004); A Neural Network Based Model for Prognosis of Early Breast Cancer. Applied Intelligence 2004;20:231-8.
[15] Daniels JE, Cayton RM. Cadosa: A Fuzzy Expert System for Differential Diagnosis of Obstructive Sleep Apnoea and Related Conditions. Expert Systems with Applications 1997;12(2):163-77.
[16] Wainer J, Sandri S. Fuzzy Temporal/ Categorical Information in Diagnosis. Journal of Intelligent Information Systems 1999;13:9-29.
[17] Obot OU, Uzoka FME. Fuzzy rule-based framework for the management of tropical diseases. Int J Med Eng Inform 2008;1(1):7-17.
[18] Obot OU. (2007); System Model for Medical Diagnosis and Therapy of Cardiovascular Diseases: A Case Study of Heart Failure. PhD Thesis. Federal University of Technology; Akure, Nigeria. 2007.
[19] Wong K, Fung CC, Myers D. An Integrated Neural Fuzzy Approach with Reduced Fuzzy Rules for Well Log Analysis. International Journal of Fuzzy Systems 2002;4(1):592-9.
[20] Takagi T, Sugeno M. Derivation of Fuzzy Control Rules from Human Operators Control Actions. Proceedings of the IAFC Symposium on Fuzzy Information, Knowledge Representation and Decision Analysis. 1993. p. 55-60.
[21] Liberatore MJ, Nydick RL. The analytic hierarchy process in medical and health care decision making: A literature review. Eur J Oper Res 2008;189(1):194-207.

Medical and Care Compunetics 6
L. Bos et al. (Eds.)
IOS Press, 2010

doi:10.3233/978-1-60750-565-5-245

Rules and Access Rights of the Estonian Integrated e-Health System

Madis Tiik MD[1]
Tartu University, Estonian E-Health Foundation

Abstract. There should be a clear understanding that when implementing an electronic health record system (EHR), one of the hardest problems we have to solve is the access rights. In Estonia this process lasted for three years and involved all stakeholders of the healthcare sector. Special ethical committee was established to advise the decision makers and doctors to help them understand the ethical dilemmas from the patient's and society's point of view. In this article you will find a short overview of the access rights of the system, roles of the healthcare systems' employees. Descriptions of some specific situations like underage patients and representation of patient with restricted active legal capacity.

Keywords. Access rights, integrated EHR, patient's rights, legislation.

Introduction

The prerequisite for realising the health information system and the Electronic Health Record (hereafter EHR) is to establish the rules for the usage of patient's health data. The purpose of this article is to analyse the principles of the system of access rights and the system of rights related to handling patient's health data from the following aspects:

- Purpose of data usage
- Roles of health care system's employees
- Patient's will
- Specific situation

This article contains descriptions of:

- Data stored in the EHR information system
- Rules of accessing patient's health data

The EHR data usage rules were created by the Estonian eHealth Foundation and it was finished on 18.03.2008. The Health Services Organization Act and Associated Acts Amendment Act[2] approved by the Estonian Parliament „Riigikogu" on 20.12.2007 has also been considered.

---

[1] Corresponding author. madis@e-tervis.ee

[2] Health Services Organization Act and Associated Acts Amendment Act (Tervishoiuteenuste korraldamise seadus ja sellega seonduvate seaduste muutmise seadus), available only in Estonian, https://www.riigiteataja.ee/ert/act.jsp?id=12909773

The Minister of Social Affairs has issued a regulation that establishes a list of documents necessary to prove the provision of health care services, and these documents have to be forwarded to the EHR system as electronic documents. From 01.01.2009 all healthcare providers are obligated to send agreed numbers of medical documents to the central database. The responsibility of the Estonian E-Health Foundations is to provide necessary services to patients and healthcare providers and secure the operation of the system.

1. Definitions used to describe the roles

1. An underage patient – individual aged 0-18 whose data is being processed in the EHR, who can carry out different types of activities in the EHR, and who has a legal representative.
2. Guardian – legal representative. Person who is making transactions and activities on behalf of patient. In the EHR system this person is considered to have a role of a representative who has maximum rights. The data of the guardian is enquired from the Population Register via online processing.
3. Information Service – data issued from the EHR information system over the X-tee standard interface (including enquiries and electronic documents).
4. Patient – person whose data is processed in the EHR information system.
5. Patient's health data – sensitive personal data containing information about patient's health condition.
6. Patient's general personal data – non-sensitive information about patient, such as address, etc.
7. Patient with restricted active legal capacity– Person who has no rights to carry out any activities or transactions in the EHR information system because their active legal capacity has been restricted by court.
8. Attending physician – health care service providers, who are treating a patient and who are registered with the Health Care Board. Midwives and medical assistants providing independent services are deemed as sub-categories, and they have the same rights as an attending physician.
9. Attending physician's assistant – employee who is assisting attending physician and who is not registered in the register of the Health Care Board. For example, attending physician's secretary.
10. Treatment setting – treatment, advising, and documenting of patient's complaints by the health care service employee registered at the Health Care Board.
11. Employee at the registry office – person who is carrying out the activities of the registry but is not an attending physician.
12. Legal representative – legal representative and guardian are the same person, i.e. legal representative has the rights of a guardian, and guardian has the rights of a legal representative.
13. Representative – person appointed by patient who has the right to carry out activities and transactions in the EHR information system. There can be representatives of two different levels of rights. Representative who has full rights is identical to patient and can proceed with all activities and transactions (including expressions of will) on behalf of patient. Representative with limited rights can view patient's data in the EHR information system but has

no other rights. The extent of the rights of a representative is determined by the authorization (expression of will) made by patient. In terms of the EHR information system legal representative is a patient's representative who has full rights. Person under guardianship can't appoint representatives – representatives are appointed on his/her behalf by guardian.

2. Data in the Electronic Health Record

Patient's health information will be submitted to the EHR by health care service providers in form of electronic documents as listed below:

- Electronic information notes
- Electronic medical documents

The electronic documents are formalised as standard HL7 CDA documents that will be stored in central database (i.e. archived electronically). The person compiling the medical document has to be identifiable: documents containing medical information or a physician's decision must have the physician's digital signature or be date-stamped by health care service provider's information system. The confirmation of the sender's information system is sufficient if the document only contains information related to the administrative or technical process (i.e. appointment confirmation).

There will be additional information associated with patient's person and health sent to the EHR:

- Orally submitted information from patient and patient's representative
    - Contact information
    - Representatives
    - Patient's expressions of will regarding their preferences of health services
        - Refusal from blood transfusion
        - Refusal from organ transplantation
        - Consent for organ donation
        - Refusal from resuscitation (treatment related will)
        - In the event of death, consent to donate a body for research and educational assignments.

2.1. Data Required for Using the Electronic Health Record Information System

The EHR information system needs and uses data:

- to authorize an attending physician
- to authorize a patient and a representative
- to enable patient to get information about their health data
- to enable physician to fill out the personal data section in documents
- to support physician in the process of medical decision making
- as an additional information source gathering/taking anamnesis

- to automatically create notes by the EHR system (the EHR information service)
- to carry out assessments related to treatment quality and health care administration

Data not submitted either by health care provider or by patient will be enquired through online processing from the organisations or administrative domains, and this data will be used to carry out a specific automated procedure. Therefore, the end-user (physician and patient) does not set access rules for this data. Each enquiry of data or storage of data in the EHR information system will be determined according to the mission-critical and informational-logistical considerations.

The data necessary for authorizing attending physicians is mission-critical since without this data no physician will be able to use the services of the EHR. Therefore, certain tables from the registers of the Health Care Board have to be duplicated and renewed after regular intervals (for instance once in every 24 hours) in the EHR information system.

2.2. Electronic documents

The electronic documents differ from the documents listed in the regulation of documents proving the provision of health care services, because electronic documents contain comprehensive information representing a specific fixed time gathered by one person.

(e.g. emergency medical care card is filled out by several physicians, and entries on this document are derived from and represent different moments in time. HL7 messages are created separately per each entry. However, because the HL7 message is comprehensive it can be decided upon this message which patient and incident is being referring to, i.e. which messages together form the total content of the emergency medical card; health care service provider can forward the electronic documents either together at one time at the end of the case or after each treatment episode. According to a general principle, the electronic documents are forwarded to the EHR information system when the patient leaves the doctor's office or health care institution that provided the treatment).

Electronic document includes additional information added by default by the health care institution's information system *(e.g. directory code used in the document for each field described by the directory, i.e. OID, value of the directory's element in coding determined by OID if the output form of the document has a name of formatting legible only to the human eye, unique identifier of a case in health care providers information system, etc.).*

Documents are marked in the EHR information system to indicate if the first time reviewing of a document has to be done together with a physician. This specific mark will be added by the physician creating the document before he/she forwards it to the EHR information system.

Types of EHR Documents Pursuant to Access to Documents

1. Documents visible to the patient and attending physician without any restrictions

2. Documents closed by the attending physician (the physician compiling the document will add a specific mark banning access to the document by patient or attending physician)
    a. Documents visible to the attending physician but visible to patient only after the first review (the attending physician will introduce the document to patient)
    b. Documents visible to the attending physician but not available for the patient to enquire from the EHR information system
    c. Documents not visible to the attending physician but what can be enquired by patient from the EHR information system
3. Documents closed by patient
    a. Documents not visible to the attending physician but visible to the patient (and representatives acting in patient's rights)
    b. Documents not visible to the representative/legal representative but are visible to the attending physician

Correcting Incorrect Data in Documents

The attending physician can invalidate a document if he/she discovers that a document with incorrect information has been forwarded to the EHR information system (attending physician will send a message to the EHR information system to inform that the status of the document has been changed). The attending physician can send a new updated version of the document to the EHR information system after the initial document has been invalidated.

If a document containing incorrect information is discovered either by patient or an attending physician, the organization responsible for creating the document has to be contacted. The document will be corrected by the organization that created the document in the first place, and the corrected version of the document will be forwarded to the EHR information system.

3. Rules on Accessing Patient's Health Data

3.1. General Principles

This chapter describes the attending physician's job in regular and emergency care situations. Information created during treatment will be first stored in health care service provider's information system, and the attending physician uses the information contained in local system. Documents forwarded to the EHR will be electronically signed by the attending physician or date-stamped by health care service provider.

Only the health care employee (the attending physician) currently associated with patient's treatment has the right to make enquiries about patient's data, i.e. the patient's attending physician or a medical assistant. Making enquires about patient's health data outside of treatment process is not allowed.

Health data will be issued to health care employees registered with Health Care Board and who are marked as the attending physician

During the first visit, the health care service provider's information system will enquire about patient's personal data

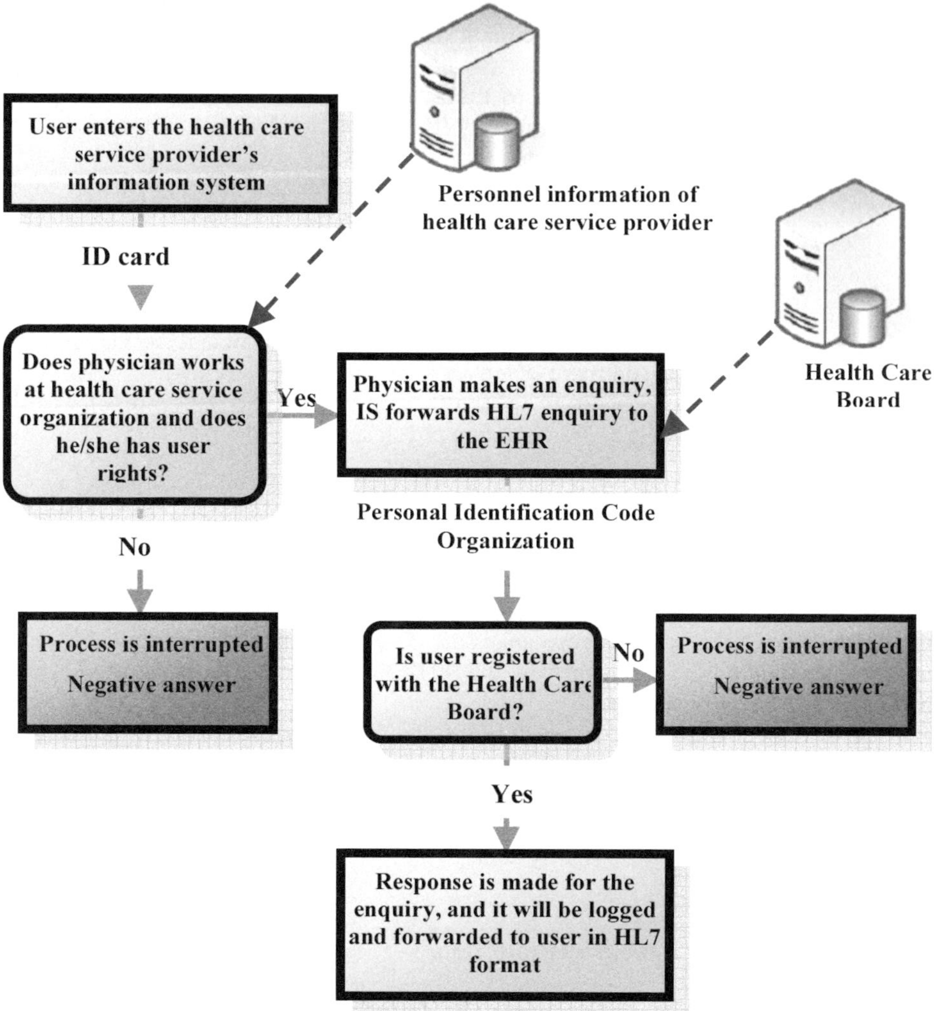

Figure 1. Authorization of health data enquiry.

- Pre-filled document's header will be compiled if possible, and the physician will orally verify the continued validity of data if necessary

Following the data usage rules provided in this document, the attending physician may choose to enquire other documents or information related to patient as the treatment process progresses. This necessity is determined by the attending physician, and he/she must be able to justify to patient the purpose of using the data in relation to providing a specific service.

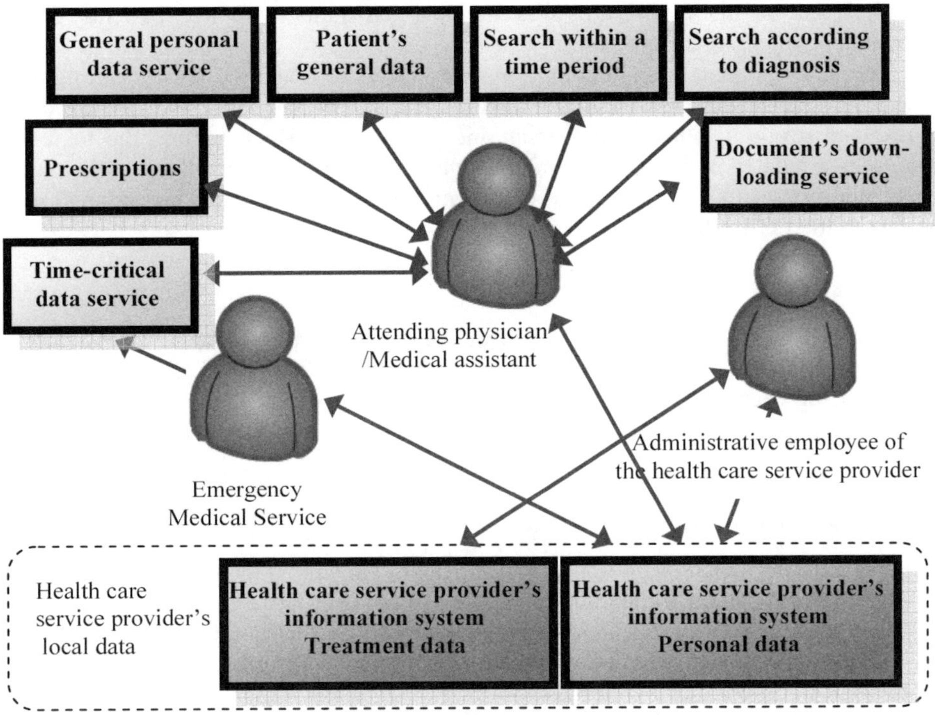

Figure 2. Services and their users.

3.2. Roles of Data Users

- Physician (health care service providers associated with patient's treatment and registered at the Health Care Board)
- Patient
- Patient's guardian (a legal representative)
- Patient with restricted active legal capacity
- Representatives – persons associated with patient
  - Representative with complete rights
  - Representative with restricted rights (can only view data)

Attending Physician

An attending physician is a health care employee registered with the Health Care Board who is currently associated with patient's treatment. A family physician is the attending physician on permanent basis to all patients in his/her practice list. The attending physician may hold different positions related to specific case (replacement physician, on-call physician, consulting physician, etc.), and regardless of the position the physician is still considered to be the attending physician. Patient's data can be enquired from the EHR information system by patient's attending physicians and assistants (excluding the enquiry about the referrals list which can also be enquired by register office's employees). The assistants will participate in treatment together with the physician or they will work as medical assistants who see patients during independent appointment times.

Acting as the patient's attending physician refers to treating a patient during a set time period beginning with the initial appointment and ending when the case of illness is resolved (excluding family physician and pathologist). Documenting the treatment process is regulated by legislation and the summary of each case of illness (ambulatory visits, duration of in-patient medical treatment, day care surgery and procedures) must be sent to the EHR information system.

Family Physician's Rights

A family physician is the attending physician on permanent basis to all patients in his/her practice list. The family physician may enquire from the EHR the electronic documents and personal data of patients listed in his/her practice list.

It is not possible to make enquires about documents to which patient has set access restrictions.

Specialty Physician's Rights

The specialty physician is entitled to enquire about patient's documents and data in the EHR if he/she is patient's attending physician.

The organisation's information system must ensure that attending physicians can be correctly established and authorized in organisation's information system and that other users could not make enquiries without proper authorization. More specifically, it has to be made sure that physicians, assistants and other employees of the organisation could not carry out any activities by using name and password of another physician or assistant.

Differences of Gaining Access for Pathologists and Forensic Medical Physicians

Pathologists and forensic medical physicians have access to patient's medical information in the EHR after patient's death (excluding documents patient has banned access to) if patient is brought for autopsy.

Pharmacist's Rights

Pharmacists have the right to make enquiries to the prescription centre about prescriptions prescribed to patients as well as prescriptions not bought out. The pharmacist can't make enquiries from the EHR.

If patient wishes, the attending physician will add names of representatives to the prescription who will have the right to buy it out from the pharmacy. The names of representatives are available in the e-prescription centre, and patient can determine his/her representatives at the time the prescription is issued. The patient can determine if a certain prescription can be bought out by a certain person, by patient himself or by anyone.

Resident's Rights

Resident is a general practitioner who in the event of patient's treatment is patient's attending physician.

School Health Care Employee's Rights

A school's health care employee is not involved in treatment process but carries out the prophylactic exams of school children. On some occasions, the school health care employee has a role of the attending physician, and in this case he/she has rights in the EHR information system equal to the rights of the attending physician.

The physician and a medical assistant both are active in school health care system, and both of them have the right to make independent referrals (physician directly to specialty physician, assistant to family physician). The decisions of other health care employees that have occurred based on these referrals will be reflected in the EHR and must be available to school's health care employee.

3.3. Restrictions

Patient's Right to Set Restrictions

The patient has a right to set access restrictions to documents, cases of illness and to all his/her information in the EHR. The access ban can be set one specific document or applied to complete data in the EHR. In the event patient has set access restrictions, users will not be able to enquire patient's documents or any data from restricted documents. There will be an indication generated dynamically in patient's general personal data sent as a response to enquiry if patient has set any restrictions to his/her data. Access to data necessary for the interoperability of different information systems can't be banned. For instance, health information system must still be able to exchange information with medical registers regardless of the fact that access to data has been closed. Therefore, the closing will only close access to the attending physician providing health care services.

The patient will be informed by information system at the time of setting the restriction that it is dangerous to patient's life and health to provide health care services based on insufficient information.

Example: If patient has set an access restriction to epicrisis then this restriction will also extend to the index of and diagnosis in the epicrisis as well as to prescribed medications, etc. Therefore, when making an enquiry to get a patient's comprehensive list of epicrisis compiled throughout their medical history, the epicrisis with restricted access will be omitted. Also, the medication indicated on this epicrisis will not be visible under the list of medications being taken by patient.

Patients with restricted active legal capacity or who have been assigned a guardian by court don't have a right to set restrictions. In case of guardianship, patient's rights will be executed by the guardian (defined by the EHR information system as a representative who has complete rights).

Ignoring the Access Restriction

The access restrictions to patient's health data in the EHR information system can't be ignored. There will be no access allowed to initial documents even in the emergency situation and the patient will take full responsibility regarding possible consequences that may arise from banning access to data.

Patient's Right to Enquire the Electronic Health Record Documents

The patient has a right to enquire all documents relating to him/her from the EHR information system that physician has not set any restrictions on.

In the event of an examination the physician ordering the examination will indicate on referral if the initial viewing of the results of the examination has to take place accompanied by the physician or if patient may view the results independently. If patient wished to see the results of the exam before the summary is created then he/she can do so at the institution were the physician who ordered the examination works, and this is where the attending physician will introduce the appropriate documents to patient.

Information deemed unnecessary at the time of creating the summary will not be forwarded to the EHR information system, and patient may examine this information at health care organisation if necessary.

The patient has a right to enquire information from the EHR information system on how his/her data has been used by attending physicians.

Rights of a Patient's Representative

The patient's representative of full rights is by default patient's legal representative (guardian for an underage patient and persons with restricted active legal capacity). The EHR information system makes enquiries via online processing about legal representatives from the Population Register. Representative with full rights has a complete authorization to act on behalf of patient.

The patient doesn't have a right to change the level of authorization of legal representative.

In addition, the patient can assign representatives authorized to make transactions on behalf of patient in the EHR information system. The authorization can be partial or comprehensive. Partially authorized representative can only view patient's data and is not allowed to make any transactions on behalf of patient. Representative with full rights:

- can get health information related to the patient from the EHR information system or from health care service provider
  - will be informed in emergency situations
  - gets information after patient dies
- executes patient's rights
  - sets or removes access restrictions on documents
  - makes expressions of will
  - assigns other representatives

The patient (excluding patients with restricted active legal capacity) has a right to change or let go of a representative (excluding legal representative). Only an adult of active legal capacity can be authorized as a representative. A representative can be the patient's attending physician who will execute patient's rights in the EHR information system according to the agreement with the patient.

Rights of an Underage Patient

The underage patient has a right to set restrictions to documents and cases of illness, i.e. his/her legal representatives and representatives can't enquire these documents or cases of illness.

The attending physician must be convinced that the underage patient is capable of responsibly assessing the pro- and con-arguments related to the provision of health care services[3]. If the underage patient is capable of such assessment, then he/she is capable of giving consent. This means that if the underage patient came to see the physician independently, then the documents associated with this particular case can only be enquired by the patient. The attending physician must ask the patient if he/she wants to disclose information to his/her legal representative. Information will not be disclosed by default. The physician has a right to disclose information to legal representative if patient or other persons would be put in danger if information is not disclosed[4].

Rights of a Person Whose Active Legal Capacity is Restricted by Court

Persons whose active legal capacity has been restricted by court do not have a right to administer their data in the EHR. The rights of a person whose active legal capacity has been restricted by court will be executed by his/her legal representative.

Patient's Right to Request Correction of Data

If patient discovers a document in the EHR information system that according to his/her assessment has incorrect information, the patient has a right to request from health care provider the forwarding of a corrected document to the EHR. Patient must turn to health care service provider in order for the document to be corrected.

3.4. Other Health Care Employees

Administrative Personnel

Administrative employees can't enquire patient's data from the EHR information system. Administrative employees will use data contained in the health care service provider's information system. Health care service provider's information system may enquire patient's non-sensitive general data from the EHR, and this information will be used by administrative personnel through their information system.

Registry office's employees can use patient's non-sensitive general data in the extent necessary to set up appointment times and prepare documents. Registry office's employee has a right to view data on referral in the extent necessary for sending the patient to an appropriate physician and to prepare documents given to the physician, and for this purpose registry office's employee can make an enquiry on referrals to the EHR information system.

Accountants can't enquire data from the EHR information system. Accountants will be created access to the organization's internal data in the extent necessary to create reports and invoices for treatment.

Since administrative employees do not have an independent right to make enquiries in the EHR information system, there will be no data enquiry access rules established for them. Administrative employees are employed on contractual basis and the organization's information system must ensure that data will be used as minimally as possible, and that the employees will only have access to data without which they

---

[3] Law of Obligations Act § 766 section 4, http://www.legaltext.ee/et/andmebaas/ava.asp?m=022
[4] Law of Obligations Act § 768 section 2, http://www.legaltext.ee/et/andmebaas/ava.asp?m=022

could not complete their work. The fulfilling of the minimal requirement will be verified by the Data Protection Inspectorate at the time of issuing the data use license.

Physicians of Defence Forces

If Defence Forces physicians are registered at the register of the Health Care Board, they will be enabled access to patient's health data through information system interfaced with the EHR. The physicians of Defence Forces are attending physicians to their patients.

Rights of a Prison Physician

If prison physicians are registered at the register of the Health Care Board, they will be enabled access to patient's health data through information system interfaced with the EHR. The prison physicians are attending physicians to their patients.

4. Summary

Implementing a nationwide integrated EHR has been one of the largest and most complex projects in the Estonian healthcare sector. During the process several parallel processes were carried out: establishing and developing responsible body – Estonian E-Health Foundation; creating a legal system; establishing access rights and rules for participants; creating integrated EHR with service oriented architecture and maintenance for the system .

Creating the rules and access rights, you must find a right balance between personal rights and social expectations for delicate data usage.

Estonia is a first country in the EU that has done it, but we still need to make a lot of efforts to receive full acceptance from medical professionals and citizens.

Medical and Care Compunetics 6
L. Bos et al. (Eds.)
IOS Press, 2010

Subject Index

Author Index